# Risk Communication
# and Public Health

# Risk Communication and Public Health

SECOND EDITION

Edited by

Peter Bennett

Kenneth Calman

Sarah Curtis

Denis Fischbacher-Smith

# OXFORD

UNIVERSITY PRESS

Great Clarendon Street, Oxford OX2 6DP

Oxford University Press is a department of the University of Oxford.
It furthers the University's objective of excellence in research, scholarship,
and education by publishing worldwide in

Oxford New York

Auckland Cape Town Dar es Salaam Hong Kong Karachi
Kuala Lumpur Madrid Melbourne Mexico City Nairobi
New Delhi Shanghai Taipei Toronto

With offices in

Argentina Austria Brazil Chile Czech Republic France Greece
Guatemala Hungary Italy Japan Poland Portugal Singapore
South Korea Switzerland Thailand Turkey Ukraine Vietnam

Oxford is a registered trade mark of Oxford University Press
in the UK and in certain other countries

Published in the United States
by Oxford University Press Inc., New York

British Library Cataloguing in Publication Data
Data available

Library of Congress Cataloging-in-Publication Data
Data available

Typeset by Cepha Imaging Private Ltd., Bangalore, India
Printed by the MPG
Books Group in the UK

ISBN 978–0–19–956284–8

10 9 8 7 6 5 4 3 2 1

# Preface

**Sir Liam Donaldson, Chief Medical Officer for England**

Personal decision-making is a peculiarly human phenomenon. Some people roll dice; others consult the stars. Some conduct extensive research; others trust their various instincts. Some value security and certainty; others enjoy risk-taking.

We are different from most other species on Earth. For them, a stimulus evokes a response without conscious interjection. We are blessed—sometimes cursed—by our self-awareness, our ability to visualize alternate futures, our higher consciousness.

Consider a 70-year-old man with cancer. Told that surgery carries a higher mortality risk than the cancer itself, he decides to decline the operation. A rigorous research study may underpin his doctor's advice, but it cannot foresee this man's particular course. Had he chosen to have the operation, he may have lived for far longer. He will never know. The previous patient in the clinic may have had an identical dilemma and made the opposite decision. There may be a number of reasons. His personal values and circumstances may be subtly different. The doctor may have delivered the information in a subtly different manner. Perhaps the patient simply misunderstood.

Consider a pedestrian in a rush to get home from work. He needs to cross a road that is busy with fast-moving traffic. Hurrying across will probably get him home more quickly, but it may end in disaster. Will he dash across, or walk to the crossing and wait? The same man regularly chooses to eat a full cooked breakfast and watch television. His wife has given up trying to feed him muesli and get him to the gym. He gets immediate pleasure from these choices, but he may die prematurely from a stroke.

Humans constantly make decisions. We balance risk and reward, often in the face of uncertainty, to decide how to act. Every one of us is different. We each place a different value on every risk and every reward. We weigh the options according to our particular personality and prior experience. Personal choices are refined over time, as we experience the effects of our previous choices, observe others' behaviour, and learn further information to add to our ever-incomplete personal knowledge base. Some of this information is factually correct, some is completely wrong. Some is presented to us in such a way that it affects our decision-making profoundly, some we barely notice. We are complex beings in a complex world.

Most public health professionals need to communicate with the public. Many hope to influence behaviour by doing so. Some aim to help individuals to make better choices. Some hope to offer reassurance. In times of crisis, the need to communicate risk arises as much from public expectation as professional need. Often there is uncertainty—prior to the Swine Flu outbreak last April, we knew that an influenza pandemic would occur at some time. But it might have started this year, next year, or a decade away. It is likely that 30 people in our region have a rare cancer, but we do not know which 30. We suspect that a particular foodstuff may be dangerous, but even experts have a poor understanding of the problem at the time when the public wants information.

This makes public health fascinating. It provides endless challenge. It is a challenge that is not getting any easier. The media through which messages are spread are increasingly complex. Chatter amongst families and neighbours has been superseded by websites, internet fora, and blogs. Rolling 24-hour news channels have changed the nature of what makes—and sustains—a story. Risk and uncertainty are complex concepts. Rates, ratios, and risks may make more sense in the abstract than when individuals try to apply them to their own circumstances. Simple figures can evoke powerful emotional responses. How do people make sense of what they are hearing, react to it, and adapt it into their world view?

Understanding the public communication of risk demands an understanding of marketing, of the media, and of the mind. This book teaches a difficult, fascinating subject. It does so superbly.

# Acknowledgement

The Editors would like to thank Kim Armstrong, Durham University, for her hard work and patience in helping us to prepare this book for publication.

# Contents

# Notes on the Editors

## Dr Peter Bennett

Following a first degree in Physics, Peter studied the logic, history and philosophy of science, obtaining his DPhil from Sussex University. He joined the Operational Research Group at Sussex before moving to Strathclyde University where he became Reader in Management Science and Director of Postgraduate Studies. At the same time, he was involved in applied research and consultancy projects for clients ranging from community groups to trans-national companies. He has retained a strong interest in decisions involving uncertainty, risk, and conflict, on which he has published widely. He joined the Department of Health as a Principal OR Analyst in 1996, and since then has been heavily involved in analyses of risks to Public Health. He produced the Department of Health guidelines on Risk Communication, and the previous OUP volume *Risk Communication and Public Health*, co-edited with Sir Kenneth Calman. He has led the production of risk assessments in several different areas, but particularly on the risks of variant CJD being spread by blood transfusion or re-use of surgical instruments. These are areas in which scientific uncertainty magnifies the challenges of effective risk communication. He now leads a cross-disciplinary team of analysts in the Health Improvement and Protection Directorate of the Department, and is acting Head of Profession for Operational Research.

## Sir Kenneth Calman

Sir Kenneth Calman is Chancellor of the University of Glasgow. He graduated in medicine (with commendation) in 1967, having obtained a number of distinctions and prizes throughout this course. He moved into the Department of Surgery in Glasgow and proceeded to the Fellowship of the Royal College of Surgeons and an MD Thesis with Honours on Organ Preservation. In 1972, he was the MRC Clinical Research Fellow at the Chester Beatty Research Institute in London and returned to Glasgow in 1974 as Professor of Oncology. He remained in that post for 10 years. In 1984 he became Dean of Postgraduate Medicine and Professor of Postgraduate Medical Education at the University of Glasgow and Consultant Physician with an interest in palliative care at Victoria Infirmary, Glasgow. In 1989 he was appointed Chief Medical Officer at the Scottish Home and Health Department and in September 1991 he became Chief Medical Officer in the Department of Health in London. He was a member of the Executive Board of the World Health Organization, and its Chairman from 1998 to 1999. He was Vice Chancellor and Warden of the University of Durham from 1998 until 2007. He was a member of the Statistics Commission from 1999 until 2007. He is a member of the Nuffield Council on Bioethics and President of the Institute of Medical Ethics. He is a member of the Board of the British Library. He was awarded a KCB in 1996. His most recent books are *A study of storytelling, humour and learning in medicine* and *Medical Education: Past, present and future.* He lives in Glasgow and on the Island of Arran.

## Professor Sarah Curtis

Sarah Curtis is Professor of Health and Risk at Durham University. She has extensive international research experience in the geography of health and health services, especially on inequalities of health and access to healthcare, healthcare needs assessment, health impact assessment, and development of healthy public policy. Her research covers topics including: adaptation of health and social care systems to changing risks of climate change (funded by EPSRC); health impact assessment of urban regeneration schemes (for the Department of Health, and other agencies); development of healthy public policy (with agencies in Canada and UK); ESRC funded research on effects of the socioeconomic environment on wellbeing and health of adults and children; research funded by the British Academy on hospital design; international research on migration, health, and wellbeing supported by ESRC; comparative research on geographical variation in psychiatric service use supported by the Office of Mental Health for New York State, US. Other experience includes: research and consultancy for UK Health Authorities, World Health Organization; Institut National de la Santé et Recherche Medicale, France; served as Non-Executive Director of an NHS Community and Mental Health Care Trust; currently Advisory Board Member for the London Health Observatory, and Board Member and Advisor for the National Collaborating Centre for Healthy Public Policy, National Institute of Public Health, Quebec, Canada. She is Senior Editor, Medical Geography for the international journal *Social Science and Medicine.*

## Professor Denis Fischbacher-Smith

Denis Fischbacher-Smith is Professor of Risk and Resilience at the University of Glasgow. His main research interests are in the areas of: organizational resilience, risk and crisis management; adverse events in healthcare; complexity and organizational performance (especially around healthcare organizations and the emergency services); human error and systems failure; and the role of embedded error cost in strategic change. Professor Fischbacher-Smith's work has been concerned with issues of risk management and business continuity, and this has been carried out over a 25-year period. His early work was concerned with the evacuation of urban areas owing to extreme events— an interest he maintains to this day. He has also undertaken research on the training and performance of crisis management teams, the production of emergency/contingency plans (and their limitations), and the processes by which vulnerability can be generated within organizations and urban 'space'. He has published widely in the area of crisis management and has been a regular consultant to a number of 'blue chip' companies as well as local authorities, the emergency services, and government. Outside of his academic activities, Professor Fischbacher-Smith has been a Director of HARM Consulting and CSC Ltd, as well as a Non-Executive Director of JMU Services, Mersey Regional Ambulance Service, St Helens RLFC and Aintree University Hospital NHS Trust. In terms of policy development, he was a member of the Ministerial Advisory Committee that produced An Organisation with a Memory for the Department of Health (England and Wales).

# Notes on other contributors

## David BaMaung

David is currently working as a Counter Terrorism Security Advisor within Strathclyde Police and provides counter terrorism protective security advice to the wider business community. He previously served as a police officer for 30 years, retiring as a Police Inspector. During his police career, he worked as Divisional Emergency Planning Liaison Officer and was a member of the multi-agency Evacuation Planning Team for Glasgow City Centre. He was also an invited external speaker on the Business Continuity Promotion course, held at the Cabinet Office Emergency Planning College. Outwith his normal role, David was a Police Support Unit Public Order and CBRN (Chemical, Biological, Radiological & Nuclear) Inspector.

In 2006, he was Project Manager for a Scottish Government-funded counter terrorism initiative 'Project Caledonia'. David became one of only three UK police officers trained in the European Union Community Mechanism for Civil Protection programme, as part of a multinational, multi-agency response force to respond to global crises. During the programme, he undertook training in Rome and Germany. He is currently undertaking a PhD in Critical National Infrastructure Resilience.

## Dr Laurence Barton

Laurence Barton is a Crisis Prevention and Response Consultant whose career spans higher education and the private sector. His clients include The Walt Disney Company, British Petroleum, DowCorning, ConocoPhillips, Emerson, Nike, KPMG, and a number of health systems and hospitals worldwide. He teaches crisis management at The FBI Training Academy and assists with organizational crisis planning and simulations.

A former Fulbright Scholar to Japan in crisis management, he has lectured in over 30 countries and led the response to over 1600 incidents worldwide, including industrial accidents, public health crises, workplace violence and threats, child abductions in hospitals, and numerous other critical incidents. His latest book, *Crisis Leadership Now* (McGraw-Hill, 2008) is the number one best selling book in the world on crisis management. He recently completed a major analysis of hospital disaster preparedness for InSpine, the international journal of spine care professionals. A former faculty member at Harvard Business School, he is President and Professor of Management at The American College, Bryn Mawr, PA, USA.

Dr Barton holds an AB, magna cum laude, from Boston College, the MALD from The Fletcher School of Law and Diplomacy, and his PhD from Boston University. He may be reached at larry@larrybarton.com.

## Dr Karen Bickerstaff

Karen is a Lecturer in Geography at King's College London. She has a research interest in the equity implications of environmental and technological risks and public understandings of, and responses to, such risks. Her work also addresses the spatial production and mediation of professional, and, specifically, scientific knowledge as well as the practice of more participatory styles of knowledge production and decision-making that aim, in various ways, to include affected publics and stakeholders. She is currently involved in a number of research projects that reflect a concern with the mundane and everyday practices through which people engage with and make sense of technological risks, as well as the equity and justice implications of energy systems.

## Dr Rachel Casiday

Rachel has research interests in the social context of risk, children's health, volunteering, and voluntary sector involvement in health provision. Her PhD research in medical anthropology (Durham University, 2005) examined concepts of risk and parental decision-making about the MMR vaccine. She worked as a Postdoctoral Research Fellow in the Durham University School of Medicine and Health, carrying out public health and risk-related research on a range of topics, including coronary heart disease prevention, irritable bowel syndrome, and child malnutrition in sub-Saharan Africa. She is currently a Lecturer in Voluntary Sector Studies at the University of Wales Lampeter, and has recently completed a systematic review commissioned by Volunteering England on the health impacts of volunteering.

## Dr Sarah Damery

Sarah is a Research Fellow in Primary Care Clinical sciences at the University of Birmingham. She holds a BA, MA, and PhD in Geography. Her research interests focus on the investigation of individual and institutional risk perceptions, framings and understandings in a range of contexts, and the manner by which the institutionalization of certain approaches and the exclusion of others impacts on the effectiveness of policies put in place to manage risk. Her work to date has been concerned with understanding the interface between 'expert' and 'public' risk framings, and the role that uncertainty plays in attempts to understand and manage risk. Most recently, she was Research Fellow on a National Institute for Health Research (Research for Patient Benefit)-funded project *Healthcare Workers' Attitudes To Working During Pandemic Influenza.*

## Sue Davies MBE

Sue is the Chief Policy Adviser at *Which?*, the UK consumer association, working on food issues. She is also a member of the Council of Food Policy Advisers and is a member of the Management Board of the European Food Safety Authority (EFSA). She has represented consumer interest on a range of government committees and working groups, including the Advisory Committee on the Microbiological Safety of Food (ACMSF), School Meals Review Panel and Food Incidents Task Force. She also currently represents BEUC, the European Consumer Organisation, on the EU's Platform on Diet, Physical Activity and Health, and represents Consumers International in discussions on international food standards at the Codex Alimentarius Commission. She was until recently Chair of EFSA's Stakeholder Consultative Platform and is also the EU Co-Chair of the Trans-Atlantic Consumer Dialogue (TACD) Food Working Group, a policy forum for EU and US consumer organizations. She was awarded the MBE in 2003 for services to food safety.

## Heleen van Dijk

Heleen obtained a Master of Science in Social Psychology with a specialization in consumer decision-making at the University of Amsterdam, The Netherlands. She is currently a PhD student in the Marketing and Consumer Behaviour Group of the Social Sciences Department of Wageningen University in the Netherlands. In her PhD research she aims to understand consumer responses to communication about both risks and benefits related to food.

## Anton Dittner

At the time of writing, Anton Dittner works for the Emerging Health Threats Forum, specializing in the field of CBRN terrorism. Anton is working in collaboration with the Health Protection Agency on the UK components of the Global Health Security Initiative's *CBRN Threats and Pandemic Influenza Early Alerting and Reporting* pilot project. Anton received his degree from Durham

University, and trained at Royal Military Academy Sandhurst. Prior to working for Emerging Health Threats Forum, Anton wrote articles for *Strategic Intelligence Review* and *Asia Intelligence.*

## Dr Heather Draper

Heather Draper is Reader at the Biomedical Ethics Centre for Biomedical Ethics Primary Care Clinical Sciences, University of Birmingham. She is a specialist in biomedical ethics whose interests range from the ethics of reproduction to, more recently, public health ethics. She was Principal Investigator on the National Institute for Health Research-funded project *Healthcare workers' attitudes to working during pandemic influenza*, which ran from Oct 2007 until March 2009. The project resulted from the work of the University of Birmingham's multidisciplinary pandemic influenza team. Although Heather is comfortable writing philosophically (e.g. Paternity fraud and compensation for misattributed paternity (*Journal of Medical Ethics* 2007)), she is primarily interested in the practical application of ethics to biomedical issues. She is therefore interested in empirical bioethics, which aims to combine empirical data with ethical analysis. She also offers ethical advice on three hospital clinical ethics committees (including recently advice on pandemic planning) as well as practical help in research ethics to researchers in her academic School at the University of Birmingham. She was Co-Editor on *Gillon's Principles of Health Care Ethics* (Wiley) which was Highly Commended in the 2008 BMA book competition under Basis of Medicine section.

## Dr Christine Dunn

Christine Dunn is a Senior Lecturer in the Department of Geography at Durham University. Her main research interests centre on exploring relationships between spatial distributions of human disease and the natural and built environments. Her work includes methodological developments in the spatial analysis of health-related data with particular emphasis on Geographical Information Systems (GIS). She has a specific interest in the conceptualization and application of Participatory GIS, and the theory and practice of spatial information technologies in the context of development in the Global South. Much of Dr Dunn's work is situated at the science–social science interface with interests in scientific and lay understandings of health risks. Her current focus is on the potential interfaces between scientific and social scientific approaches to understanding patterns of malaria in Africa. She is currently Chair of the Royal Geographical Society (with the Institute of British Geographers) Geography of Health Research Group and was awarded the 2009 Royal Geographical Society Cuthbert Peek Award for her work on advancing geographical knowledge of human impact on the environment through the application of contemporary mapping methods.

## Dr Eva Elliott

Dr Eva Elliott is a UK Research Council Academic Fellow in Social and Economic Change at the Cardiff Institute of Society Health and Ethics at Cardiff University School of Social Sciences. She also project manages the Welsh Health Impact Assessment Support Unit. More recently she has developed an active interest in the meanings and processes of urban and rural regeneration, in the context of a global neo-liberal economy, in addressing the consequences of health inequality. She has also written, with Gareth Williams, on the role of public sociology in developing forms of civic intelligence through activities such as health impact assessment.

## Dr Moira Fischbacher-Smith

Moira is a Senior Lecturer in Strategic Management in the Centre for Health, Environment and Risk Research, Department of Management, University of Glasgow. After graduating in business studies, she worked for 3 years for Health Protection Scotland (then the Communicable Diseases Surveillance Unit). During this time, she began her PhD at the University of Glasgow. She moved to work at the University in 1995, where her research interests were, and continue to be, focused on networks and organizational performance in healthcare and local government. She is also interested in public–private partnerships, service design, and the role of public health in dealing with mass emergencies. Moira's interests in public health have been furthered through commencing part-time study in 2007 for a Masters in Public Health. Her research has also developed more recently into considering the role of networks within risk management. The research projects that Moira has been involved in at Glasgow University have been funded through the UK Design Council, the Scottish Government, and the Engineering and Physical Sciences Research Council. She is on the editorial advisory board of *Risk Management: An International Journal* and, until recently, was on the advisory board of the *European Management Journal*. She has published in journals, including *Public Money and Management, Financial Accountability and Management, Palliative Medicine,* and *The British Journal of General Practice*.

## Dr Arnout R. H. Fischer

Dr Fischer is Assistant Professor in the Marketing and Consumer Behaviour Group of the Social Sciences Department of Wageningen University in the Netherlands. He aims to understand public behaviour through social psychological approaches. He currently investigates methods for early detection of new and emerging food-related health risks. He also studies communication of risks and benefits to existing and new foods and food production methods. He has published on risk communication and consumer behaviour in relation to food safety in academic books and peer-reviewed journals.

## Professor Simon French

Simon French is Professor of Information and Decision Sciences at Manchester Business School. He has an international reputation in decision analysis, risk assessment, and Bayesian statistics. In all his work, the emphasis is on multi-disciplinary approaches to solving real problems and the innovative use of technology in supporting decision-making. In 1990–92 he was a member of the International Chernobyl Project, leading the team which looked at the issues driving decision-making in the aftermath of the accident, running five decision conferences within the Soviet Union. It was this experience that led him to realize the paramount importance of including good information management and communication as an integral part of risk management, especially in relation to crisis response. Since then he has worked, often in collaboration with John Maule, in many multidisciplinary, national and European projects which address major societal risk management. Currently he is working on e-democracy and e-participation and wider contexts of societal decision-making. Since the Chernobyl project, he has maintained a strong interest in crisis management and was recently awarded the first Information Systems for Crisis Response and Management (ISCRAM) community's award for Lifetime Achievement.

## Professor Lynn J. Frewer

Professor Frewer has a background in Psychology. Lynn is currently Professor of Food Safety and Consumer Behaviour at the University of Wageningen in the Netherlands. Previously she was Head of the Consumer Science Group at the Institute of Food Research in the UK.

Lynn has research interests focused on understanding societal and individual responses to both risk and benefit, in particular linked to the agrifood sector. Current research activities focus on understanding how people make decisions about the risks and benefits associated with different dietary choices and how to develop effective communication about these issues, understanding citizen attitudes to emerging technologies such as nanotechnology, and developing best practice in stakeholder and citizen consultation linked to risk governance.

Other activities include research directed towards understanding the impact of legislative changes on the food chain actors (for example, the impact of traceability legislation on both consumer and producer perceptions of food safety) as well as the broad socioeconomic impact of some important public health issues (for example, food allergy or domestic food hygiene preparation practices). A particular focus of Lynn's research relates to developing interdisciplinary activities between the social and natural sciences.

## Dr Sara Fuller

Sara Fuller is a Research Associate in the Department of Geography at Durham University. Her research focuses on environmental justice, democracy, and multilevel environmental governance in both the UK and EU, and she has been involved in a number of recent research projects looking at these issues, including a literature review on risk communication funded by the Health Protection Agency. She previously completed her PhD at the University of Sheffield which focused on environmental NGOs and their activities in relation to large scale infrastructure projects in Eastern Europe. Sara has also worked as a researcher on several research projects at the Centre for Sustainable Development, University of Westminster, exploring the interfaces between social exclusion and the environment in deprived communities.

## Emily Harrop

Emily Harrop is a final year PhD student in the School of Social Sciences, Cardiff University. Her PhD was set up under the ESRC's CASE Studentship scheme, in collaboration with the Wales Centre for Health, and is titled: 'Contested knowledge in the assessment of public health risks: A case study of the Nant-y-Gwyddon landfill site in the Rhondda Valley, South Wales' (Award No. PTA-033-2006-00062). Before starting the studentship she worked as a Research Assistant at Cardiff Institute of Society, Health and Ethics, Cardiff University.

## Professor Karen Henwood

Karen is Professor of Social Sciences at Cardiff University and a Principal Investigator on the 'Timescapes' ESRC network where she leads the project 'Masculinities, Identities and Risk: Transition in the Lives of Men as Fathers'. Her research interests concern the ways in which differences in identity and subjectivity are forged in relation to biography, relationships, social context, and cultural issues; troubled and troubling identities; social constructions and lived experiences of gender, risk, embodiment, and wellbeing. She also has a range of methodological interests, including the use of interpretive thematic approaches (such as grounded theory); discursive and narrative methods; the development of qualitative longitudinal methodology; innovative, collaborative approaches to data sharing, archiving and secondary analysis; and combining different qualitative and qualitative and quantitative methods. For further information see: http://www.cf.ac.uk/socsi/contactsandpeople/academicstaff/G-H/professor-karen-henwood-overview.html.

## Dr Patricia Hewitt

Dr Hewitt is Consultant Specialist in Transfusion Microbiology, National Blood Service, NHS Blood and Transplant. She has worked within the English blood service for over 20 years, is Lead Clinician within NHS Blood and Transplant (NHSBT) for Transfusion Microbiology clinical matters and is also Chair of the Transfusion Microbiology Clinical Group. She is responsible for the management within the blood service of donors (of blood, tissues, and cord blood stem cells) who are found to be positive for infections during the routine testing of donations. She has overall responsibility for the investigation of cases of infection thought to have been transmitted by blood transfusion.

Dr Hewitt is Chair of the UK Standing Advisory Committee on Transfusion Transmitted Infection and a member of the Serious Hazards of Transfusion (SHOT) Steering Group. She is a Principal Investigator in a joint surveillance study with the National CJD Surveillance Unit looking at the relationship between blood transfusion and CJD. She is a member of the CJD Clinical Incidents Panel, set up by the Department of Health to advise on the management of cases who might have been exposed to CJD through medical procedures. Throughout her career, Dr Hewitt has had a special interest in communication, risk, and ethical/medicolegal issues relating to donors.

## Professor Ray Hudson

Ray Hudson is Professor of Geography and Pro-Vice-Chancellor at Durham University, with particular responsibility for the University's regional engagement strategy. Prior to taking the PVC post, he was Director of the interdisciplinary Wolfson Research Institute, which specializes in work on health and wellbeing. He has a BA, PhD, and DSc from the University of Bristol, and an Honorary DSc from Roskilde University. His main research interests lie in political–economic geography, particularly geographies of economies, the politics and policies of territorial development, and the social and health consequences of economic decline. He is author or editor of over 20 published books and numerous papers. His work has been recognized by the Royal

Geographical Society via the award of the Edward Heath Award and the Victoria Medal. He is an elected Fellow of the Academy of the Social Sciences, the British Academy, and Academia Europaea. He is actively involved in practical regeneration work in north-east England via his links with the Regional Development Agency and membership of a number of economic development organizations in County Durham and the Tees Valley. He has also advised the EU and other regions outside the north-east on these issues and served as Special Advisor to the House of Commons Select Committee on coalfields regeneration.

## Jonathan Ives

Jonathan is a Lecturer in Behavioural Science at the University of Birmingham. He holds a BA and MPhil in Philosophy, and a PhD in Biomedical Ethics and Law. Jon teaches medical sociology, medical ethics and qualitative research methods to undergraduate and postgraduate students. His research interests are varied, but focus on public health ethics and pandemics, the ethics and philosophy of fatherhood and the family, theory and methods of empirical bioethics and research ethics.

## Dr Fu-Meng Khaw

Meng Khaw is Director of Public Health at North Tyneside Primary Care Trust and Honorary Senior Lecturer in Epidemiology and Public Health at Newcastle University. Meng has research experience across a broad range of health-related issues, including: outcomes of joint replacement surgery, decision-making in healthcare, perception of barriers to testing for hepatitis C amongst prisoners, correlation of air pollutants and their impact on health, and most recently, risk communication for communicable diseases. He completed an MD on the integration of hip implants in vivo, which was funded by a Surgical Fellowship from the Royal College of Surgeons of England. He worked as a Consultant in Health Protection in the Health Protection Agency, scoping risk-related research on communicable diseases. In his current role, he is maintaining an interest in research on the factors influencing the perception of risk from environmental hazards.

## Professor John Maule

John Maule is Professor of Human Decision Making and Director of the Centre for Decision Research at Leeds University Business School. He has spent many years undertaking research on how people make judgements and take decisions, and how we can use this knowledge to improve the effectiveness of these activities. He has published widely on risk and decision-making, and is currently involved in research projects concerned with: modelling and communicating risk across the food chain; perception and communication of terrorist risk; communicating the risk of side effects in medicines leaflets, and the effects of emotion on risk-taking.

He has a very strong commitment to applying academic theory and research on human decision-making to professional and work contexts. He has collaborated on the development of a training course to identify and overcome the factors that inhibit security awareness, acted as a consultant on risk and risk communication for government agencies and run courses on this topic for private and public sector organizations. He has also developed many research-led courses designed to help people understand and improve their decision-making, including courses on strategic thinking, risk, and decision-making for senior managers, bankers, doctors, senior police officers, and security professionals.

## Professor Hugh Pennington

Hugh Pennington trained in medicine and microbiology at St Thomas's Hospital Medical School, London. He was Professor of Bacteriology at the University of Aberdeen from 1979 to 2003, and Dean of Medicine there from 1987 to 1992. His research interests have focused on virus protein synthesis and the molecular typing and epidemiology of bacterial pathogens. Among other organisms, he has worked on Newcastle disease, smallpox and vaccinia viruses, MRSA, *Neisseria meningitidis*, and *E. coli* O157. In 1996–97 he chaired an inquiry for the government into the Central Scotland *E. coli* O157 food poisoning outbreak, and he chaired the Public Inquiry into the 2005 South Wales *E. coli* O157 outbreak. From 2000 to 2005 he was a member of the BBC Broadcasting Council for Scotland, from 2003 to 2006 President of the Society for General Microbiology, and from 2002 to 2007 a member of the United Nations University World Food Program Technical Advisory Group. He was a founder member of the Food Standards Agency Scottish Food Advisory Committee. His *When Food Kills, BSE, E. coli, and Disaster Science* was published in 2003, and he writes from time to time on microbiological issues for the *London Review of Books*.

## Professor Judith Petts

Professor Petts is Pro-Vice-Chancellor, Research and Knowledge Transfer, University of Birmingham, and was Head of the School of Geography, Earth and Environmental Sciences, from 2001 to 2007. She is also Director of the

Centre for Environmental Research and Training, and holds the Chair of Environmental Risk Management.

Judith has 30 years' applied research and advisory work on environmental risk management. Her research spans three primary areas: environmental governance and policy-making, science–society relationships, and perceptions, responses and behaviour. Her particular area of interest is in risk communication and public engagement in decision-making, and she has been involved in the development and evaluation of innovative forms of engagement in key policy areas. Her research has engaged with a variety of risks—from incineration to flooding, from MMR to climate change. As such, she has extensive experience of working with government departments and local authorities. Judith's current external appointments include membership of the Royal Commission on Environmental Pollution, and of EPSRC's Societal Issues Panel.

## Professor Nick Pidgeon

Nick Pidgeon is Professor of Environmental Psychology at Cardiff University and ESRC Professorial Fellow in Climate Change. His research looks at how public attitudes, public trust, and institutional responses form a part of the dynamics of a range of risk controversies. Issues he has studied include GM agriculture, nuclear power, climate change, and nanotechnologies. He is co-author (with B. Turner) of the book *Man-Made Disasters* (2nd edn 1997) and (with R. Kasperson and P. Slovic) of *The Social Amplification of Risk* (Cambridge, 2003). For further information see: http://www.understanding-risk.org.

## David Pryer

David joined Kent Police in 1974. Within his service, his focus was on command band training for many senior police officers, and he himself retired as the Commander of the North Kent Area in 2003. This work involved him leading on many sensitive issues, including developing the organization's diversity strategy following the Macpherson Report into the murder of Stephen Lawrence. One of his many roles as a police commander was that of community leader where he chaired groups such as the Crime Reduction Partnership and local multiracial liaison group.

In 2004, he commenced work as a board member with a Primary Care Trust developing a vocational interest in health service provision, monitoring performance with the health service, value for money, and resolution of service failure. He also made an active contribution to the widespread mergers of Primary Care Trusts in 2006. He was also an active member of a board managing health and leisure provision within the Gravesham area.

In January 2005, he was appointed Chairman of the CJD Incidents Panel, dealing with incidents of exposure to all forms of CJD. He has had a central role in leading the Panel on its work to introduce measures to protect the public from the potential risks of person-to-person infection. He has also chaired numerous organizations, including the Regional Audience Council for the BBC, and been an active member of the Associated Audience Council for England.

## Professor Pat Troop CBE

Professor Troop has spent 30 years in public health, working at the local, regional, national, and international levels, taking in all aspects of public heath. From 1999 to 2003, she was the Deputy Chief Medical Officer for England, where she had responsibility for public health, especially health protection and international health. From 2003 until her retirement in 2008, Professor Troop was the founding Chief Executive of the Health Protection Agency, which she established as a leading public health organization, with over 3000 staff, covering infections and environmental hazards, including chemicals and radiation, and emergency preparedness and response. Since her retirement, Professor Troop continues to be involved in a number of public health activities, including work with the World Health Organization.

Professor Troop is a Visiting Professor at the London School of Hygiene and Tropical Medicine, an Honorary Professor at City University, and received Honorary Doctorates from the Universities of East Anglia and Cranfield. She was awarded the Outstanding Alumna of the Year from Manchester University in 2007 and a CBE for services to public health in 2000.

## Professor Gareth Williams

Gareth Williams has been a Professor of Sociology in the School of Social Sciences at Cardiff University since 1999. He is Co-Director of the Regeneration Institute (a joint initiative with the School of City and Regional Planning), Associate Director of the Cardiff Institute of Society Health and Ethics, and Director of the Welsh Health Impact Assessment Support Unit. He has published widely in academic and professional journals and has written and edited a number of books, including *Community Health and Wellbeing: Action Research on Health Inequalities* (with Steve Cropper *et al.*), published by Policy Press in 2007.

# Risk, communication, and the public understanding of uncertainty in public health

Chapter 1

# Understanding public responses to risk: policy and practice

Peter Bennett (Department of Health, London), Kenneth Calman (University of Glasgow), Sarah Curtis (Durham University), & Denis Fischbacher-Smith (University of Glasgow)

## Introduction: the challenge of risk communication

The need to communicate about risks to public health—whether real, alleged or potential—is widespread throughout government, the NHS, local authorities, and the private sector. Many campaigning groups, charities, and other organizations are also engaged in debates about risk. Long-established policy areas include the control of infectious diseases, risks from pollutants or technological hazards, and safety of foods and medicines. 'Natural' hazards such as flooding can generate long-term issues even after their immediate impact has subsided. Transport has its own set of safety issues, as have work-related risks. Then there are debates over the so-called 'lifestyle' risks that relate to smoking, poor diet or even dangerous sports. Many of the risks that we face are both ill-defined—and in some instances, ill-understood—and interconnected. This is particularly the case for those related to health. The resulting debates are not limited to the public health agenda but may have widespread implications for different facets of government. Controversies about health risks seldom stem *solely* from issues of communication, but poor communication is very often a factor in allowing concerns to escalate and opposing groups to become polarized. From one point of view, 'the public'—spurred on by the media—may be accused of ignoring perfectly sensible and scientifically sound advice. From another perspective, those 'in charge' may be seen as untrustworthy, secretive, or prone to unwarranted 'nannying'. This collection of essays seeks to explore the landscape within which these controversies are located and to consider some of the underlying challenges around risk communication.

There has been progress in understanding the various responses to risk, and their implications for communication and conflict resolution. The precursor to this volume (Bennett & Calman, 1999) gave some indication of the state of play within the academic and practice communities about 10 years ago. Since then, the field has moved on. For example, the following issues have emerged.

- Some specific issues have risen in prominence. For example, the events of 11th September 2001 obviously increased concerns about threats from terrorist attack. The threat of a global influenza pandemic has been attracting increasing attention for several years, and as this volume goes to press (late May 2009), international attention is focused on the potential for the outbreak of human 'swine flu' originating in Mexico to create just such a pandemic. Whatever the outcome, there will undoubtedly be lessons both for risk management and communication. Meanwhile, increasing concern about obesity has highlighted issues around the role of government in influencing 'lifestyle' choices. Hospital-acquired infections such as MRSA and *C. difficile* have regularly made headlines in the UK and, in some cases, resulted in senior health service managers losing their positions

- At the same time, few of the topics that were prominent 10 years ago have gone away, so new risk communication issues compete for attention with more longstanding concerns. Some of the more obvious examples include variant CJD, the MMR vaccine or genetically modified crops. The topics covered in later chapters of this collection reflect this rich mix of concerns and conflicts

- Research into the processes of risk perception and communication has continued. Examples include the role and nature of trust, and the interplay between individual beliefs of risks and social dynamics. There has been progress in several key areas and this is outlined in various chapters. There are also further insights that can be gained from related disciplines—with the increased influence of social marketing and the processes around networks being notable examples

- At the same time, there have been significant organizational changes in the way potential risks to public health are managed. Prominent in the UK has been the establishment of the new Food Standards Agency, which was just about to be set up when the previous volume was written. The new agency has been able to bring a much more open and transparent approach to the field. This has been paralleled by steps to open up scientific advisory committees to wider scrutiny and participation. Analogous developments in other countries have led in the same direction of greater transparency

- Technology has continued to develop, perhaps most importantly the technology of communication itself. Although the internet was already a powerful factor in 1999, its use and significance has expanded dramatically. Not only has it served as an ever-increasing source of information and opinion—often difficult to distinguish—but the popularity of blogs, social networks, and a range of online forums has led to huge participation in the sharing and discussion of views, going far beyond mere access

◆ These developments have posed challenges to the established centralized media, whose role as mediators of public perceptions looks less secure. One immediate consequence has been the need to meet the increasing demands of a 24-hour rolling news agenda, at a time of severe cutbacks in journalistic resources. For media professionals, having time to research—or even check—stories before broadcast has become an increasingly scarce luxury (Davies, 2008; Rosenberg and Feldman, 2008). Such pressure increases the likelihood of anything with the characteristics of a 'good story' being repeated and recycled, regardless of accuracy. It has also arguably left the mass media more open to deliberate manipulation.

Given these changes, some of the 'established knowledge' of 10 years ago may look less well established—or at least less significant—now. However, much of what seemed to be emerging in the first edition has been borne out by subsequent developments. This opening chapter aims to set out some of these (relatively) enduring fundamentals. Subsequent chapters cover the most recent research and either bring previous examples up to date or provide insights into new issues. The final chapter attempts to pull some of these additional threads together, and looks to the current agenda for research and for risk communication practice.

## Risk communication and its limitations

To set the discussion in context, the emphasis throughout this volume is on risks to *public* health, with an implied need to communicate with substantial numbers of people (if not the *whole* population, perhaps everyone who may have been exposed to a specific hazard). Nevertheless, some of the principles that apply to one-to-one communication are relevant. The encoding of information, the manner in which it is transmitted, and the processes used to decode it are central to all forms of communication. The frameworks that we use to make sense of the information that we receive and the manner in which that sense-making process is undertaken are also important. Many communication problems occur because elements of this process break down. In some instances, public and individual communication becomes operationally intertwined. The course of a public health episode, for example, may depend critically on whether the individuals most affected (who may well have a strong public voice) feel they were kept properly informed and their concerns were dealt with, and how they report those feelings. The interplay between individual and mass communication figures strongly in several of the chapters in this volume.

Public reactions to risk often appear to be at odds with scientific estimates. Although risk may technically be defined as 'probability times severity of harm', the suggestion that a hazard poses an annual risk of death of 'one chance in x' (or '1 in $10^x$') may cause anything from near-panic to virtual indifference. But such reactions are not totally unpredictable—or *necessarily* unreasonable. Over the past 40 years, an extensive body of research into the various responses to risk has established some useful insights into public reactions to such warnings. It is important, however, to note a progressive change both in the research literature and in the practice of risk communication that has led us:

- From an original emphasis on 'public misperceptions of risk', which tended to treat all deviations from expert estimates as products of ignorance or stupidity
- Via investigation of what actually does cause concern and why
- To approaches which promote risk communication as a two-way process in which both 'expert' and 'lay' perspectives should inform each other.

At the same time, there has been an increasing acknowledgement of the political context within which risk communication takes place, and where the nature of scientific evidence itself may be disputed. Risk itself is increasingly seen as a social construct. These themes are taken up in more detail in the next chapter, and are illustrated in many of the subsequent contributions.

The need to acknowledge and engage with a variety of defensible views on risk has thus been increasingly recognized by government and policy- makers. This is not to deny that misperceptions still exist—people may sometimes be most fearful of the 'wrong' hazards—but rather that a more effective (and, some might argue, equitable) environment exists within which to debate those hazards. More fundamentally, there is a greater awareness that everyone— public and 'expert' alike—is fallible when thinking about risk, and fallible in some predictable ways. From this perspective, better processes of risk communication will not provide a panacea to the conflicts around hazard and uncertainty: it will not necessarily resolve conflict, guarantee understanding or cause people to behave in ways with which one agrees. However, effective risk communication can help to:

- Clarify the nature of disagreements, and restrict their scope (for example, by identifying which points might be resolved by factual research, and which reflect fundamental differences in values)

◆ Enable people to make more considered (and perhaps more informed) decisions

◆ Lessen the resentment caused by people feeling excluded from decisions that affect them by providing a mechanism and framework within which they can articulate their concerns.

Even these limited aims call for long-term efforts across responsible organizations, rather than being amenable to a 'quick PR fix'. Nevertheless, there are specific pitfalls to be avoided. Their immediate consequences can be all too clear: warnings that fail to warn (or cause unforeseen panic), reassurances that fail to reassure, and advice that is discounted.

We also need to distinguish between those communication failures in which a 'correct' message is misunderstood or disbelieved and those in which the message itself is flawed. In taking a broad view of risk communication, it is important not to dwell exclusively on success or failure in 'getting the message across'. Sometimes the intended message is itself mistaken—even if honestly believed—or is overturned by later scientific information. If so, there may have been a failure to allow sufficiently for uncertainty in developing the initial policy: a more precautionary approach might have been beneficial. Consider, for example, the communication issues around the potential risk to humans from BSE ('mad cow disease') in cattle and the safety of the MMR vaccine— both discussed in later chapters. In the early stages of both controversies, the most pressing need from a governmental perspective may have appeared broadly similar: that of providing a credible message of reassurance. The initial 'problem' in both cases was that not everyone believed the message. For the MMR vaccine, this definition of the problem remains relevant, given that further evidence supports the vaccine's safety. With BSE, the much more fundamental problem was that subsequent evidence showed the initial message to be plainly mistaken—there *was* a risk to human health. Both examples reinforce the point about not considering communication in isolation: unless the underlying evidence base around risk assessment is robust, then effective communication may only serve to drive home an ultimately flawed message with greater impact.

## Understanding responses to risk

For present purposes, some basic research findings can conveniently be grouped under four headings:

◆ Risks are different

◆ People are different

- Probabilities can be difficult to interpret
- Debates about risk are conditioned by their social / political context.

## Risks are different

Why do some risks trigger so much more alarm, anxiety or outrage than others? One way of looking at this question (sometimes referred to as the psychometric approach) concentrates on how different attributes of risks affect individual attitudes—for example, using survey-based research. This has been the topic of a large volume of research (see, for example, Fischhoff, 1995), the results of which can be broadly summarized by the 'fright factors' shown in Box 1.1, which combine the most significant items from several existing analyses. Note that these relate to perceptions of risk. What matters here is not whether a risk is *really* involuntary, but whether it is seen in that way. Debate remains as to which factors are most important in particular circumstances: the factors listed should be regarded as rules of thumb rather than precise predictions. They may well also be interdependent rather than simply additive. Nevertheless, there is little disagreement that factors of this type are important much of the time. It should come as no surprise when risks scoring highly against fright factors provoke a strong public response. These are the classic

---

### Box 1.1 Fright factors

Risks are generally more worrying (and less acceptable) if perceived:

1 To be *involuntary* (e.g. exposure to pollution) rather than voluntary (e.g. dangerous sports or smoking)

2 As *inequitably distributed* (some benefit while others suffer the consequences)

3 As *inescapable* by taking personal precautions

4 To arise from an *unfamiliar* or *novel* source

5 To result from *manmade, rather than natural* sources

6 To cause *hidden and irreversible* damage, e.g. through onset of illness many years after exposure

7 To pose some particular danger to *small children or pregnant women* or more generally to *future generations*

**Fright factors** (continued)

8 To threaten a form of death (or illness/injury) arousing *particular dread*

9 To damage *identifiable rather than anonymous victims*

10 To be *poorly understood by science*

11 As subject to *contradictory statements* from responsible sources (or, even worse, from the same source).

ingredients for a 'scare'. Conversely, it will be difficult to direct attention to low scoring risks.

The qualitative differences between hazards have particular implications for the use of *risk comparisons*. One popular communication tactic is to juxtapose data on different risks (both in terms of the consequences and the probabilities associated with them), a typical example being shown in Box 1.2. Sometimes comparisons have been put together to make risk 'scales' or 'ladders'. The rationale is twofold. Firstly, small probabilities are difficult to conceptualize and so numerical comparisons might help clarify which risks justify most attention (Paling, 1997). More controversially, comparisons have been seen as a means of *correcting* perceptions. This has been partly prompted by evidence that people tend to *overestimate* deaths owing to unusual or dramatic causes while *underestimating* those due to common killers such as heart disease (Fischhoff *et al.*, 1981).

However, the implications of such findings—for example, when seen as 'proving' the public's inability to make sensible judgements about risks—have been hotly debated. Similarly, risk comparisons have acquired a checkered reputation as aids to communication. Typically omitting both the effects of fright factors and the values of intended audiences, they often miss the point. For example, the common yardstick of a one-in-a-million chance of death in Box 1.2 is thought-provoking, but the table juxtaposes voluntary and involuntary risks and wildly different forms of death (accident, cancer). Furthermore, the numbers can give a false impression of precision. There is no indication that the figures may be highly uncertain, hotly contested or both. Where, the sceptic may ask, do the numbers come from, and why should I trust them? Such concerns led the authors of one widely cited source of comparative data (Covello *et al.*, 1988) to add a repeated 'health warning' to the effect that *use of these comparisons can seriously damage your credibility*.

## Box 1.2 (Mis)use of risk comparisons

Risks 'estimated to increase the annual chance of death by 1 in one million'

| Activity | Cause of death |
|---|---|
| Smoking 1.4 cigarettes | Cancer, heart disease |
| Spending 1 hour in a coal mine | Black lung disease |
| Living 2 days in New York or Boston | Air pollution |
| Travelling 10 miles by bicycle | Accident |
| Flying 1000 miles by jet | Accident |
| Living 2 months in Denver (rather than New York) | Cancer (cosmic radiation) |
| One chest X-ray in a good hospital | Cancer (from radiation) |
| Eating 40 tbs. of peanut butter | Liver cancer (aflatoxin B) |
| Drinking 30 12-oz cans of diet soda | Cancer (from saccharin) |
| Living 150 years within 20 miles of nuclear power plant | Cancer (from radiation |

(Source: Wilson, 1979)

Clearly, comparisons are most relevant when they refer directly to alternative choices: nobody has to choose between going down a mine and living in Denver, but many people make choices about whether to fly or go by train. Otherwise, caution is advisable. There is little solid evidence to show when comparisons might work well (Roth *et al.*, 1990; Johnson, 2003). If the aim is to convey a rough order of magnitude, familiar comparators such as 'about one person in a small town' for '1 in 10 000' may be more helpful (Calman and Royston, 1997). In any case, a clear distinction should be made between simply providing a sense of perspective and using comparisons to imply acceptability: 'you are irrational to worry about *this* risk when you happily accept *that* greater one'. The latter is likely to backfire, especially if involuntary and voluntary risks are juxtaposed.

### People are different: the primacy of values

Though fright factors may sometimes lead people to exaggerate certain types of risk, there is no basis for dismissing them as unreasonable per se. At least some of the time, they may reflect fundamental and important *value judgements*. Even the most extreme of examples—that of the risk of death—points to the difficulties in making comparisons. For example, it would be perverse to insist that a fatal cancer *should* carry no more dread than the prospect of being struck by lightning. Similarly, a willingness to accept voluntary risks may reflect the value placed on personal autonomy rather than a concern about the probability of harm. Risk often has attractions: mountaineers and racing drivers take precautions to limit the risks they take, but facing *some* risk is undeniably part of the attraction.

Responses to risk are dependent not only on context, but on personal values, political and moral beliefs, attitudes toward technology, and so on. All help determine which fright factors most frighten and what sources (and forms) of information are trusted. Clearly, people's beliefs and values differ widely. Although fright factors may be quite a good guide to the overall public response to risks, *individual* reactions may depend more strongly on approval or disapproval of the source of risk on other grounds. Those who love (or hate) the motor car anyway are usually more (or less) sanguine about its health risks. Similarly, debates about nuclear power are about more than just risk, or even risk plus fright factors. At the other end of the scale, emphasizing the dangers of drug abuse will have no effect on those who relish personal risk—any more than teenagers playing chicken on the railway line will be deterred by the sober revelation that it is dangerous.

Though the last may be an extreme example, all highlight the further point that perceived *benefits* matter. Possible negative outcomes are, after all, usually only half of the equation. Benefits need not be material goods—'intangible' examples include convenience (open-platform buses are popular, despite the acknowledged risks). Indeed, there is evidence that people often respond to safety measures (e.g. more effective brakes on cars) by taking benefits that return their risk to its previous level (driving faster). This phenomenon of 'risk compensation' is extensively discussed by Adams (1995). However, its plausible existence in some contexts does not imply that all safety measures are ineffective—even for voluntary risks. For example, people may inadvertently be putting themselves at greater risk than they realize.

The primacy of individual values has also been emphasized in the context of doctor–patient communication, especially over the last decade or so (see, for example, Meryn, 1998). Different patients faced with the 'same' choices may weight relevant risks quite differently against each other, and against potential benefits, hence increasing support for shared decision-making. However, individuals also differ in their beliefs *about responsibility for choice*. Some still see this as part of the professional's duty, while others wish to become 'expert' in their own disease and feel frustrated if not helped to do so. Analogous issues can be seen in a public health context—for example, on the responsibility for deciding that a child's vaccination is sufficiently safe (see Chapter 9).

The public health sphere presents the additional difficulty of communicating with many people at once. Rather than simply considering the public as a homogeneous mass, it is essential to consider the possible values held by key stakeholders or audiences. One attempt to categorize overall attitudes to risk is that of cultural theory (Douglas & Wildavsky, 1982; Rayner, 1992). This distinguishes between:

- Egalitarians, who tend to see the balance of nature as fragile, to distrust expertise and strongly favour public participation in decisions
- Individualists, who want to make their own decisions and see nature as robust
- Hierarchists, who want well established rules and procedures to regulate risks and tend to see nature as 'robust within limits'
- Fatalists, who see life as capricious and attempts at control as futile.

Such views are also confirmed and reinforced through social interactions, whether between egalitarian members of a campaigning group, hierarchists working as risk regulators or fatalists seeking mutual sympathy. People seldom conform *consistently* to any of the four ideal types, and are also usually members of varied social groups. Most are capable of putting on individualist, hierarchist, egalitarian or fatalist 'spectacles'. It is therefore better to think of these in terms of archetypes, rather than as characterizing individual people. Despite such caveats, cultural theory may provide a useful heuristic: for example, by prompting one to consider how a strong individualist (or egalitarian, say) would react to a proposed message, and seeking arguments to counter major objections.

The differentiation (or segmentation) of different potential audiences is a major theme of social marketing. This seeks to apply or adapt principles already used in commercial marketing to achieve social goals. Founded in the early 1970s (Kotler & Zaltman, 1971), social marketing has enjoyed a recent upsurge in interest and has exerted considerable influence within health promotion (Kotler and Roberto, 2002; Hastings, 2007). It starts from the proposition that those seeking to influence behaviour for the public good need to know their (multiple) audiences, just as commercial organizations such as supermarkets need a clear profile of their multiple types of customer. A good deal of effort therefore needs to go into investigating who one is trying to influence, and designing messages and their means of delivery accordingly. This approach has had a strong influence, for example, on recent road safety campaigns: messages are specifically targeted at particular types of driver liable to indulge in specific types of unsafe behaviour. Furthermore, the messages are based on research into the beliefs and values that produce that behaviour, and explicit hypotheses about what might trigger change. For example, there appears to be a significant group who strongly see themselves as good drivers—and may indeed be skilled at fast driving—but overestimate their ability to control risks. They will not hear any message about being a 'bad driver' as applying to them, but may be more persuaded by the need to allow for *other* drivers' failings. The underlying categorization is generally inductive, investigating what characteristics typically cluster together, rather than imposing a single 'top-down' classification as in cultural theory. It is complemented by more quantitative demographic research into age, geography, income, etc., to help indicate the numbers to be expected within each category. Use of social marketing raises some interesting questions as to the ethical limits of using (potentially) manipulative methods in a 'good cause'. Nevertheless, its basic message of the need to know one's audience can hardly be faulted.

## Understanding probability: heuristics, biases, and framing

Risk is essentially bound up with the concept of chance—the likelihood of an unwelcome outcome being realized. The accepted measure of likelihood is probability, and probabilities obey well known mathematical laws. However, a key problem within risk perception is that simplified ways of managing information (or *heuristics*), which serve well enough in most situations, can give misleading results in others (Tversky & Kahneman, 1974). Left unchecked, they lead to various common biases in dealing with probabilities. Some of the most relevant are as follows:

- Availability bias—events are perceived to be more frequent if examples are easily brought to mind, so memorable events seem more common even if they only occur rarely

- Confirmation bias—once a view has been formed, new evidence is generally made to fit: contrary information is filtered out, ambiguous data interpreted as confirmation, and consistent information seen as proof- positive. One's own actions can also make expectations self-fulfilling

- Overconfidence—we think our predictions or estimates are more likely to be correct than they really are. This bias appears to affect almost all professions, scientific or otherwise, as well as the lay public. The few exceptions are those who, like weather forecasters, receive constant feedback on the accuracy of their predictions.

Estimating the effect of *combining* probabilities presents further challenges. One issue of particular importance is illustrated in Box 1.3, concerning the interpretation of screening tests, in this case for a hypothetical disease called Smee's syndrome.

Given the information presented, most people seriously overestimate the chance of having the disease—the correct answer being just under 1% (1 chance in 100). The pitfall is to put too much weight on the reliability of the test

## Box 1.3 Screening for Smee's syndrome

Smee's syndrome is a disease carried by about 6000 people in the UK. Once symptoms have developed, it is generally too late for effective treatment, and death can be slow and painful. If caught early, there is an effective cure—but at that stage there are no warning symptoms.

Fortunately, a screening test has been developed, which has been made available to anyone who wants to be tested. The test is highly reliable, in that virtually everyone carrying the disease will test positive (there are no false negatives), while 99% of those without Smee's will test negative.

Suppose you have tested positive for Smee's syndrome. What is the chance that you actually carry the disease?

(the 99%) and not enough on the small prevalence of the disease, i.e. the chance of an individual having Smee's prior to being tested. Given that the population of the UK is roughly 60 million, the prevalence is roughly 1 in 10 000. Although the test is indeed quite reliable, the number of false positive results will still greatly outnumber the true positives.[1] Although we have used a hypothetical example, the interpretation of screening results causes real problems (Gigerenzer, 2002). At an individual level, patients and those advising them may place far too much weight on test results. This applies in particular to screening of wide populations for asymptomatic and relatively uncommon diseases: the situation is very different if there are other reasons for concern, e.g. an individual at higher risk for genetic or lifestyle reasons, or with some symptoms requiring explanation. At a public health level, a realistic appreciation of the consequences of test results is essential in determining the costs and benefits of any given testing scheme. Yet there may be public and commercial pressure to introduce testing on the assumption that 'screening can only do good'. A particular issue at present is the possible introduction of a vCJD screening test for blood donors, where there is the

---

1 The answer in this case can be explained as follows: consider 10 000 people taking the test. On average, one of them will actually have Smee's syndrome, and will reliably test positive for it. Of the other 9999 who do not have Smee's, we should expect 1% also to test positive. To the nearest whole number, that means that there are 100 false positives for every true positive result. So if you test positive for Smee's you are 100 times more likely to have had a false positive result than a true positive.

additional complication of the true prevalence of infection being unknown. Any such test will raise considerable challenges for risk communication: encouragingly, there is evidence to show that screening test results can be explained in ways that promote a real appreciation of their significance (Wilkinson *et al.*, 1990; Woloshin *et al.*, 2007).

*Framing* refers not so much to bias, but more to the point that any situation can be construed in alternative ways, in terms of how the available information is mentally arranged. This can have a major—and often unrealized—effect on the conclusions reached. A common example is that outcomes may be measured against different reference points—as with the glass half-full or half-empty. The practical impact on decisions can be demonstrated by presenting people with the same choice in different ways.

To take a public health example, consider a choice of how to prepare for the anticipated outbreak of a hypothetical disease. If nothing is done, 600 people can be expected to die. There are two alternative ways of preparing for the outbreak. Suppose the effectiveness of plan A is moderate and predictable, but that of plan B depends on the strain of the disease, which will not be known in advance. Plan B will either be completely effective or (more probably) completely ineffective. Given further information on outcomes, the resulting choice can be framed in either of two ways, as in Boxes 1.4a and 1.4b.

| | |
|---|---|
| **Box 1.4a Public health options framed in terms of losses** | **Box 1.4b Public health options framed in terms of gains** |
| If nothing were done, all 600 people at risk would die. | If nothing were done, none of the 600 people at risk would be saved. |
| • If plan A is chosen, 400 people will die for certain | • If plan A is chosen, 200 people will be saved for certain |
| • If plan B is chosen, there is a one in three chance that nobody will die, but a two in three chance that all 600 will still die. | • If plan B is chosen, there is a one in three chance of saving all 600, but a two in three chance of saving nobody. |
| **Which plan would you choose?** | **Which plan would you choose?** |

The figures have been chosen so that the two plans have the same *expected* benefit as each other, but plan B is 'riskier'. More importantly, the two boxes describe precisely the same outcomes in different ways. Yet the two descriptions elicit markedly different responses. When the choice is presented as in 1.4 a, plan B is usually much more popular. The certainty of 400 deaths seemingly gives a powerful incentive to avoid A, even though the more probable outcome of B is even worse. The choice presented as in 1.4 b generally receives a much more mixed response, with plan A often proving more popular than B. Neither way of looking at the problem is *wrong*, but the results are strikingly different. Framing can have quite subtle effects, but this example illustrates one simple point. Like gamblers who bet more wildly to recoup losses—people tend to make riskier choices if all alternatives are framed in terms of losses, but 'play safe' if choosing between alternative gains. Similar effects have been found when comparing individual health outcomes (McNeil *et al.*, 1982). Perhaps most strikingly, they can be just as pronounced for experts: physicians, or those studying public health, as for the general public.

Obviously, framing can be seen as a means of manipulation, but very often the point is simply to avoid accidental mismatches in framing, either because the possibility has not been considered, or because too little is known. Ways of avoiding this include consultation exercises, small-scale piloting of messages, workshops to promote 'assumption busting', and direct research on public beliefs. An open communication process should also ensure exposure to alternative ways of framing an issue. To present choices in as neutral a way as possible, the best approach is probably to give information about both losses and gains throughout, e.g. 'If plan A is adopted, 200 people will die *and* the other 400 at risk will be saved', despite the potential accusation of wasting words.

More generally, it is worth reiterating the point that people can approach risks from completely different frames of reference. If a regulator sets some allowable maximum level for a pollutant, is it protecting the public from a risk, or legitimizing one? Are we engaged in a negotiation, or a search for the best technical solution?

## Societal and political perspectives

Dealing with risk communication issues at the societal and political levels also generates some significant issues for policy- makers and managers. The issues here centre on the manner in which trust is generated and sustained, the processes around the amplification of concerns about specific forms of hazard, and the role of the media in both of these processes. The challenges of dealing with risk perception and risk communication are increased by the multi-channel nature of the communication processes and the difficulty of gaining feedback verification for messages disseminated to wide audiences.

## Trust

In many circumstances, messages are initially judged not by content but by source: *who is telling me this, and can I trust them?* (Renn & Levine, 1991). *Any* message from a source seen as untrustworthy is liable to be disregarded, no matter how well intentioned and well delivered. Indeed, well presented arguments from distrusted sources may actually have a negative effect—as if people conclude that the sender is not only untrustworthy but cunning.

Many studies document a decline in trust in scientific expertise. Reliance on scientific credentials *alone* is therefore unlikely to work. There are no known ways of generating instant trust, but the literature does offer some strong clues as to how it may be won or lost. Firstly, actions often do speak louder than words: judgements about trust will depend on what is done as well as what is said. This applies not only to the actions actually being taken to deal with a risk, but also to the *manner* adopted. Organizational 'body language' is important: appearing to act only under pressure, for example, can be fatal.

Though trust is easily lost, building it is a long-term cumulative process. Short of a reputation for infallibility, the single most important factor in building trust is probably *openness*. This involves not only making information available, but giving a candid account of the evidence underlying decisions. If there are genuine reasons for non-disclosure of data, the reasons need to be given both clearly and early on. The point is that there should be a *presumption* in favour of disclosure. There is also a need to consider the openness of the decision *process*. Can outsiders see how decisions are reached? Who is to contribute, and at what stage? There is a reluctance to trust any system that looks like a 'closed shop'. People need to know that their own concerns—and their own understandings of the risk in question—can be heard, and be taken seriously. Those who feel belittled, ignored or excluded are liable to react with hostility even to full disclosure of information.

It is not hard to find studies featuring distrust of government. Doctors start with much higher credibility, but reactions to high-profile incidents (e.g. HIV-positive surgeons) show how fragile even this can be. However, research has also shown trust to be multifaceted, with relevant factors including perceived competence, objectivity, fairness, consistency, and goodwill. Particular sources may score differently on these dimensions. For example, industrial and commercial sources are frequently seen as competent but potentially biased. Perceptions can also depend on the issue at stake. For example, there is evidence of government bodies being rather *highly* trusted when it comes to radiological safety—more so than environmental campaigners (Hunt *et al.*, 1999). The stated level of trust may also fail to match actual effects on behaviour. The overall point is that black-and-white judgements are not inevitable. There are plenty of cases in which a fair degree of trust has been maintained even in difficult circumstances. However, there is strong evidence that if trust *is* lost, re-establishing it is a long and uphill task.

Many of these points were already well accepted when the previous version of this book was published. However, some findings are more novel. For example, it appears that in at least some circumstances, the *prior* trustworthiness of an information source may be of little consequence. Rather, those with strong beliefs about a particular topic tend to 'reverse engineer' their judgements on trust. Consciously or otherwise, they choose to trust those who support their initial beliefs (Frewer *et al.*, 2003). Trust in a source is thus contingent on prior beliefs on a given topic rather than being an independent factor, with new information then subject to confirmatory biases (White *et al.*, 2003; Poortinga & Pidgeon, 2004). Such research is starting to integrate the insights available from several of the different strands of work just outlined.

## The 'social amplification' of risk

Though individual beliefs are important, people are not isolated actors but operate in a social context. Responses to risk also need to be understood at a societal level. At that level, events to do with risk can be likened to a stone dropping in a pool. Sometimes there is little more than the initial splash. Sometimes the *indirect effects*—caused, as it were, by the distant ripples—can far exceed the direct ones. Hence the idea of social amplification of risk (Kasperson *et al.*, 1988). This is most obvious with events such as accidents: it has been remarked that although no one died at Three Mile Island, the nuclear malfunction there had huge indirect effects on the industry worldwide. An event gains significance not so much because of what has happened, but because of what it seems to portend. A classic example is seen in the *New Yorker*'s editorial of 18th February 1985 on the Bhopal disaster:

> What truly grips us . . . is not so much the numbers as the spectacle of suddenly vanishing competence, of men utterly routed by technology, of fail-safe systems failing with a logic as inexorable as it was once—indeed, right up to that very moment—unforeseeable. And the spectacle haunts us because it seems to carry allegorical import, like the whispery omen of a hovering future.

The event thus becomes a *signal*—a warning that assurances are always untrustworthy, or that technology is out of control. What is less clear is why some events acquire such significance, out of all those that *could* do so.

Risk *communication* can itself have its own indirect effects. If a health warning is issued on a prominent variety of cheese or wine, rival producers may rejoice at first. But their glee is typically cut short as they find that consumers also (unfairly!) shun *their* products. They may be forced to close or to lay off staff, with further indirect effects. Then there may be expensive attempts to restore confidence, political recriminations—perhaps international in scope—and so on. The social system has reacted in a way that *amplifies* the impact of the original risk. Conversely, risks that one might expect to gain more prominence may be 'socially attenuated' and have little public impact. Social amplification research has been criticised for allegedly assuming that some objective measure of risk exists, which is then amplified, attenuated or distorted. The alternative view is of risk as a social construct, not an objective reality (Irwin & Wynne, 1995). The current state of the debate, and its practical implications, is summarized in Chapter 4 (Pidgeon & Henwood).

## The mass media

As to when social amplification is likely to be most pronounced, the fright factors noted before will again be relevant. However, additional features come into play once we consider the social system rather than only individual perceptions. The mass media clearly play a major role. Reportage affects both perceptions of risk in general and how specific issues are initially framed. Then as an episode develops, reports of people's reactions to the original risk feed the indirect effects. However, the mass media are not *all-important*. Professional (e.g. medical) networks are often also significant, as are informal networks of friends and acquaintances—the classic grapevine.

People typically trust the goodwill of family and friends more than any institutional source, while access to decentralized media such as the internet increases the influence of self-organized networks. In any case, to blame 'sensationalist reporting' for exaggerated fears is largely to miss the point. Media coverage may well amplify the public's interest in dramatic forms of mishap, but it does not *create* it. A 'good story' is one in which public and media interest reinforce each other. It is difficult to see how this could be otherwise.

Research continues on why some particular stories about health risks take off spectacularly.

Alongside the previous fright factors, the media triggers shown in Box 1.5 provide additional (though less thoroughly researched) indicators. Nor are these effects necessarily accidental. Interest groups of all sorts have a natural interest in shaping media definition and coverage of issues, and increasingly sophisticated ways of doing so, e.g. mounting eyecatching and newsworthy

## Box 1.5 Media triggers

A possible risk to public health is more likely to become a major story if the following are prominent or can readily be made to become so:

1 Questions of *blame*

2 Alleged *secrets and attempted cover-ups*

3 *Human interest* through identifiable heroes, villains, dupes, etc. (as well as victims)

4 Links with *existing high-profile issues or personalities*

5 *Conflict*

6 *Signal value*: the story as a portent of further ills *(What next?)*

7 *Many people exposed* to the risk, even if at low levels *'It could be you!'*

8 Strong *visual impact* (e.g. pictures of suffering)

9 Links to *sex* and/or *crime*.

events. Nevertheless, deliberate attempts to influence will still be working with or against the grain of likely public concern and media interest, as represented by fright factors and media triggers. Stories also sometimes have an incubation period: interest can erupt some time after the actual event, catching out the unwary. Mechanisms for this are again interesting, e.g. national media picking up an old local story and magnifying it (Davies, 2008).

Of the triggers listed, there is some evidence that the single most important is *blame*, particularly in keeping a story running for a long period. However, each case may be affected by many factors, including chance, e.g. a shortage or glut of competing stories. Once a story is established, the very fact that there is interest in the topic becomes a related story. The result can be that reportage snowballs as media compete for coverage.

Put crudely, a good story may require villains and heroes. But the casting need not be fixed in advance.

## Conclusions

Our aim in this opening chapter has been to set out some of the parameters for the chapters that follow. Inevitably, we have touched upon issues without developing them in detail or necessarily providing closure. Subsequent chapters will provide further illustration and argument, although it is important to note that considerable controversies remain. This book does not, and indeed cannot, provide a consensus on all the key issues. For the time being, differing perspectives and the insights offered by the various cases of risk communication provide us with elements of the wider mosaic with which we have to contend. Where there are areas of conflict, these may provide the reader with insights into new possibilities for analysis and research. They also highlight the problems that policy- makers face in walking the tightrope that is so often typified by risk communication in the public health arena.

## References

Adams, J. (1995). *Risk*. London, University College London Press.

Bennett, P. G. & Calman, K. C. (1999). *Risk Communication and Public Health*. Oxford, Oxford University Press.

Calman, K. C. & Royston, G. H. D. (1997). Risk language and dialects. *British Medical Journal*, 313: 799–802.

Covello, V. T., Sandman, P. M. & Slovic, P. (1988) *Risk Communication, Risk Statistics and Risk Comparisons; a Manual for Plant Managers*. Washington DC, Chemical Manufacturers' Association.

Davies, N. (2008). *Flat Earth News*. London, Chatto & Windus.

Douglas, M. & Wildavsky, A. B. (1982). Risk and culture: An essay on the selection of technical and environmental dangers. Berkeley, University of California Press.

Fischhoff, B. (1995). Risk perception and communication unplugged: twenty years of process. *Risk Analysis*, 15(2), 137–45.

Fischhoff, B., Lichtenstein, S., Slovic, P., Derby, S. L. & Keeney, R. L. (1981). *Acceptable Risk*. Cambridge, New York, Cambridge University Press.

Frewer, L. J., Scholderer, J. & Bredahl, L. (2003). Communication about the risks and benefits of genetically-modified foods: the mediating role of trust. *Risk Analysis*, 23 (6): 1117– 33.

Gigerenzer, G. (2002). *Reckoning with risk: learning to live with uncertainty*. Allen Lane, Penguin Press.

Hastings, G. (2007). *Social marketing: why should the devil have all the best tunes?* London, Butterworth–Heinemann.

Hunt, S., Frewer, L. J. & Shepherd, R. (1999). Public trust in sources of information about radiation risks in the UK. *Journal of Risk Research*, 1: 167–81.

Irwin, A. & Wynne, B. (eds) (1995). *Misunderstanding science? The public reconstruction of science and technology*. Cambridge, New York, Cambridge University Press.

Johnson, B. R. (2003). Are some risk comparisons more effective under conflict? A replication and extension of Roth *et al. Risk Analysis*, 23(4): 767–80.

Kasperson, R. E., Renn, O., Slovic, P. *et al.* (1988): The social amplification of risk: a conceptual framework. *Risk Analysis*, 8: 177–87.

Kotler, P. & Roberto, E. L. (2002). *Social marketing: improving the quality of life*. Thousand Oaks, CA, Sage.

Kotler, P. & Zaltman, G. (1971). Social marketing: an approach to planned social change. *Journal of Marketing*, 35: 3–12.

McNeil, B. J., Pauker, S. G., Sox, H. C. & Tversky, A. (1982). On the elicitation of preferences for alternative therapies. *New England Journal of Medicine*, 306: 1259–62.

Meryn, S. (1998). Improving doctor–patient communication: not an option, but a necessity. *British Medical Journal*, 316: 1922.

Paling, J. (1997). *Up to your armpits in alligators? How to sort out what risks are worth worrying about*. Gainesville, Risk Communication and Environmental Institute.

Poortinga, W. & Pidgeon, N. (2004). Trust, the asymmetry principle and the role of prior beliefs. *Risk Analysis*, 24(6): 1475–86.

Rayner, S. (1992). Cultural theory and risk analysis. In S. Krimsky & D. Golding (eds). *Social Theories of Risk*. Westport, CT, GD Praeger.

Renn, O. & Levine, D. (1991). Credibility and trust in risk communication. In R. E. Kasperson and P. J. M. Stallen (eds). *Communicating Risks to the Public*. Kluwer, Dordrecht, International Perspectives.

Rosenberg, H. & Feldman, C. S. (2008). *No time to think: the menace of media speed and the 24-hour news cycle*. New York, Continuum International Publishing.

Roth, E. M., Morgan, M. G., Fischhoff, B. *et al.* (1990). What do we know about making risk comparisons? *Risk Analysis*, 10: 375–87.

Tversky, A. & Kahneman, D. (1974). Judgement under uncertainty: Heuristics and biases. *Science*, 185: 1124–31.

White, M. P., Pahl, S., Buehner, M. & Haye, A. (2003). Trust in risky messages: The role of prior attitudes. *Risk Analysis*, 23(4): 717–26.

Wilson, R. (1979). Analysing the daily risks of life. *Technology Review*, 81(4): 40–6; 403–15.

Wilkinson, C., Jones, J. M. & McBride, J. (1990). Anxiety caused by abnormal result of cervical smear test: a controlled trial. *British Medical Journal* 300: 440.

Woloshin, S., Schwartz, L. M., Welch, G. (2007). The effectiveness of a primer to help people understand risk. *Annals of Internal Medicine* 146: 256–65.

Chapter 2

# Bringing light to the shadows and shadows to the light: risk, risk management, and risk communication

Denis Fischbacher-Smith (University of Glasgow), Alan Irwin (Brunel University), & Moira Fischbacher-Smith (University of Glasgow)

## Introduction

> Human beings are meaning-seeking creatures. Unless we find some pattern or meaning in our lives, we fall very easily into despair. Language plays an important part in our quest (Armstrong, 2007, p. 1).

This opening quotation suggests that language is a key element in our development of understanding and, as such, can be seen to play a major role in contemporary debates around risk and the processes of risk communication. 'We moderns' (Latour, 1993; 1999; 2005) tend to look for patterns in 'data' and 'knowledge' in an attempt to make sense of the world in which we operate. We try to impose some kind of order upon events which otherwise could appear dangerously meaningless, random, and uncertain. We seek to reduce uncertainty where possible and this tendency is a key component of many public health debates. Since the data and knowledge that underpin our understanding are likely to be partial at best, this drive towards both sense- and meaning-making can produce uncertainties, contradictions, and anxieties over the future. We live in the so-called 'risk society' (Beck, 1986; 1992) not because the risks of life have become numerically greater, but because of our increased awareness that the tools we use to deal with risk (science, modernization, rational calculation) are both insufficient and generative of further risks as the technologies we develop in the name of progress—nuclear energy, transportation systems, oil-intensive consumer products—become sources of threat in themselves. This means too that the inevitable tendency in western societies, like old generals forever fighting the previous battle, is that we tend to look backwards so as to predict the future state(s) of the world in which we live. Indeed, the business of risk assessment itself can be seen as such a 'backward'-looking process. In this way also, risk assessment can be viewed as an attempted colonization of the future (Giddens, 1990), or, put another way, the wish to impose some kind of structure, predictability, and order upon events which have yet to occur (and may indeed never occur). The result is the generation of a complex mosaic of issues within which we try to make sense of the fragmented information that we can piece together and use our equally fragmented knowledge as a means of interpreting the world around us. Add to this the limitations and boundaries of the various interpretive 'lenses' that we use in the sense-making process and it is clear that the problems that we face in our understanding of risk are both considerable and complex (Weick, 1993; 1995; 2001).

The challenge for these processes of order- (and meaning-) making comes when decision-makers (and the wider society in which they are located) are confronted with an issue that is outside of their experience base and yet which is (at least potentially) sufficiently significant as to require action to mitigate its effects or, in the case of unacceptable risks, to prevent the activity taking place. In certain cases, a precautionary approach will be taken to prevent the generation of harm, even where the evidential basis for that decision is weak (Calman & Smith, 2001). Here, a balance has to be found between regulation (and the constraints that it imposes on behaviour), risk acceptability and, under certain circumstances, the nature and timescale of the precautionary approach. At the heart of this process lies the manner in which information and knowledge come together to generate a 'burden of proof' and so legitimize the rejection, modification, or acceptance of a set of risks. BSE and the mobile phone masts debates are useful recent examples of these issues.

## The 'problem' of risk in public health

Public health issues provide one of the most contentious areas in which risk acceptability debates occur and where the pressures for a precautionary approach can be seen to be most significant. The problems in this arena centre on the manner in which various public groups seek to impose meaning across a range of risk issues and look to 'science' (and its 'expert' representatives) as the conduit through which that meaning will be constructed, mediated, and (potentially) provided. There have been many debates around public health-related risks such as thalidomide (Stephens & Brynner, 2001), BSE (Phillips, 2000), smoking (Ferber, 2004; Gray, 1997; Schroeder, 2002; Tansey *et al.*, 2004), and HIV/AIDS (Griffin, 2000; Hooper, 2000). Problems also arise in the context of new and 'emergent' forms of disease where there is little, if any, prior experience and evidence to help formulate the probabilistic element of any risk assessment. In this setting, the consequences of the hazard are focused on by the public and the media, even though the potential for that hazard being realized is scientifically unknown at that point in time. In fact, it may also be the case that the consequences of the hazard are also unknown as the evidence base that is available at the time leads scientists and policy-makers to the wrong conclusion. Each of these knowledge 'states' has generated conflicts around expertise, scientific evidence, interpretation, and understanding. Difficulties arise when meaning—invariably expressed in terms of a cause and effect relationship—is not agreed upon and where the resultant contested problem domain is filled with conflicting theories, speculation, and conjecture on the basis of a relatively weak and challenged evidence base. The contested ground of such debates becomes dominated by technical experts, who seek to provide guidance to the 'shadow spaces' (Pelling *et al.*, 2008) that can surround these issues. Expertise is seen as a potential means of bringing light to the shadows and, in so doing, aiding in the sense-making process and reducing uncertainty.

It is in these 'shadow spaces' (Pelling *et al.*, 2008) that many of the contentious debates around public health risk are to be found. Of course, we also know that it is often in the shadows that new possibilities and opportunities arise, removed from the harsh glare of scientific culture and the drive to reduce complex issues of culture, value, and meaning into causal relations focused narrowly on 'risk' alone. Activist organizations and groups of sufferers can also play an important positive role in developing new knowledge and understandings, pushing scientific institutions forward when organizational paralysis occurs in the face of radical uncertainty, competing priorities, and costly research and development. Frequently also, discussion in the 'shadow spaces' reveals that risk is not the only issue at stake, but there are also a range of issues around power, wealth, the limits of expertise, and reputation (Miller, 1999; Redfern *et al.*, 2000; Shermer, 2001; Smith & McCloskey, 2000; Stephens & Brynner, 2001; Taylor, 2003). Thus, in the UK debate over genetically modified (GM) foods, the wider public concerns over the future of British agriculture, the likely benefits to consumers, and the perceived over-dominance of North American food producers were rigidly converted into a 'risk' issue by government bodies for whom the only 'rational' question was whether there were long-term health and environmental consequences from the growth of GM crops in the UK. A similar situation occurs now over civil nuclear power as a range of anxieties relating to nuclear proliferation, loss of civil liberties, under-development of alternative energy sources, and restrictions on future generations become reduced to the abacus of risk. Other examples of debates that have occupied these shadow spaces can be found around the issues associated with BSE, thalidomide, and the MMR vaccine, where the ensuing debates illustrated the potential for conflict over scientific issues. This is especially the case where there is no 'clear' burden of proof—especially when 'evidence' was taken out of the laboratory and applied within the real world context—and no real understanding of the likely damage pathways and contagion processes associated with disease transmission. Despite the lack of scientific evidence in a real world context, science is often required to provide comment on the nature of the risks and the potential strategies that might be available for mitigation. It is here that the role of expertise in dealing with the demands of shadow spaces becomes problematic. Perhaps the most celebrated example of the politicization of the process can be found in the case of BSE and the risks associated with its transmission to humans in the form of variant Creutzfeldt–Jakob disease (vCJD). In an attempt to prevent a crisis within the UK's farming industry, the then Secretary of State for agriculture (John Gummer) attempted to reassure the British public that British beef was safe by feeding his daughter a beef burger in front of the media. (This tactic was later repeated by the corresponding French minister to 'prove' that French beef was safe, though in this case he was to eat the beef that he had just bought. This episode was also shown on television.) Whilst the scientific community (or at least parts of it) was attempting to determine what the evidence was for the hazard—an invariably slow process—politicians and policy-makers were demanding information quickly to quell growing public concerns (see Chapter 11). This difficulty of the mismatch between the objectives and timescales held by scientists and policy-makers pervades many fields of endeavour and is a constant source of difficulty.

The core premise of this chapter is that the manner in which risk-based information is constructed, tested, communicated, and validated is a multidimensional and multi-channel process. The 'shadows' presented within risk debates are invariably not controlled by any group, and no single group has the ability to bring the requisite amount of illumination to the debates to 'prove' a particular outcome. Thus, there is an indeterminate policy position in which debates range and a 'solution' is not made available by science or where the 'error cost' of decisions is considerable (Collingridge, 1984; 1992; Collingridge & Reeve, 1986). One way of capturing this new understanding of risk and risk communication is by reflecting a little on the last three decades of institutional action, practical experience, and academic investigation of these issues. In this chapter, we will make a modest attempt at this task starting, firstly, with some of the 'classic' accounts of the 1970s (specifically Rowe's attempt to schematize the processes of risk assessment) and, secondly, by presenting a tentative list of some of the developments in our awareness of risk, risk management, and risk communication since that time. Inevitably, such a listing implies a 'cleaner' break with history—and a sharper and over-simplified temporal shift—than has actually occurred. However, we would argue that these undeniable difficulties should not deny the importance of critical reflection over these issues.

## 'Life on Mars'—risk management from a 1970s perspective as the 'classical' paradigm

The UK television series, 'Life on Mars', saw a man return to the 1970s following a car accident and explored his attempts to deal with the social norms and expectations of the time as he struggled to make sense of the world around him. In many respects, a return to the 1970s for a 'modern' risk analyst might well have similar characteristics. The late 1960s into the 1970s represented the emergence of what we can term the 'classical' paradigm for risk management. Of course, there are many 'origin myths' for risk management. Risk is believed, for example, to be amenable to tracking through the notion of a wager or investment in a financial context, discerned in the need to make decisions in the face of the potentially lethal uncertainties of military combat, and identified in law and the requirements of evidence. However, the modern management of risk has significant origins in the discipline of engineering, which has sought to provide tools and techniques around the identification and estimation of risk, along with an assessment of the consequences associated with those hazards. Risk seen formally from this perspective is a product of the probability of a particular hazard being realized and the consequences associated with that hazard.

As Lowrance presented this in his classic text, *Of Acceptable Risk* (Lowrance, 1981), risk assessment should be divided into two categories: the *measurement of risk* (an essentially objective and scientific activity) and the *judgement of safety* (which he presented as a normative and political activity). According to this framework, calculations of probability and consequence belong in the first stage, whilst public debates, political balances, and value judgements are restricted to the second. Employing slightly different terminology, at around the same time Rowe presented a similarly idealized representation of the risk assessment process which saw risk assessment being composed of the processes of risk analysis (risk identification, estimation, and consequence modelling) and the processes that determine the acceptability of those 'scientifically determined' levels of risk (Rowe, 1977). Figure 2.1 shows this process and

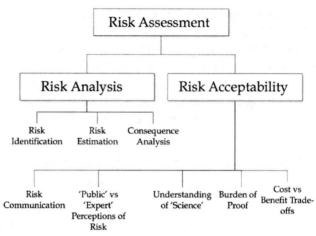

**Fig. 2.1** The process of risk assessment (after Rowe).

also highlights some of the issues that invariably fall into the shadows that surround risk debates.

The risk analysis process as presented by Rowe appears, on the surface, to be ideally suited to those events for which there is a reasonably high frequency of failure and where failure pathways and their consequences are well understood. This a priori data allows the process of risk analysis to calculate failure modes and effects and ascribe probabilities to those 'pathways' that are both robust (owing to the availability of frequency data) and have a reasonable-to-high degree of predictive validity around failure rates. Even so, the probability estimates will be bounded by uncertainty and this should ideally be specified in terms of confidence limits on the data. Where uncertainty around the data is high, or where there is little, if any, a priori evidence of previous failures and their associated consequences, then this process breaks down. For low probability–high consequence events ($P_LC_H$), or for those events where there is no prior experience of the hazard or its consequences, then there are (or should be) significant doubts around the validity that decision-makers should grant to risk analytical calculations.

As presented in Rowe's 'classical' model, risk analysis is a technical process that seeks to identify hazards (as the source of risk), determine the probabilities of those hazards, and model the consequences of those hazards within the context of the population that is 'at risk'. However, this process is invariably mediated by technical experts and can create difficulties around the burden of proof, error cost, and the exercise of powerful interests (Collingridge, 1992;

Collingridge & Reeve, 1986; Smith, 1990; 1991; Smith & Elliott, 1992). Whilst there are well established tools and techniques for the calculation of risk and the determination of consequences, the evidential basis for such determinations and the extent to which the findings have predictive validity have proved to be areas of debate. Problems occur with $P_LC_H$ events where, owing to the low frequency of occurrence, the data that is available to make effective judgements is insufficient. In such cases, experts' best estimates have been used as a means of bridging the information gap (Smith, 1990). The problem in these cases is that the final determination of probabilities, on which policy-makers will make decisions, does not always highlight the degree of uncertainty and ambiguity in the data that is used.

A useful illustration of the problems in dealing with probabilities, uncertainty, and ambiguity is that of bird flu. Whilst it is clear that there is a risk of H5N1 being transmitted from birds to humans via a process of virus mixing, there is little or no a priori data on which to base probabilistic models of that mutation. The assumption is made that the virus will migrate. At this point, normal disease spread models can be used to calculate the rate and spread of the disease within a given population. However, these models have a great deal of sophistication built into their analytical architectures, they will only perform around the parameters and assumptions that the analysts build into them. Organizations seeking to develop their contingency plans for an H5N1 outbreak must then factor in their own assumptions around the information that emerges from any scenario model of the outbreak. Thus at any point in time, there are multiple sources of uncertainty that feed into the model.

The case of bird flu can also be used to challenge the fundamental distinction between risk analysis and risk acceptability made by authors such as Lowrance and Rowe. To develop one point already hinted at, any risk analysis must be 'framed' by the initial questions being asked and the assumptions made by those who will be investigating the process. This act of 'framing' must of course be influenced by policy and political concerns as well as the requirements of technical measurement. Is the question to be answered one that is about the relative risks of different methods of poultry farming or the risks to the general public from wildlife exposure? Is the question about the vulnerability of certain social and demographic groups or the population as a whole? Should the question assume (in a form of 'naïve sociology') that regulatory requirements and control systems will actually be adhered to and that the carefully controlled conditions of the laboratory safely mirror the real world? How then do questions about ethics, benefits, and societal need factor into these calculations? Whilst the analysis/acceptability dichotomy appears solid, it is open to challenge on a number of grounds.

At this point, we can begin to consider some of the factors that make the Rowe model unhelpfully misleading. Many of these factors have emerged in the light of three decades of practical experience with risk, decades that have witnessed the accidents at Three Mile Island, Chernobyl, and Bhopal. The BSE saga has also had longlasting repercussions through national and international regulatory processes, especially in terms of science public relations with regard to risk. Controversy over GM food and nuclear power has highlighted the importance of societal assessments of risk, assessments that can explicitly bring together the very factors that the classical engineering models of risk seek to keep apart. Our point is not that these incidents and reactions have in themselves created a change in the 'mood music' around risk—the BSE case, for example, could be interpreted in a number of ways apart from the influential conclusions of the Phillips report (Phillips, 2000). However, the political and public aftermath of such cases has created a sense of institutional vulnerability in the face of risk (especially when confronting new areas of innovation and technological development), a need to find new ways of dealing with and communicating risk, and a sense that the 'classical' model of risk assessment with its clear distinctions and sense of centralized control is no longer sufficient. We can start our discussion by considering the very notion of risk itself as a definable entity.

## Risk revisited—challenges to the classical model

### Risk, uncertainty, and indeterminacy

At the core of the contemporary treatment of sociotechnical challenges can be found a degree of confusion over three increasingly problematical categories of risk (Felt & Wynne, 2008; Wynne, 2002). If 'risk' implies a known entity that (based on previous experience and well tested empirical models) can be granted a probability and scale of consequences, many of today's challenges suggest a much higher degree of *uncertainty*. Thus, the risk to consumers from eating British beef could be defined in 1989 as tiny since there was no known mechanism by which contaminated cows could generate human health problems. This statement of risk, however, concealed significant scientific uncertainties— and not least since the non-identification of a mechanism could not be taken as proof that no such mechanism existed (this being a time before prions were understood). Building such radical uncertainties into risk calculations represents a substantial challenge since, as has often been pointed out since BSE, the absence of evidence certainly cannot be taken to imply evidence of absence.

Going further, it may be that in many areas of risk we are facing not simply radical uncertainties—mechanisms, causal factors, and consequences which are not so far understood—but also fundamental *indeterminacies* (the 'unknown unknowns' of Donald Rumsfeld's now infamous formulation). How can we know (and therefore calculate) the consequences of entities (the products of nanotechnology or synthetic biology, for example) which have never previously existed? How can we put a probability on something we have not imagined and for which no established models exist? In other words, how can we know what we don't know? To label such risks as 'uncertain' implies that there should be confidence limits to our understanding. The more radical (and troublesome) possibility is that such risk categories cannot be understood since they present potentialities that we do not—and cannot—envisage. Risk analysis appears a very restricted tool for the expression of such radical doubt.

In addition, there is every possibility that such uncertainties can be open to manipulation and selective presentation. Perhaps the archetypal example of such conflict concerns the manner in which the tobacco companies sought to use their expert and financial power to shape debates around risk (Ferber, 2004; Gostin, 2007; Gray, 1997; Ramsay, 2002). This particular case is well documented and it does raise several issues that are important in our present discussions. One of the key characteristics of the tobacco 'wars' was the manner in which technical expertise was used to undermine the opposition—especially around detailed technical issues of addiction. In this way, the construction of uncertainty became a tool to diminish the possibilities of regulatory closure (a similar situation seems to occur with regard to climate change). The manner in which this information is then judged by policy- and decision-makers becomes crucial. Such discussions are also important for the communication of risk and uncertainty.

## Science, citizen science, and public knowledge

There is an increasing recognition that those possibly affected by various hazards may have insights into the nature of the issues that belie their apparent lack of scientific credentials in a conventional sense. The concept of 'citizen science' (Irwin, 1995), or public knowledgeability, does not imply that members of the public are likely to possess the developed technical skills in a specific field of a qualified 'expert'. However, it does suggest that public groups may be more than *tabula rasa*: empty vessels waiting to be filled by the knowledges and understandings of science. To return to the case of BSE in the UK, it might seem only reasonable that scientific advice to separate the brain and spinal column of cattle from the carcasses sold to the meat industry should draw (and be tested) upon the insights and understandings of those in abattoirs that actually conduct such operations on a regular basis. This, however, was not seen as relevant during the mid-1990s. Instead, the tendency is to view non-scientific sources of advice, experience, and insight as secondary to the calculations of science. Equally, when it comes to risk communication, the tendency is still to summon up the 'deficit model' (Irwin & Wynne, 1996) of an ignorant and ill-informed public—an approach that can fail to understand the basis of public concerns and provoke feelings of antagonism and rejection. Of course, the analysis/acceptability distinction fails to recognize the potentially multiple sources of knowledge around risk issues.

## Transparency, trust, and accountability

Very strikingly, the last decade in particular has witnessed a strong emphasis on the need to open up the processes of scientific advice to external scrutiny, to set new standards of transparency, and to 'engage' with the wider publics. The Phillips inquiry into BSE in Britain was not the first such statement (coming after, for example, the 1998 Royal Commission on Environmental Pollution report on setting environmental standards), but it did represent the challenge to the governmental control of risk in an especially direct fashion. As the report summarized its main finding:

> The Government did not lie to the public about BSE. It believed that the risks posed by BSE to humans were remote. The Government was preoccupied with preventing an alarmist over-reaction to BSE because it believed that the risk was remote. It is now clear that this campaign of reassurance was a mistake. When on 20 March 1996 the Government announced that BSE had probably been transmitted to humans, the public felt that they had been betrayed. (Phillips, 2000, Vol. 1, Section 1)

The need to rebuild public trust in scientific governance lies at the heart of this new emphasis on engagement, openness, and communication (Irwin, 1995; 2006). Of course, this new approach raises many new challenges—not least questions about whether limited exercises in transparency will actually engender trust or its very opposite. However, the trend towards enhanced accountability suggests a very different playing field for risk than the closed calculations of the 1970s. In this spirit also, recent years have witnessed a series of high profile engagement exercises concerning risk-related issues—with the UK GM Nation exercise being one of the prime examples. Such exercises characteristically raise as many questions about the relationship between science, risk, and governance as they actually answer (Irwin, 2006). However, such initiatives do indicate the new context for risk governance and the need to avoid any appearance of secrecy or absence of democratic accountability.

## Risk, identity, and culture

One recurrent finding from social scientific investigations into risk concerns the close relationship between everyday culture and the kinds of risk which are identified (Douglas & Wildavsky, 1983). Thus, there are geographical areas in which the nature of the public health problem (and its attendant underlying causes) is the very thing that is integral to that area's identity and is a part of its history. An example of this comes from work carried out in the East End of Glasgow around Community Health Partnerships (Fischbacher *et al.*, 2009) where the comments made by an addictions worker set out some of these issues:

> The East is unique . . . there is nearly twice as much child protection, there is nearly twice the number on the child protection register, there is more criminal justice, a higher level of mental health problems . . . and addiction is the biggest in the city. The problem in the East is, in some respects, what gives the East its identity.

In this context, the assessment of risk and the policies put in place to deal with those risks cannot be separated out from the underlying structures and urban fabrics that are interwoven with, and serve as causal agents to, the problem. Failures to address the situational context in which risks are generated and to ignore the insights that citizens have on the nature of those risks will prove problematic in trying to implement solutions to the issues. From a public health perspective this raises some important issues around intervention, as illustrated by a further comment from an addictions worker in Glasgow (Fischbacher *et al.*, 2009):

> . . . we have to understand the population we serve better, and that means we have to have different responses to the issues that are there . . . the culture's different in the East . . . the territory is marked in the East. So when we construct services we need to understand that, because there's no point putting a service there, because we know these folk won't go . . . these kind of cultures, they're actually palpable . . . Generations of ten, twenty years . . . it's what they do. And with all that, with all the culture is unemployment and disability and addictions and alcohol and poverty and deprivation and poor housing, you know, and poor self worth, and all that . . .

The problems in this case are clearly embedded in the area that serves to create the very risks that have to be managed by 'public health'. The obvious difficulty rests in the manner in which this vicious circle is broken into and by whom. Urban areas often display interactions between social, economic, and health problems that produce a complex mosaic of issues that require policy interventions around 'risk'. Such interventions need to be introduced in a manner that does not disenfranchise the very people who are deemed to be 'at risk'. Many of these problems are often labelled as 'lifestyle risks' and involve alcohol, drugs, and sexually related disease. Yet such a label serves to mask the underlying causal factors that help to generate the conditions that might move people to engage in these activities. The underlying social and economic factors that serve to create the conditions in which such health problems are generated are often overlooked in favour of processes of risk communication, lifestyle education, and medical intervention. The latter are seen as more tractable processes of intervention.

A further example of the complex dynamics of the problem centres on the manner in which environmental impacts may be concentrated in particular (often the least affluent) communities with the associated health implications that such environmental degradation can bring. These impacts can be both spatially determined in clearly defined areas (with the associated hazard range of the impact being clearly seen) or occupationally concentrated (with its attendant class-related implications). In both cases, the abilities of those at risk to extricate themselves from the source of the hazard will be constrained by the same social and economic factors that trapped them in the situation in the first place.

## Communicating risk

What is clear from research undertaken to date is that the language used to communicate complex scientific issues is important in helping to shape the nature of the debate and the attendant understanding that comes with it. As we have already noted, communication initiatives in the 1970s and 1980s tended to take a more paternalistic approach to dealing with the various publics around such debates. The view was simply that if these groups were 'better educated' then they would be in a position to understand the issues. Meanwhile, it was considered better to play up the certainties of risk assessment (what the Phillips report memorably termed 'leaning into the wind') when dealing with public groups rather than openly acknowledging areas of uncertainty. Whilst this approach still has currency in some areas, there is also a widespread acceptance that the diverse publics can often have a significant understanding of the issues and may also have insights that can challenge the dominant views held by elements of the scientific communities.

There are several hurdles that need to be overcome when addressing the role of expertise in risk debates and the manner in which uncertainty in risk information is communicated. Of particular importance is the manner in which all forms of knowledge construction have their limitations when taken out of the specific context in which the knowledge was developed. Scientific knowledge, especially that knowledge which is based on work carried out within the laboratory and then applied to a 'real world' setting, will invariably have problems around predictive validity and the burden of proof. This will be especially the case in those contexts where the real world setting brings with it a large number of intervening variables that generates uncertainty around causal pathways. Knowledge based within communities may suffer from the manner in which the assumptions of that knowledge are tested and validated. This public understanding may, however, provide empirical evidence that undermines the theoretical assumptions that are embedded within more formal, scientifically based forms of knowledge. In addition, there are potential problems around the manner in which powerful economic interests can help to shape the landscape of debates around risk by determining what knowledge is legitimate or at least acceptable. The debates that raged in the USA around tobacco and its associated health effects serve again to illustrate this process (see, for example, Barnes & McCaffree, 2002; Gostin, 2007; Ramsay, 2002; Schroeder, 2002; Susser, 1997; Tansey *et al.*, 2004).

The other side of this issue is that without some checks on the knowledge claims made by some 'experts', then the potential for 'junk' science to prevail within such debates is increased. Thus the construction of a 'legitimate' scientific claim is the first major hurdle in dealing with the shadow spaces around public health risk debates. Many of the debates around risk fall into the category of the 'symbolic bun fight' in which different interests in the debates seek to portray their assessment of complex and often non-linear risk issues as 'safe' or 'unsafe'. Both of these states are inherently bounded by uncertainty and in a way that ensures that there is often no clear 'burden of proof' owing to the lack of robust a priori evidence that would allow for a more conventional form of risk assessment. At the very least, we can say that communicating risk in such circumstances is not only a matter of offering persuasive messages to the public—and indeed such explicit attempts at persuasion can risk appearing inauthentic and untrustworthy. Instead, communication needs to be considered as an open and two-way process with the institutions under scrutiny as much as the messages they deliberately seek to convey.

## Conclusion—risk, risk management, and the communication of complexity

These new characteristics and challenges certainly suggest a different intellectual paradigm for risk than was offered in the 1970s. Whilst Lord Rothschild could call in 1978 for an 'index of risks' (drawing upon earlier analysts, notably Starr, 1969) which would allow risk comparisons to be made as a guide to acceptability, now the risks of everyday life are seen to embrace wider uncertainties, demand public engagement and accountability, and acknowledge diverse forms of knowledge and understanding. Risk has been recognized as being more complex that hitherto thought. It is not easily reducible to core elements that can be managed within a reductionist model of science. The shadow spaces around risk are those where emergent properties arising from the interaction of the various components of the issues generate problems that beguile those who seek to manage them. Risk management does not conform to the neat prescriptions of cause and effect relationships and the debates and the issues are certainly not linear. Meanwhile, it does seem that we live in more anxious times—times also where any accident or incident leads to the pursuit of the search for causality and increasingly the process of scapegoating. The determination of who is 'to blame' is often seen to be important—whether the scapegoat is a social or medical worker, a police officer, a government department or a chemical company—and this scapegoating process has become a core element of the 'management of risk'. In such circumstances, the defence that a full risk assessment was conducted is unlikely to be sufficient, even if this requirement to analyse 'risk' has also created a whole 'risk' industry in its own right—as health service and social workers, police, and local government employees will testify.

These are complex and demanding problems for risk management, risk communication, and relations between institutions and the wider publics. In particular, there is a need to avoid letting the complexity of risk create organizational paralysis whilst still being open to contingencies, indeterminacies, and re-interpretations of the evidence. Meanwhile, public support and trust may be built not by retreating into the old certainties, but by communicating openly about what is both known and unknown, reliably tested and conditional, flexible and fixed. This would seem to require new forms of risk management and, specifically, risk leadership. In particular, the challenge is to engender a leadership style which recognizes inevitable complexity and legitimate uncertainty, draws upon multiple sources of evidence and expertise, robustly tests the often implicit framing assumptions built into risk calculations, and recognizes that frameworks of risk cannot sit apart from wider cultures of identity creation and meaning. Risk communication from this perspective is not a separate branch of risk management but a constituent part of its very enactment. Quite clearly also, the new conditions of risk require a much wider range of technical, business, organizational, and social intelligences than has been the case in past. Only by recognizing the wide and diverse requirements generated by risk debates can we hope to illuminate the shadows that typify many policy areas.

## References

Armstrong, K. (2007) *The bible: a biography*. Berkeley, CA, Grove Press (Grove/Atlantic).

Barnes, R. & McCaffree, D. R. (2002). Tobacco wars—the physician's role in public health advocacy. *Journal of the Oklahoma State Medical Association*, 95(3): 120–5.

Beck, U. (1986). *Risikogesellschaft: Auf dem Weg in eine andere Moderne.* Frankfurt, Suhrkamp Verlag.

Beck, U. (1992). *Risk society. Towards a new modernity* (M. Ritter, Trans.). London, Sage.

Calman, K. & Smith, D. (2001). Works in theory but not in practice? Some notes on the precautionary principle. *Public Administration*, 79(1): 185–204.

Collingridge, D. (1984). *Technology in the policy process—the control of nuclear power.* London, Francis Pinter.

Collingridge, D. (1992). *The management of scale: Big organizations, big decisions, big mistakes.* London, Routledge.

Collingridge, D. & Reeve, C. (1986). *Science speaks to power: the role of experts in policy-making.* London, Francis Pinter.

Douglas, M. & Wildavsky, A. (1983). *Risk and culture.* Berkeley, University of California Press.

Felt, U. & Wynne, B. (eds) (2008). *Taking European knowledge seriously. A report of the expert group on science and governance.* Brussels, European Commission.

Ferber, D. (2004). Tobacco wars—research on secondhand smoke questioned. *Science*, 306(5700): 1274.

Fischbacher, M., Mackinnon, J. & Pate, J. (2009). *Improving population health in Glasgow: Managing partnerships for health improvements (Phase II).* Glasgow, Glasgow Centre for Population Health.

Giddens, A. (1990). *The consequences of modernity.* Cambridge, Polity Press.

Gostin, L. O. (2007). The "tobacco wars"—global litigation strategies. *Journal of the American Medical Association*, 298: 2537–9.

Gray, C. (1997). Tobacco wars—the bloody battle between good health and good politics. *Canadian Medical Association Journal*, 156(2): 237–40.

Griffin, G. (2000). *Representations of HIV and AIDS—visibility blue/s.* Manchester, Manchester University Press.

Hooper, E. (2000). *The river: a journey back to the source of HIV and AIDS.* Harmondsworth, Penguin.

Irwin, A. (1995). *Citizen science: A study of people, expertise and sustainable development.* London, Routledge.

Irwin, A. (2006). The politics of talk: coming to terms with the 'new' scientific governance. *Social Studies of Science*, 36(2): 299–320.

Irwin, A. & Wynne, B. (eds) (1996). *Misunderstanding science? The public reconstruction of science and technology.* Cambridge, Cambridge University Press.

Latour, B. (1993). *We have never been modern.* London, Harvester Wheatsheaf.

Latour, B. (1999). On recalling ANT. In: J. Law & J. Hassard (eds). *Actor Network Theory and after.* Oxford, Blackwell/The Sociological Review, pp. 15–25.

Latour, B. (2005). *Reassembling the social. An introduction to Actor-Network Theory.* Oxford, Oxford University Press.

Lowrance, W. W. (1981). Of acceptable risk: science and the determination of safety. San Francisco, CA, W. Kaufmann.

Miller, D. (1999). Risk, science and policy: definitional struggles, information management, the media and BSE. *Social Science and Medicine*, 49: 1239–55.

Pelling, M., High, C., Dearing, J. & Smith, D. (2008). Shadow spaces for social learning: a relational understanding of adaptive capacity to climate change within organisations. *Environment and Planning A*, 40: 867–84.

Phillips, J. (2000). *The BSE Inquiry. The report of the inquiry into BSE and variant CJD in the United Kingdom*. London, HMSO.

Ramsay, C. (2002). Tobacco wars: Inside the California battles. *Journal of Health Politics Policy and Law*, 27(3): 525–7.

Redfern, M., Keeling, J. & Powell, E. (2000). *The Royal Liverpool Children's Inquiry Report*. London, The Stationery Office.

Rowe, W. D. (1977). *An anatomy of risk*. New York, Wiley.

Schroeder, S. A. (2002). Conflicting dispatches from the tobacco wars. *New England Journal of Medicine*, 347(14): 1106–9.

Shermer, M. (2001). *The borderlands of science. Where sense meets nonsense*. Oxford, Oxford University Press.

Smith, D. (1990). Corporate power and the politics of uncertainty: Risk management at the Canvey Island complex. *Industrial Crisis Quarterly*, 4(1): 1–26.

Smith, D. (1991). The Kraken wakes—the political dynamics of the hazardous waste issue. *Industrial Crisis Quarterly*, 5(3): 189–207.

Smith, D. & Elliott, P. (1992). Hazardous waste and risk assessment. *European Environment*, 2(1): 1–4.

Smith, D. & McCloskey, J. (2000). History repeating itself? Expertise, barriers to learning and the precautionary principle. In: E. Coles, D. Smith & S. Tombs (eds). *Risk Management and Society*. Dordrecht, Kluwer, pp. 101–24.

Starr, C. (1969). Social benefit versus technological risk. *Science*, 165: 1232–8.

Stephens, T. & Brynner, R. (2001). *Dark remedy. The impact of thalidomide and its revival as a vital medicine*. Cambridge, Mass, Perseus Publishing.

Susser, M. (1997). Goliath and some Davids in the tobacco wars. *American Journal of Public Health*, 87(10): 1593–5.

Tansey, R., White, M. & Collins, J. (2004). Is smoking as deadly as you think? A research methods perspective. *Interfaces*, 34(4): 280–6.

Taylor, I. (2003). Policy on the hoof: the handling of the foot and mouth disease outbreak in the UK 2001. *Policy and Politics*, 31(4): 535–46.

Weick, K. E. (1993). The collapse of sensemaking in organizations: The Mann Gulch Disaster. *Administrative Science Quarterly*, 38: 628–52.

Weick, K. E. (1995). *Sensemaking in organizations*. Thousand Oaks, Sage.

Weick, K. E. (2001). *Making sense of the organization*. Oxford, Blackwell.

Wynne, B. (2002). Risk and environment as legitimatory discourses of reflexivity: Reflexivity inside out? *Current Sociology*, 50(3): 459–77.

# Chapter 3

# Consumer perceptions of the risks and benefits associated with food hazards

Lynn Frewer, Heleen van Dijk, & Arnout Fischer (University of Wageningen)

## Introduction

Perceived risks are considered to be an important determinant of consumer behaviour (Fischhoff et al., 1978; Kahneman & Tversky, 1979; Slovic, 1987). As a consequence, there is an extensive research literature focused on the perceived risks associated with food, food-related hazards, and food production technologies (Pennings et al., 2002; Setbon, 2005; Verbeke, 2001).

More recently, research in the food area has focused on situations where both risks and benefits are associated with consumption of specific foods. Research in risk assessment has been extended to risk–benefit assessment. Assessment processes are now providing increased understanding of situations where both risk and benefit are potentially associated with specific food choices, in line with these changes in risk (benefit) assessment frameworks (Verbeke et al., 2008). As a consequence, there is currently increased emphasis on research directed towards understanding risk–benefit communication and risk perception rather than just risk issues. Such combined risk–benefit approaches include information on optimal nutrition, functional foods and nutrigenomics, as well as traditional food safety issues.

Initial research in the area of risk perception and risk communication focused on understanding why lay people had different risk perceptions from 'expert' risk assessments. This seminal research identified different 'psychological' dimensions of risk perception (Fischhoff et al., 1978; Slovic, 1987; 1992; Slovic et al., 1982). It was found that the extent to which a risk is perceived to be *unnatural, potentially catastrophic*, or to which an individual perceives exposure to be *involuntary* influences their responses to specific hazards to a greater extent than assessments provided by technical experts. It has also been shown that consumers tend to be suspicious of new foods, a phenomena known as food neophobia (Pliner & Hobden, 1992). These psychological dimensions are reliable predictors of people's responses to potential risks across different hazard domains, including that of food hazards.

Individual differences in consumer responses to domestic food hazards, and communication about the associated risks, has also been a focus of empirical investigation. For example, risk perceptions, food safety-related behaviours, consumer responses to food safety scares, and consumer use of information are dependent on consistent personality characteristics as well as other background variables (Berg, 2004; Dosman et al., 2001; Fischer & Frewer, 2008; Kornelis et al., 2007; Parry et al., 2004; Verbeke, 2002).

New insights into integrated risk and benefit assessment of foods have underlined the importance of communication about risk and benefit at the same time. However, risk and benefit information may not be interpreted independently by people receiving integrated risk–benefit messages, as illustrated by a consistent negative correlation between risk and benefit perception, implying further research is required to understand the fundamental mechanisms underlying consumer decision-making under circumstances where both health risks and benefits are associated with food choices.

Another concept that has been extensively studied in relation to consumer perceptions of food safety, and food risk management in general, is the concept of trust and/or consumer confidence in food safety (Berg, 2005; de Jonge et al., 2007; 2008; Frewer & Miles, 2003; Saba & Messina, 2003; Siegrist, 2000; van Kleef et al., 2006). Consumer trust in different actors and institutions responsible for consumer protection, as well as trust in the information provided by different information sources, is considered to be important in terms of consumer responses to risk communication and risk governance activities (van Kleef et al., 2006).The extent to which consumer risk perception, together with trust in different information sources, and trust in regulation and risk governance activities, predicts consumer acceptance of the products of these technologies has also been a focus of empirical study (Bredahl, 2001; Eiser et al., 2002; Poortinga & Pidgeon, 2005; Siegrist, 2000). The influence of specific food safety incidents on consumer risk perceptions and behaviour (e.g. in a 'crisis' context) have also been examined (Eiser et al., 2002; Henson & Northen, 2000; Pennings et al., 2002; Rozin et al., 1999; Verbeke & Viaene, 1999).

## Drivers of risk perception: natural versus technological food hazards

The early 20th century was associated with considerable changes in the range of technologies utilized in agricultural and food production. The international application of intensive farming methods (for example, the introduction of chemical fertilizers and pesticides) has been termed 'the green revolution', for the most part occurring in the middle and latter years of the 20th century (Evenson & Gollin, 2003). However, societal concerns have emerged about the negative effects of exposure to agrochemicals (whether from environmental exposure or consumption of 'contaminated' foods) on human health and the environment. An important landmark in this debate was signalled by the publication of the book *The Silent Spring* by Carson in 1962, which contributed to the development of the environmentalist movement after its publication. More recently, societal concerns have arisen regarding the replacement of natural ecosystems with novel agricultural practices (for example, the destruction of natural rainforest and replacement by monocultures). Other societally controversial applications of technology in the agrifood sector have included the introduction of irradiated foods (Bruhn, 1995), the development and introduction of genetically modified foods and crops (Frewer *et al.*, 2004), and, more recently, the introduction of bionanotechnology into agricultural practices and food production (Siegrist *et al.*, 2007). Whilst societal negativity associated with technological innovation is not unique to the agrifood sector (Flynn & Bellaby, 2007), there is evidence to suggest the existence of domain-specific societal sensitivity towards the use of technology in food production, as compared to, for example, medical or pharmaceutical developments (Kessler, 1995).

The societal demand for traditional approaches to food (van Rijswijk *et al.*, 2008), coupled with demand for 'naturalness', is a factor which appears to be valued by consumers in the context of food choice (Frewer *et al.*, 1997), a factor which supports the perception of healthiness and safety of organic production, even while health assessments do not support this (Saba & Messina, 2003). Cultural and historical variation across different regions and social contexts of course implies that the extent of differences in consumer variation in their acceptance of technology in the agrifood sector may be prone to cross cultural differences, and individual differences in consumer evaluations of risks (Kornelis *et al.*, 2007; Morris *et al.*, 2005). None the less, there is evidence to suggest that consumers are less concerned about 'natural', or familiar food risks, and for this reason may make inappropriate and unhealthy food choices (Fife-Schaw & Rowe, 2000) or take inappropriate risks regarding (for example) domestic food hygiene practices. From this, it is important to discuss both behavioural changes and consumer responses to public health information, and consumer perceptions of risk and benefit associated with specific food choices. These will be discussed and illustrated using case studies in the following sections.

## Behavioural change—the case of improving domestic food handling practices

Food poisoning represents an important public health issue (Havelaar *et al.*, 2004). Food safety objectives have been introduced to promote public health through reduction in the number of cases of foodborne illnesses. However, it is difficult, if not impossible, to legislate for consumer behaviour. Inappropriate storage, food preparation, and cross-contamination may result in illness, even though products are safe for consumption at the point of sale. The goal of improving public health can only be obtained through implementation of appropriate and effective information interventions (Fischer *et al.*, 2007).

Internationally, there has been disagreement at what point in the food chain the food safety objectives should be set—at the point of sale of food products or at the moment of consumption. From the perspective of public health, it is far more useful to set food safety objectives at the point of consumption, as this is the point where microbial load determines the probability of illness occurring (Nauta *et al.*, 2008). The problem is that public health therefore is ultimately contingent on the, non-enforceable, safety level of food preparation practices adopted by the consumer. Nevertheless, placing food safety objectives at the point of consumption has currently been agreed by a recent meeting of the codex alimentarius (Codex Alimentaris Committee, 2004; Zwietering & van Asselt, 2005). This implies that more effective approaches have to be developed to optimize domestic hygiene practices relevant to food preparation. From this, it is important to conduct research to understand potential barriers to the elimination of unhealthy food preparation by consumers, and to apply this understanding to the implementation of effective intervention strategies specifically focusing on influencing consumer behaviour.

Domestic food preparation involves a frequently repeated behaviour embedded in an individual's routine activities associated with 'lifestyle' choices (Fischer & De Vries, 2008). An important factor which needs to be taken into account in any discussion of lifestyle risks is that of *optimistic bias* or *unrealistic optimism* (Weinstein, 1980). People tend to rate their own personal risks from a particular lifestyle hazard as being less than those experienced by an 'average' member of society, or in comparison to another individual with similar demographic characteristics (for a review in the food area, see Miles & Scaife, 2003). Optimistic biases are much greater for lifestyle hazards (such as food poisoning contracted in the home, or illness experienced as a consequence of inappropriate dietary choices) compared to technologies applied to food production (Frewer *et al.*, 1994). At the same time, people perceive that they know more about the risks associated with lifestyle choices when compared to other people, and are in greater control over their personal exposure to specific hazards. As a consequence, people tend to perceive that information about risk reduction is directed towards other individual consumers who are more at risk from the hazard, who have less control about their personal exposure to the associated risks, and who possess less knowledge regarding self-protective behaviours. People exhibiting optimistic bias may not take precautions to reduce their risk from a hazard (Perloff & Fetzer, 1986; Weinstein, 1987; 1989). The risks of food poisoning are typically prone to optimistic bias (Frewer *et al.*, 1994). Some empirical research has succeeded in developing interventions to reduce optimistic bias, including increasing perceived accountability associated with an individual's risk judgement. This can be achieved through providing information about actual risk-taking behaviours (McKenna & Myers, 1997), or through making people compare themselves with an individual similar to themselves (Harris *et al.*, 2000), or an individual identified similar to the receiver of the risk information (Alicke *et al.*, 1995). To date there has been varied success in reducing optimistic bias through cognitive approaches (Miles & Scaife, 2003). Although targeting information to those individuals most at risk may optimize use of available resources, an important first step is to differentiate or segment consumers who are most at risk, as a consequence of both attitudinal factors and their vulnerability to the risks.

To promote consumer health, it is important that consumers prepare potentially risky meals safely to reduce potential microbial contamination. The development of effective health interventions (for example, targeted risk communications or information campaigns focused on the needs of those consumers most at risk), is contingent upon understanding what constitutes safe behaviour. Understanding social psychological factors which determine behaviour is likely to be important if consumer protection is to be optimized, as domestic food preparation practices are influential in determining consumer health risks (Fischer *et al.*, 2005). Most consumers are aware of the risks of cross-contamination, and that heating food thoroughly is an important part of illness prevention when prompted. However, not all consumers spontaneously mention such issues as important, nor do these same participants show sufficiently safe behaviour, indicating a lack of motivation to cook safely (Fischer *et al.*, 2007). Habitual cooking, i.e. preparation of foods without conscious thought, also militates against adoption of novel food safety practices (Fischer & Frewer, 2008).

To further interpret individuals' motivations to cook safely, a series of food preparation behaviours was combined into a single measure for food safety practice using a Rasch model (Fischer *et al.*, 2006). The outcomes of this model allowed the prediction of potential risks of different groups of people (where young single males fit the expectation by being least motivated and most likely to create a contaminated meal). Hence, differences in likelihood of conducting safe domestic hygiene practices across the population suggest that stratified risk communication strategies represent an important element of targeting risk communication to those who need it most (Fischer *et al.*, 2006), delivered in a way that makes it most likely they will use it (Kornelis *et al.*, 2007).

To overcome the problem of domestic food poisoning, two approaches were compared against a control condition. The first approach demonstrated that information which included relevant emotions (disgust) in the message content increased both consumer awareness of risks and their motivation to counter the problem of food poisoning; less relevant emotions (anger) only showed awareness compared to neutral communication (Nauta *et al.*, 2008). In addition, the most successful (disgust) information campaign had no significant effect on actual food preparation 1 week after it had been provided. Against this, a neutral reminder regarding the prevention of cross-contamination in the recipe did provide a measurable and relevant reduction of bacterial contamination (Nauta *et al.*, 2008). This last finding provides additional evidence of habitual behaviour in the situation where food safety attitudes are not active. The message in the recipe activated an existing attitude to produce a positive effect in terms of consumer health protection. One conclusion from this research is that consumers possess more knowledge about safe food preparation than they use, and breaking habits and activating this knowledge at the same time the behaviour is being conducted is important (Nauta *et al.*, 2008).

## Communicating the risks and benefits—the case of fatty fish

Food consumption often involves consumers making a trade-off between the risks and benefits associated with the consumption of a particular food product. For example, fish represents a product where consumers have to balance the health benefits of eating fish (e.g. beneficial effects associated with omega 3 fatty acids) against possible safety risks (e.g. adverse effects associated with contamination) (Mozaffarian & Rimm, 2006; Verbeke *et al.*, 2005). If consumers are to make informed consumption choices, they will need to base these decisions on information about both risks and benefits (Burger & Gochfeld, 2006).

In concordance with this, risk assessment, as well as regulatory decision-making, is increasingly focused on risk *and* benefit associated with a specific food issue (EFSA, 2006; Wentholt *et al.*, in press). To assess the balance between the risks and benefits associated with a particular food, an integrated risk–benefit assessment is required, which converts risks and benefits into a common measure of net health impact (Hoekstra *et al.*, 2008; Ponce *et al.*, 2000). In recent years, various methods have been developed which have the capacity for evaluating the impact of *both* risks and benefits on public health and wellbeing simultaneously (e.g. Disability-Adjusted Life Years, Quality-Adjusted Life Years), which has resulted in the need to develop effective risk–benefit communication with consumers (Verbeke *et al.*, 2005; 2008).

In an exploratory study, consumer perceptions of the adequacy of current information provision about risks and benefits related to fish consumption, together with consumer preferences regarding information about the *net* health impact of both risks and benefits on life expectancy, quality of life and disability-adjusted life years (DALYs) were examined. The results indicated that current risk–benefit communication is perceived as confusing, and is not trusted. Most participants found information about the combined health impact on both life expectancy and quality of life the most meaningful on which to base their decision to choose the product. However, the integration also introduced complexities, with DALYs in particular being too complicated for consumers to interpret. Increased transparency about any uncertainties and scientific ambiguousness associated with combined risk–benefit communication had the potential to increase perception of honesty associated with the information source, whilst at the same time reduced the effectiveness of information regarding change in consumption behaviours and negatively influenced perceptions of healthiness associated with the food under consideration.

Other research on the communication of both risk and benefits related to food has shown that the order in which the information is provided may influence the relative impact of information. That is, only information provided first may influence consumer attitude towards the food (Verbeke *et al.*, 2008), especially if the consumer determines the amount of information accessed (Fischer & Frewer, 2009, in press). The impact of communication about both risks and benefits may also be affected by prior attitudes toward the product. For example, research has shown that strong, non-ambivalent attitudes towards different food production methods are less likely to be changed by additional information about risks and benefits; and that existing attitudes can even polarize after provision of balanced risk and benefit information.

## The role of trust in developing effective risk–benefit communication

Consumer trust in different actors and institutions responsible for guaranteeing and controlling food safety, as well as trust in the information provided by different information sources that communicate about food safety or food-related risks, is an important part of developing consumer confidence regarding food safety. Whilst the role of trust in this context has been extensively studied (de Jonge *et al.*, 2007), it has an important relationship with evaluation of the efficacy of food risk management practices (inter alia van Kleef *et al.*, 2006). The question arises as to what constitutes optimal risk management practices from a consumer perspective. Results from qualitative studies (Houghton *et al.*, 2006; Krystallis *et al.*, 2007; van Kleef *et al.*, 2006) have provided insight into which underlying psychological factors have the potential to influence consumer evaluations of risk management practices (van Kleef *et al.*, 2007). Initiation of preventative risk management activities by risk regulators, strict enforcement of, and communication about, relevant regulations, transparency associated with regulatory activities, and information provision about the application of control systems and their performance were shown to be essential indicators for consumer perceptions of high quality food risk management. Country-specific factors included scepticism regarding the practice of risk assessment and management. Whilst consumers, regardless of nationality, expected that food risk managers would have a high level of expertise, the extent to which consumers perceived risk managers to be honest did not have a significant impact on the perceived quality of risk management, perhaps because of lack of variability in consumer perceptions regarding perceived honesty (Frewer *et al.*, 1996). Certainly, perceived honesty of risk managers increased in relevance when the survey was replicated in Russia, probably in response to consumer perceptions derived from the historical political context of the Russian situation (Popova *et al.*, in press). One conclusion can be made—communication with the public about how risks are managed is an important part of effective risk analysis, as is communication about risk assessments.

Although the topic of trust would warrant a chapter, or a whole book on its own, public involvement exercises as a method to regain consumer and societal trust will be specifically discussed, as these are currently seen as a solution to overcome societal reluctance to adopt technological innovations and regulatory activities. In recent years, there has been a growing trend in many societies to involve a wider range of stakeholders in policy decisions than has traditionally been the case in the past. Such stakeholders *may* include the public, or at least, representatives of the public, as well as consumer, environmental, and industry interest groups (amongst others). Besides regaining trust, various other reasons have been proposed to explain the recent popularity of stakeholder involvement. These include acquisition of political efficacy, enhancement of democracy, acceptance of decisions associated with policy development and implementation, and improvement of policy decisions (Walls *et al.*, in press). The assumption of these benefits is unquestioned, as much in the area of food risk governance as in other areas, leading to research being directed towards understanding at what stages in the decision-making process should the public and other stakeholders be involved (Wentholt *et al.*, in press).

To achieve the goal of 'greater participation', a series of methodologies has been developed to facilitate public and stakeholder involvement; these roughly divide into 'consultation' and 'participation'. *Consultation* utilizes traditional opinion solicitation methods, where the opinion of the public or other stakeholder group is collected in the *absence* of interaction with sponsors or policy communities. Information about public opinion is provided to the expert community, and from thence onwards the process is separated from the public. The information flow has only one direction—from the public to the experts—usually at one point in time. The second group of methods, which can be classified as *participation*, consists of methods which actively aim to engage participants in an ongoing dialogue with sponsors, and which aim to be truly interactive.

It is important to differentiate between the different aims of consultation and engagement exercises. Furthermore, the exercise itself should be independently *evaluated against criteria associated with process and impact* (Rowe & Frewer, 2000). Public engagement associated with food technology development or other technological or societal initiatives, such as bionanotechnology or genetic modification of foods, affect society more broadly in terms of technology development, implementation, and commercialization. Independent evaluation or peer-reviewed publication of consultations and public engagement exercises is rare, which leads to much repetition of the activities, and obscures the impact of involvement on the strategic development of technology development, implementation, and regulation instead of making it more transparent (Rowe & Frewer, 2005), thus resulting in less, rather than more trust.

In conclusion, various challenges for improving public health behaviour in the coming years can be identified. These include further understanding of unconscious, habitual, behaviours, research into how risk–benefit communication influences attitudes and knowledge, and subsequently has an impact on consumer behaviour, and futher research evaluating the efficacy of different approaches to building trust in food safety, food-related innovation, and regulatory frameworks.

## References

Alicke, M. D., Klotz, M. L., Breitenbecher, D. L., Yurak, T. J. & Vredenburg, D. S. (1995). Personal contact, individuation, and the better-than-average effect. *Journal of Personality and Social Psychology*, 68: 804–25.

Berg, L. (2004). Trust in food in the age of mad cow disease: a comparative study of consumers' evaluation of food safety in Belgium, Britain and Norway. *Appetite*, 42: 21–32.

Berg, L. (2005). Trust in food safety in Russia, Denmark and Norway. *European Societies*, 7: 103–29.

Bredahl, L. (2001). Determinants of consumer attitudes and purchase intentions with regard to genetically modified food—results of a cross-national survey. *Journal of Consumer Policy*, 24: 23–61.

Bruhn, C. M. (1995). Consumer attitudes and market response to irradiated food. *Journal of Food Protection*, 58: 175–81.

Burger, J. & Gochfeld, M. (2006). A framework and information needs for the management of the risks from consumption of self-caught fish. *Environmental Research*, 101: 275–85.

Carson, C. (1962). *The Silent Spring*. Boston, MA, Houghton Mifflin.

Codex Alimentaris Committee. (2004). ALINORM 04/27/13.

de Jonge, J., van Trijp, H. C. M., Renes, R. J. & Frewer, L. J. (2007). Understanding consumer confidence in the safety of food: its two-dimensional structure and determinants. *Risk Analysis*, 27: 729–40.

de Jonge, J., van Trijp, J. C. M., van der Lans, I. A., Renes, R. J. & Frewer, L. J. (2008). How trust in institutions and organizations builds general consumer confidence in the safety of food: A decomposition of effects. *Appetite*, 51: 311–17.

Dosman, D. M., Adamowicz, W. L. & Hrudey, S. E. (2001). Socioeconomic determinants of health- and food safety-related risk perceptions. *Risk Analysis*, 21: 307–18.

EFSA (2006). *Risk-Benefit Analysis of Foods: Methods and Approaches*. Website (retrieved November 2007): http://www.efsa.europa.eu/EFSA/Scientific_Document/comm_colloque_6_en.pdf

Eiser, J. R., Miles, S. & Frewer, L. J. (2002). Trust, perceived risk, and attitudes toward food technologies. *Journal of Applied Social Psychology*, 32: 2423–33.

Evenson, R. E. & Gollin, D. (2003). Assessing the impact of the Green Revolution, 1960 to 2000. *Science*, 300: 758–62.

Fife-Schaw, C. & Rowe, G. (2000). Extending the application of the psychometric approach for assessing public perceptions of food risks: some methodological considerations. *Journal of Risk Research*, 3: 167–79.

Fischer, A. R. H. & Frewer, L. J. (2008). Food-safety practices in the domestic kitchen: Demographic, personality, and experiential determinants. *Journal of Applied Social Psychology*, 38: 2859–84.

Fischer, A. R. H. & Frewer, L. J. (2009). Consumer familiarity with foods and the perception of risks and benefits. *Food Quality and Preference*, in press.

Fischer, A. R. H. & de Vries, P. W. (2008). Everyday behaviour and everyday risk: An exploration how people respond to frequently encountered risks. *Health, Risk and Society*, 10: 385–97.

Fischer, A. R. H., de Jong, A. E. I., de Jonge, R., Frewer, L. J. & Nauta, M. J. (2005). Improving food safety in the domestic environment: The need for a transdisciplinary approach. *Risk Analysis*, 25: 503–17.

Fischer, A. R. H., Frewer, L. J. & Nauta, M. J. (2006). Towards improving food safety in the domestic environment: A multi-item Rasch scale for the measurement of the safety efficacy of domestic food handling practices. *Risk Analysis*, 26: 1323–38.

Fischer, A. R. H., de Jong, A. E. I., van Asselt, E. D., de Jonge, R., Frewer, L. J. & Nauta, M. J. (2007). Food safety in the domestic environment: An interdisciplinary investigation of microbial hazards during food preparation. *Risk Analysis,* 27: 1065–82.

Fischhoff, B., Slovic, P. & Lichtenstein, S. (1978). How safe is safe enough? A psychometric study of attitudes towards technological risks and benefits. *Policy Sciences,* 9: 127–52.

Flynn, R. & Bellaby, P. (eds) (2007). *Risk and the Public Acceptability of New Technologies.* Hampshire, UK, Palgrave.

Frewer, L. J. & Miles, S. (2003). Temporal stability of the psychological determinants of trust: Implications for communication about food risks. *Health, Risk and Society,* 5: 259–71.

Frewer, L. J., Shepherd, R. & Sparks, P. (1994). The interrelationship between perceived knowledge, control and risk associated with a range of food-related hazards targeted at the individual, other people and society. *Journal of Food Safety,* 14: 19–40.

Frewer, L. J., Howard, C., Hedderley, D. & Shepherd, R. (1996). What determines trust in information about food-related risks? Underlying psychological constructs. *Risk Analysis,* 16: 473–86.

Frewer, L. J., Howard, C. & Shepherd, R. (1997). Public concerns in the United Kingdom about general and specific applications of genetic engineering: risk, benefit, and ethics. *Science, Technology, & Human Values,* 22: 98–124.

Frewer, L. J., Lassen, J., Kettlitz, B., Scholderer, J., Beekman, V. & Berdal, K. G. (2004). Societal aspects of genetically modified foods. *Food and Chemical Toxicology,* 42: 1181–93.

Harris, P., Middleton, W. & Joiner, R. (2000). The typical student as an in-group member: eliminating optimistic bias by reducing social distance. *European Journal of Social Psychology,* 30: 235–53.

Havelaar, A. H., Nauta, M. J. & Jansen, J. T. (2004). Fine-tuning food safety objectives and risk assessment. *International Journal of Food Microbiology,* 93: 11–29.

Henson, S. & Northen, J. (2000). Consumer assessment of the safety of beef at the point of purchase: A pan-European study. *Journal of Agricultural Economics,* 51: 90–105.

Hoekstra, J., Verkaik-Kloosterman, J., Rompelberg, C. *et al.* (2008). Integrated risk-benefit analyses: Method development with folic acid as example. *Food and Chemical Toxicology,* 46: 893–909.

Houghton, J., van Kleef, E., Rowe, G. & Frewer, L. (2006). Consumer perceptions of the effectiveness of food risk management practices: A cross-cultural study. *Health, Risk and Society,* 8: 165–83.

Kahneman, D. & Tversky, A. (1979). Prospect theory: An analysis of decision under risk. *Econometrica,* 47: 263–92.

Kessler, D. A. (1995). The evolution of national nutrition policy. *Annual Review of Nutrition,* 15: 13–26.

Kornelis, M., de Jonge, J., Frewer, L. J. & Dagevos, H. (2007). Consumer selection of food-safety information sources. *Risk Analysis,* 27: 327–35.

Krystallis, A., Frewer, L., Rowe, G., Houghton, J., Kehagia, O. & Perrea, T. (2007). A perceptual divide? Consumer and expert attitudes to food risk management in Europe. *Health, Risk and Society,* 9: 407–24.

McKenna, F. P. & Myers, L. B. (1997). Illusory self-assessments—can they be reduced? *British Journal of Psychology,* 88: 39–51.

Miles, S. & Scaife, V. (2003). Optimistic bias and food. *Nutrition Research Reviews,* 16: 3–19.

Morris, M. G., Venkatesh, V. & Ackerman, P. L. (2005). Gender and age differences in employee decisions about new technology: An extension to the theory of planned behavior. *IEEE Transactions on Engineering Management,* 52: 69–84.

Mozaffarian, D. & Rimm, E. B. (2006). Fish intake, contaminants, and human health. *Journal of the American Medical Association,* 296: 1885–99.

Nauta, M. J., Fischer, A. R. H., van Asselt, E. D., de Jong, A. E. I., Frewer, L. J. & de Jonge, R. (2008). Food safety in the domestic environment: The effect of consumer risk information on human disease risks. *Risk Analysis,* 28: 179–92.

Parry, S. M., Miles, S., Tridente, A. & Palmer, S. R. (2004). Differences in perception of risk between people who have and have not experienced *Salmonella* food poisoning. *Risk Analysis,* 24: 289–99.

Pennings, J. M. E., Wansink, B. & Meulenberg, M. T. G. (2002). A note on modelling consumer reactions to a crisis: The case of mad cow disease. *International Journal of Research in Marketing,* 19: 91–100.

Perloff, L. S. & Fetzer, B. K. (1986). Self-other judgments and perceived vulnerability to victimization. *Journal of Personality and Social Psychology,* 50: 502–10.

Pliner, P. & Hobden, K. (1992). Development of a scale to measure the trait of food neophobia in humans. *Appetite,* 19: 105–20.

Ponce, R. A., Bartell, S. M., Wong, E. Y. *et al.* (2000). Use of quality-adjusted life year weights with dose-response models for public health decisions: A case study of the risks and benefits of fish consumption. *Risk Analysis,* 20: 529–42.

Poortinga, W. & Pidgeon, N. F. (2005). Trust in risk regulation: Cause or consequence of the acceptability of GM food? *Risk Analysis,* 25: 199–209.

Popova, K., Frewer, L. J., de Jonge, J., Fischer, A. R. H. & van Kleef, E. (2009). Consumer evaluations of food risk management in Russia. *British Food Journal,* in press.

Rowe, G. & Frewer, L. J. (2000). Public participation methods: A framework for evaluation. *Science, Technology & Human Values,* 25: 3–29.

Rowe, G. & Frewer, L. J. (2005). A typology of public engagement mechanisms. *Science, Technology & Human Values,* 30: 251–90.

Rozin, P., Fischler, C., Imada, S., Sarubin, A. & Wrzesniewski, A. (1999). Attitudes to food and the role of food in life in the U.S.A., Japan, Flemish Belgium and France: Possible implications for the diet–health debate. *Appetite,* 33: 163–80.

Saba, A. & Messina, F. (2003). Attitudes towards organic foods and risk/benefit perception associated with pesticides. *Food Quality And Preference,* 14: 637–45.

Setbon, M. (2005). Risk perception of the "mad cow disease" in France: Determinants and consequences. *Risk Analysis,* 25: 813–26.

Siegrist, M. (2000). The influence of trust and perceptions of risks and benefits on the acceptance of gene technology. *Risk Analysis,* 20: 195–204.

Siegrist, M., Wiek, A., Helland, A. & Kastenholz, H. (2007). Risks and nanotechnology: The public is more concerned than experts and industry. *Nature Nanotechnology,* 2: 67.

Slovic, P. (1987). Perception of risk. *Science,* 236: 280–5.

Slovic, P. (1992). Perceptions of risk: Reflections on the psychometric paradigm. In: S. Krimsky & D. Golding (eds). *Social Theories of Risk.* New York, USA, Praeger: pp.117–52.

Slovic, P., Fischhoff, B. & Lichtenstein, S. (1982). Why study risk perception? *Risk Analysis*, 2: 83–93.

van Dijk, H., Fischer, A. R. H., de Jonge, J., Rowe, G. & Frewer, L. J. (submitted). The impact of balanced risk-benefit information and prior attitudes on post-information attitudes towards food production methods.

van Dijk, H., van Kleef, E., Owen, H. & Frewer, L. J. (submitted). Consumer preferences and information needs regarding integrated risk-benefit messages related to the consumption of food.

van Kleef, E., Frewer, L. J., Chryssochoidis, G. M. *et al.* (2006). Perceptions of food risk management among key stakeholders: Results from a cross European Study. *Appetite*, 47: 46–63.

van Kleef, E., Houghton, J. R, Krystallis, T. *et al.* (2007). Consumer evaluations of food risk management quality in Europe. *Risk Analysis*, 27: 1565–80.

van Rijswijk, W., Frewer, L. J., Menozzi, D. & Faioli, G. (2008). Consumer perceptions of traceability: A cross-national comparison of the associated benefits. *Food Quality And Preference*, 19: 452–64.

Verbeke, W. (2001). Beliefs, attitude and behaviour towards fresh meat revisited after the Belgian dioxin crisis. *Food Quality and Preference*, 12: 489–98.

Verbeke, W. (2002). Impact of emotional stability and attitude on consumption decisions under risk: the Coca-Cola crisis in Belgium. *Journal of Health Communication*, 7: 455–72.

Verbeke, W. & Viaene, J. (1999). Beliefs, attitude and behaviour towards fresh meat consumption in Belgium: empirical evidence from a consumer survey. *Food Quality and Preference*, 10: 437–45.

Verbeke, W., Sioen, I., Pieniak, Z., van Camp, J. & de Henauw, S. (2005). Consumer perception versus scientific evidence about health benefits and safety risks from fish consumption. *Public Health Nutrition*, 8: 422–9.

Verbeke, W., Vanhonacker, F., Frewer, L. J., Sioen, I., de Henauw, S., & van Camp, J. (2008). Communicating risks and benefits from fish consumption: impact on Belgian consumers' perception and intention to eat fish. *Risk Analysis*, 28: 951–67.

Walls, J., Rowe, G. and Frewer, L. J. (2009). Stakeholder engagement in food risk management: evaluation of an iterated workshop approach. *Public Understanding of Science*, in press.

Weinstein, N. D. (1980). Unrealistic optimism about future life events. *Journal of Personality and Social Psychology*, 39: 806–20.

Weinstein, N. D. (1987). Unrealistic optimism about susceptibility to health problems: Conclusions from a community-wide sample. *Journal of Behavioral Medicine*, 10: 481–500.

Weinstein, N. D. (1989). Optimistic biases about personal risks. *Science*, 246: 1232–3.

Wentholt, M., Rowe G., Konig, A, Marvin, H. & Frewer, L. (2009) The views of key stakeholders on an evolving food risk governance framework: Results from a Delphi study. *Food Policy*, in press.

Zwietering, M. H. & van Asselt, E. D. (2005). The range of microbial risks in food processing. In: H. L. M. Lelieveld, M. A. Mostert & J. T. Holah (eds). *Improving Hygiene in Food Processing*. Cambridge, UK, Woodhead: pp. 31–45.

Chapter 4

# The social amplification of risk framework (SARF): theory, critiques, and policy implications

Nick Pidgeon (School of Psychology, Cardiff University) & Karen Henwood (School of Social Sciences, Cardiff University)

## Introduction

The question of how and when to engage in systematic communication and dialogue about risks with the public and other stakeholder groups has today become a central concern of many institutions, regulators, and administrators (US National Research Council, 1989; Royal Society, 1992; Cabinet Office, 2002). As a field of science policy risk communication evolved out of earlier basic social science work conducted in the 1970s and 80s on risk perceptions, which aimed to map the cognitive and social processes underlying both lay and expert conceptualizations of risk (Pidgeon & Beattie, 1998). Risk perception researchers have demonstrated how judgements about perceived risk and its acceptability are a function of (1) a wide range of qualitative aspects of hazards, such as levels of perceived control and voluntariness, or the catastrophic potential of a hazard; and sometimes (2) cultural, political, and institutional affiliations; and (3) aspects of the local geographical or social context within which a risk issue arises. Some of the wider policy implications of this work for risk management are only now beginning to be explored (e.g. US National Research Council, 1996; Renn & Walker, 2008).

Risk and its perception remains a distinctly interdisciplinary area of inquiry. However, in theoretical terms both the risk perception and risk communication literatures remain fragmented—for example, between the classic psychometric (Slovic, 2000) and the cultural interpretive approaches to risk perception to (Lupton, 1999; Henwood et al., 2008), or across disciplinary lines such as psychology, anthropology, human geography, or disaster sociology. To date there have been very few genuine attempts to provide an overarching theoretical framework through which to approach risk perception and communication issues systematically. A recent exception to this is the social amplification of risk framework (SARF) proposed by Kasperson *et al.* (1988). Their thesis is that certain aspects of hazard events and their portrayal in mediated and other sources interact with psychological, social, institutional, and cultural processes in ways that might attenuate (decrease) or amplify (increase) perceptions of risk and, through this, shape behaviour. There is considerable evidence now that risk attenuation and intensification phenomena have occurred in America and Europe in recent years, raising the question of whether the SARF might inform our understanding of basic risk communication processes and lead to improved practice in health communication and in related areas such as environmental policy.

## The social amplification of risk framework

The theoretical and empirical foundations of SARF are discussed in detail in Kasperson *et al.* (2003) and Kasperson & Kasperson (2005). The basic theoretical ideas for SARF were first developed in the late 1980s by Roger and Jeanne Kasperson and colleagues (see Kasperson *et al.*, 1988; Renn, 1991; Kasperson, 1992). The ideas arose out of an attempt to overcome the fragmented nature of the risk perception and communication fields in an *integrative theoretical framework* capable of accounting for findings from a wide range of studies. It is also used, more narrowly, to describe the various dynamic *social processes* by which certain hazards and events seen to be relatively low in risk by experts can become a particular focus of concern and sociopolitical activity within a society (risk intensification), while other more serious hazards receive comparatively less attention (risk attenuation). Examples of significant hazards subject to social attenuation of risk perceptions might include smoking, radon gas, or climate change. Social intensification of risk perceptions appears to have been a feature of a range of health and other risk crises over the past 20 years in many nations across the globe: for example, the risks posed by the 'mad cow' bovine spongiform encephalopathy (BSE) crisis, radiological and chemical contamination events, responses to the Y2K 'millennium bug', child protection failures, and major transport and terrorist disasters (Pidgeon *et al.*, 2003).

The theoretical starting point of the social amplification framework is the assumption that 'risk events', which might include actual or hypothesized accidents and incidents, will be largely irrelevant or localized in their impact unless they are communicated to society more generally (Renn, 1991). As a key part of that communication process, risk events and their characteristics become portrayed through various risk signals (images, signs, and symbols) which in turn interact with a wide range of psychological, social, institutional or cultural processes in ways that intensify or attenuate perceptions of risk. Within such a framework, risk experience can only be properly defined through the *interaction* between the potential harms attached to a risk event and the social and cultural processes which shape interpretations of that event. An advantage of SARF is that it is clear in foregrounding an essential epistemological and ontological tension, often implicit within many risk studies, that, while hazards are real enough, our knowledge of them can only ever be socially constructed (Rosa, 2003; Pidgeon *et al.*, 2008).

The metaphor of amplification is derived from classical communications theory, and is used to describe the way in which risk signals are received, interpreted, and passed on by a variety of social agents. Kasperson *et al.* (1988) argue that such signals are subject to predictable transformations as they are filtered through various social and individual 'amplification stations'. Such transformations can involve increase or decrease in the volume of information about an event, selection to heighten the salience of certain aspects of a message, or reinterpretation and elaboration of the available symbols and images, leading to a particular interpretation and response by other recipients of these messages. Amplification stations can include both individuals and social units; for example, scientists or scientific institutions, reporters and the mass media, politicians and government agencies, or other stakeholder groups and their members.

In a second stage of the framework, directed primarily at risk intensification processes, Kasperson *et al.* (1988) argue that social amplification can also account for the observation that some events will lead to spreading 'ripples' of secondary consequences, which may go far beyond the initial impact of the event, and may even impinge upon initially unrelated hazards. Such secondary impacts include market impacts (perhaps through consumer avoidance of a product or related products), calls for regulatory constraints, litigation, community opposition, loss of credibility and trust, stigmatization of a facility or community, and investor flight.

In Renn's (1991) interpretation of the basic model, the organizational structure of risk communication within a society is comprised of sources, transmitters, and receivers, as shown in Figure 4.1.

This figure presents, of course, a much simplified characterization of what is, in reality, an exceedingly complex set of relationships. Feedback can and does occur between the various groupings, as is shown, reflecting the fact that communication is almost always a process of two-way exchange or dialogue between parties (Pidgeon *et al.*, 1992). Also, scientists and agency representatives are members of the general public too, members of the public in turn

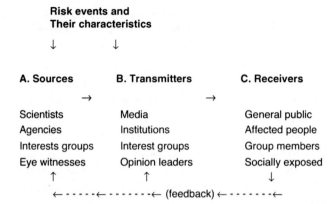

**Fig. 4.1** The organizational structure of risk communication. From Renn (1991).

receive and interpret information about risks from sources such as family and friends. In short, risk communication in the real world is better characterized, to use Krimsky & Plough's (1988) terms, as a 'tangled web' of signs, symbols, and messages.

## Critiques of the framework

A number of general critiques of SARF have been raised, principally in the set of peer review commentaries that accompanied the original 1988 article in *Risk Analysis*. While most of these authors welcomed social amplification as a genuine attempt to provide more theoretical coherence to the field, they have also highlighted points of contention, as well as avenues for further research.

One drawback of the framework, despite its apparent face validity, is that it may be too general to be subjected to any direct empirical test, particularly one of outright falsification. As emphasized in the 1988 article, the SARF is not a theory, properly speaking, but . . . 'a fledgling conceptual framework that may serve to guide ongoing efforts to develop, test, and apply such a theory to a broad array of pressing risk problems' (Kasperson *et al.*, 1988, p. 180). A theory, viewed in scientific terms as Machlis & Rosa (1990, p. 164) have emphasized, would require specification and explication of linked concepts, including the application of correspondence rules for converting abstract or inexact concepts into exact, testable ones. Its originators now concede (Kasperson *et al.*, 2003; also Rosa, 2003) that social amplification may not represent a theory in the classical sense, but rather serves as a useful analytical tool for describing and organizing relevant phenomena, for exploring and integrating relationships between rival constituent theories concerning risk perception and its

communication, and for deriving new hypotheses about the societal processing of risk images, framings, and signals. Certainly the framework does provide a template for integrating partial theories and research, and to encourage
more interactive and holistic interpretations. Kasperson (1992) has previously
cited three potential contributions of such an integrative framework: to bring
competing theories and hypotheses out of their 'terrain' and into direct conjunction (or confrontation) with each other; to provide an overall framework
in which to locate a large array of fragmented empirical findings; and to generate new hypotheses, particularly hypotheses geared to the interconnections
and interdependencies among particular concepts or components. For example, Gowda (2003) successfully draws upon the theory of policy windows
(Kingdon, 1984) and SARF to describe how policy choices became shaped in
the aftermath of the 'Megan's law' debate in the USA about child protection.

It can also be argued that, despite the recognition of important mechanisms
and routes of feedback such as depicted in Figure 4.1, the communications
engineering model on which the approach is founded places the dominant
emphasis upon too simple a conceptualization of risk communication, as a
*one-way* transfer of information, i.e. from risk events and sources, through
transmitters, and then on to receivers. As noted above, the development of
social risk perceptions is always likely to be the product of more interactive
processes between the parties to any risk communication (Jasanoff, 1998;
Murdock *et al.*, 2003). The US National Research Council (1989), character-
izes risk communication as:

> ... an interactive process of exchange of information and opinion among individuals,
> groups and institutions. It involves multiple messages about the nature of risk and
> other messages, not strictly about risk, that express concerns, opinions, or reactions to
> risk messages or to legal and institutional arrangements for risk management (p. 21).

A more radical interpretation of risk communication is that it provides first
and foremost a vehicle for *empowerment* of citizen groups in relation to government and other institutional interests, and this view underlies the development and use of new participation fora, such as planning cells and citizens'
juries, in the risk and public policy field (Renn *et al.*, 1995). Furthermore,
while it is relatively easy to point to an unreceptive or irrational public or an
ill-informed or sensationalist media as the originators of risk communication
problems, the communicator is also a key part of the process (Kasperson &
Stallen, 1991).

A further point of critique concerns the two-stage nature of the original
model, and the existing evidence to support each stage. Stage I posits that signals
from risk events become transformed to influence perceptions of risk and
thereby have an impact on first order behavioural responses. There is now a

relatively extensive set of findings from the risk perception literature to suggest that this is the case, although much remains to be done to investigate the *specific contexts* under which intensification or attenuation will occur. Stage II involves a direct link between amplification of risk perceptions and secondary consequences such as calls for stricter regulation, market impacts, and a generalization of response to other similar risk events and hazards. In many respects it is stage II which is the most important for health and environmental policy, given the potential for large economic and social impacts. To take just one example of this, not only has 'affect' and worry been found to be an important predictor of travel intentions following recent terrorist atrocities (Fischhoff *et al.*, 2004), but Gigerenzer (2006) illustrates how, in the US following the September 2001 attacks, the shift of people from travelling by air to (relatively riskier) forms of road transportation led to an estimated net increase in lives lost of 1500 in the year following the attacks.

A number of criticisms have also been raised of the amplification metaphor itself. First, that it might be taken to imply that there exists a baseline or 'true' risk readily attached to risk events, which is then distorted in some way by the social processes of amplification. It is quite clear that the proponents of the framework do not wish to imply that such a single true baseline always and unproblematically exists, particularly in many of the heavily politicized transscientific settings (Funtowicz & Ravetz, 1992) where amplification is most likely to occur. Their conceptualization of the amplification process in terms of transformation of signs, symbols, and images is compatible with the view that *all* knowledge about risk entails some elements of social construction (Johnson & Covello, 1987; Holzheu & Wiedemann, 1993; Rosa, 2003). Here, the observation that experts and public sometimes disagree about risks is compatible with the claim that different groups might filter and make salient different aspects of an event. Nevertheless, as Kasperson *et al.* (2003) note, risk perceptions can have real *consequences*, and these may be direct, as are usually treated in technical risk analyses, or may result indirectly from the secondary processing of risk information (such things as stigmatization, social conflict, and loss of confidence in products or markets).

Secondly, Rip (1988) observes that not all amplification effects might be undesired (see also Machlis & Rosa, 1990), as when sufficient political pressure for regulation of a previously neglected (attenuated) but very serious hazard is finally generated. To cite just one example, Behrens (1983) gives an account of the legislative changes which followed the fire which began in the eighth floor workrooms of one of New York's 'loft' clothing factories at the Triangle Shirtwaist Company in 1911. By the year of the disaster, over half of the city's 500 000 workers worked above the seventh floor, many in poorly maintained and equipped buildings, and all beyond the reach of effective fire department rescue. The fire led to the deaths of 146 clothing workers, many of whom became trapped and attempted to escape by jumping from the upper stories of the burning building. Although, according to Behrens, the initial public outrage at the factory management's disregard for safety eventually subsided, in the short term it was the stimulus for much needed reform of fire and workplace safety regulations in the city. Behrens concludes that 'in the immediate aftermath of major disasters, groups and individuals interested in reform are given unexpected opportunities to effect reforms that normally would take years to effect' (p. 372; see also Gowda, 2003).

The converse of risk amplification is the extreme attenuation of certain risk events so that, despite serious consequences for the risk bearers and society more generally, they pass virtually unnoticed and untended, often continuing to grow in effects until reaching disaster proportions. For example, Lorenzoni *et al.* (2005) suggest that, until quite recently, the issue of climate change could be viewed in this way. Kasperson & Kasperson (1990) describe such highly attenuated risks as 'hidden hazards' and map out five ways in which these might be sustained.

- *Global elusive hazards* involve a series of complex processes (regional interactions, slow accumulation, lengthy time lags, diffuse effects). Their incidence in a politically fragmented and unequal world tends to mute their signal power in many societies

- *Ideological hazards* remain hidden principally because they lie embedded in a societal web of values and assumptions that attenuates consequences, elevates associated benefits, or idealizes certain beliefs

- *Marginal hazards* befall people who occupy the edges of cultures, societies, or economies where they are exposed to hazards that are remote from or concealed by those at the centre or in the mainstream. Many in such marginal situations are already weakened or highly vulnerable while they enjoy limited access to entitlements and few alternative means of coping

- *Amplification-driven hazards* have effects that elude conventional types of risk assessment and environmental impact analysis and are often, therefore, allowed to grow in their secondary consequences before societal intervention occurs

- Finally, *value-threatening hazards* alter human institutions, lifestyles, and basic values, but because the pace of technological change so outstrips the capacity of social institutions to respond and adapt, disharmony in purpose, political will, and directed effort impede effective responses and the hazards grow.

Hidden hazards are important as they represent examples of how uncertainty (and ignorance; see Bammer and Smithson, 2008) become discursively constructed within a wider web of social and political relationships.

## Organizational attenuation of risk

An important emerging issue in the health risk domain is the role of organizations and institutions in the social processing and generation of risk. Organizational failures are known to occur in a variety of healthcare settings (e.g. Chief Medical Officer, 2000). Pidgeon and O'Leary (1994) have suggested that linking ideas about risk amplification (or attenuation) to the considerable empirical base of knowledge concerning organizational processes intended to prevent large scale failures and disasters would be an important extension of the framework. Most contemporary risks originate in sociotechnical systems rather than natural phenomena so that risk management and internal regulatory processes governing the behaviour of institutions in identifying, diagnosing, prioritizing, and responding to risks are key parts of the broader amplification process. As Short (1992) points out, large organizations such as healthcare institutions increasingly set the context and terms of debate for society's consideration of risk. Understanding amplification dynamics, then, requires insight into how risk-related decisions relate to organizational self-interest, messy inter- and intra-organizational relationships, economically related rationalizations, and 'rule of thumb' considerations that often conflict with the view of risk analysis as a scientific enterprise (Short, 1992, p. 8). Since major accidents are often preceded by smaller incidents and risk warnings, how signals of incubating hazards are processed within institutions and communicated to others outside the institution do much to structure society's experience with technological and industrial risks.

Noting the relative void of work on organizational risk processing, Freudenburg (1992) has examined characteristics of organizations that serve to attenuate risk signals and ultimately to *increase* the risks posed by technological systems. These include such attributes as the lack of organizational commitment to the risk management function, the bureaucratic attenuation of information flow within the organization (particularly concerning 'bad news'), specialized divisions of labour that create 'corporate gaps' in responsibility, amplified risk-taking by workers, the atrophy of organizational vigilance to risk as a result of a myriad of factors (e.g. boredom, routinization), and imbalances and mismatches in institutional resources. Freudenburg concludes that these factors often work in concert to lead even well meaning and honest scientists and managers to underestimate risks. In turn, such organizational attenuation of risk communication serves systematically and repeatedly to amplify exposure to health and environmental risks that the organization is entrusted to anticipate and to control.

Other studies of organizational handling of risk confirm Freudenburg's analysis and provide further considerations. In her analysis of the *Challenger* accident in the US, Vaughan (1997) found communication and information issues to be critical but argued that structural factors, such as pressures from a competitive environment, resource scarcity in the organization, vulnerability of important subunits, and characteristics of the internal safety regulation system were equally important. Several theoretical perspectives on organizational processing of risk can be drawn upon within the amplification/attenuation framework. Evidence of a range of broad social and organizational preconditions to large scale accidents is available in the work of Turner (Turner & Pidgeon, 1997). As a result of a detailed analysis of 84 major accidents in the UK, Turner concluded that such events rarely come about for any single reason. Rather, it is typical to find that a number of undesirable events accumulate, unnoticed or not fully understood, often over a considerable number of years, which he defines as the *disaster incubation period.* Preventive action to remove one or more of the dangerous conditions or a *trigger event,* which might be a final critical error or a slightly abnormal operating condition, bring this period to an end. Turner focuses in particular upon the information difficulties, which are typically associated with the attempts of individuals and organizations to deal with uncertain and ill-structured safety problems, during the hazard incubation period. Despite these valuable explorations, our knowledge on risk amplification and attenuation in different types of institutions remains thin and eclectic. Systematic application of the amplification framework in a comparative study of health organizations and institutions might well yield highly useful results, particularly how signals are denied, de-emphasized, or misinterpreted.

## Policy and research priorities

The objective of providing policy-makers with sound guidance on risk communication, let alone evaluating the effectiveness of existing communication practice, will be no simple matter (Fischhoff, 1995). That objective is only likely to be met by a sustained and systematic research effort, drawing upon knowledge from a range of studies together with research that illuminates the socio-political context of risk communication in its full complexity. However, there is scope to apply the SARF in ways that begin to address this agenda. These are considered briefly under three headings: mapping the institutional context of

risk communications; providing tools for policy; and amplification and attenuation in public and stakeholder participation.

## Mapping the institutional context of risk communications

Much of the research on risk communication, and in particular the existing
empirical work directly focused on the social amplification of risk, reflects
North American experience (for exceptions see contributions to Pidgeon *et al.*,
2003). There is clearly a need to conduct basic investigation of the transferabil-
ity of the existing findings, as well as the ways in which different cultural contexts uniquely shape risk communication and amplification effects. Once
again this sets a formidable task, particularly if we consider the multiple actors
present in Figure 4.1. Breakwell & Barnett (2003) draw upon the observation
that amplification and attenuation processes are complex dynamic social phenomena which almost always involve several levels (or layers) of social process,
and accordingly of potential evidence. They describe a new approach—the
layering method—that can be used to further develop and test the empirical
claims of SARF, and hence to increase the predictive power of models designed
to understand risk amplification, using it with data collected in relation to BSE
and AIDS/HIV.

If we start from the standpoint of the key mediators of much risk information—the media—then the framework should be capable of describing and
organizing the amplification rules used by these institutions in their role
between government and sections of society. How the media interface with the
different institutional players in the 'risk game' (Slovic, 1998; also Murdock
*et al.*, 2003) seems a key issue here. There is also the question of whether different institutional arrangements can be characterized as operating with predictable sets of amplification or attenuation rules (see Renn, 1991, p. 300), and
whether there is evidence for a link between such institutional behaviour and
subsequent societal impacts. The influence of both regional (e.g. EU) and
national legal frameworks, as overarching societal constraints to amplification,
would seem critical here too.

## Providing tools for policy

We have argued that the SARF should not be viewed as a theory, yielding simple and direct predictions, but as an analytical framework. Taken together with
the inherent complexity of risk communication issues noted above, it is clear
that the framework cannot be expected to yield simple or direct predictions
regarding which issues are likely to be the subject of amplification/attenuation
effects in advance. A parallel problem—which has in part epistemological and
in part practical roots—is met when researchers attempt to use knowledge of

the human and organizational causes from past technological accidents and disasters to predict the likelihood of future failures (Turner & Pidgeon, 1997, Chapter 11). Here some practitioners have adopted more holistic methods, seeking to diagnose vulnerability in large organizational systems through screening against broad classes of risk management factors. In a similar way, knowledge of the factors likely to lead to amplification effects, and the socio-political contexts in which they might operate, could possibly be used as a *screening device* for evaluating the potential for such effects, particularly with respect to any synergistic effects found between factors.

## Amplification and attenuation in public and stakeholder participation

Inviting the public to be a part of the decision-making process in risk management issues has, of course, been a major recent objective in European and North American health policy arenas. As a consequence, deliberative and participatory mechanisms have become increasingly important in the risk communication arena, and look set to be so for the foreseeable future, particularly with the application of new and emerging technologies to health (see, for example, Pidgeon & Rogers-Hayden, 2007). Participation can be seen as a vehicle for appropriate two-way risk communication between policy-makers and public, as a discursive device that empowers communities, as a means of incorporating public values in ethical decisions or sometimes as a combination of all of these. The US National Research Council report on *Understanding Risk* (1996) develops a detailed set of proposals for stakeholder engagement in relation to risk issues. They define the resultant analytical deliberative process as combining sound science and systematic uncertainty analysis with deliberation by an appropriate representation of affected parties, policy-makers, and specialists in risk analysis. According to the authors, dialogue and deliberation should occur throughout the process of risk characterization, from problem framing through to detailed risk assessment and then on to risk management and decision implementation. The National Research Council report argues here that failure to attend to dialogue at the early stages of problem framing can be particularly costly, for if a key concern is missed in subsequent analysis the danger is that the whole process may be invalidated. Seen in developmental terms, the risk characterization proposals of the National Research Council can also be viewed as the outcome of a growing transition from traditional forms of one-way 'risk communication', to more dialogic or discursive fora which have the potential to empower people in the processes of decision-making about risks (Pidgeon *et al.*, 1992; Fischhoff, 1995; see also Fuller et al, Chapter 17, this volume).

However, the current popularity of such concepts obscures the challenge of how to put these worthwhile objectives into practice. Renn addresses this considerable challenge in work drawn from the extensive experience of the Centre of Technology Assessment at Baden-Württemburg in participatory processes in Germany. In particular, Renn (2003) argues that people can experience both amplification and attenuation of risk perceptions in participatory settings. His argument draws upon material from two case studies: first, that of solid waste incinerator siting, and, second, of health benefits of noise reduction. Renn draws the important inference that risk amplification and attenuation can be made a *deliberate* subject of discursive activities within participatory risk management procedures. Such discourse helps people to realize that it is normal, but also detrimental to prudent judgement, if one selects and transmits only those pieces of information that one approves, if one amplifies signals that support one's own view, and attenuates those that do not. This holds out hope that greater understanding—if not necessarily consensus over—competing positions can be arrived at in conflicted risk debates.

## Concluding comments

In conclusion, we reiterate the important point that social amplification of risk should not be viewed as a theory but as an analytical framework. In this role it nevertheless provides a basis for organizing findings that can sensitize policy-makers in the health domain to the important human, social, and cultural factors to take into account when designing risk communications, participatory processes, and in responding to the dynamics of unfolding risk issues. This longer term objective might be best achieved by synthesizing theory and findings from several perspectives, rather than taking any singular theoretical standpoint, and plurality is a particular strength of the social amplification framework. By bringing social, cultural, and audience-relevant issues to bear on what might otherwise remain framed by the various existing technical approaches to risk assessment and management, the risk amplification model makes a genuine contribution to policy and practice in the field of risk communication and its management.

## References

Bammer, G. & Smithson, M. (eds) (2008). *Uncertainty and risk: Multidisciplinary perspectives*. London, Earthscan.

Behrens, E. G. (1983). The Triangle Shirtwaist company fire of 1911: a lesson in legislative manipulation. *Texas Law Review*, 62: 361–87.

Breakwell, G. & Barnett, J. (2003). Social amplification of risk and the layering method. In: N. F. Pidgeon, R. K. Kasperson & P. Slovic (eds). *The Social Amplification of Risk*. Cambridge, CUP, pp. 80–101.

Cabinet Office. (2002). *Risk: Improving government's capability to handle risk and uncertainty*. London, HMSO.

Chief Medical Officer. (2000). *An Organization with a Memory: Report of an Expert Group on Learning from Adverse Events in the NHS*. London, Department of Health.

Fischhoff, B. (1995). Risk communication and perception unplugged: twenty years of process. *Risk Analysis*, 15: 137–45.

Fischhoff, B., Bruine de Bruin, W., Perrin, W. & Downes, J. (2004). Travel risks in a time of terror: judgements and choices. *Risk Analysis*, 24: 1301–9.

Freudenburg, W. R. (1992). Heuristics, biases and the not so general public: expertise and error in the assessment of risks. In: S. Krimsky & D. Golding (eds). *Social Theories of Risk*. Praeger, Westport CT, pp. 229–50.

Funtowicz, S. O. & Ravetz, J. R. (1992). Three types of risk assessment and the emergence of post-normal science. In: S. Krimsky & D. Golding (eds). *Social Theories of Risk*. Praeger, Westport CT, pp. 251–74.

Gigerenzer, G. (2006). Out of the frying pan into the fire: behavioural reactions to terrorist attacks. *Risk Analysis*, 26: 347–51.

Gowda, M. V. R. (2003). Integrating politics with the social amplification of risk framework: insights from an exploration in the criminal justice context. In: N. F. Pidgeon, R. K. Kasperson & P. Slovic (eds). *The Social Amplification of Risk*. Cambridge, CUP, pp. 305–325.

Henwood, K. L., Pidgeon, N. F., Sarre, S., Simmons, P. & Smith, N. (2008). Risk, framing and everyday life: methodological and ethical reflections from three sociocultural projects. *Health, Risk and Society*, 10: 421–38.

Holzheu, F. & Wiedemann, P. (1993). Introduction: perspectives on risk perception. In: Bayerische Rück (ed.) *Risk is a Construct*. Knesebeck, Munich, pp. 9–20.

Jasanoff, S. (1998). The political science of risk perception. *Reliability Engineering and System Safety*, 59: 91–100.

Johnson, B. B. & Covello, V. T. (eds) (1987). *The Social and Cultural Construction of Risk*. Dordrecht, The Netherlands, Reidel.

Kasperson, J. X. & Kasperson, R. E. (2005). *The Social Contours of Risk Volume 1: Publics, Risk Communication and the Social Amplification of Risk*. London, Earthscan.

Kasperson, J. X., Kasperson, R., Pidgeon, N. F. & Slovic, P. (2003). The social amplification of risk: assessing fifteen years of research and theory. In: N. F. Pidgeon, R. K. Kasperson & P. Slovic (eds). *The Social Amplification of Risk*. Cambridge, CUP, pp. 13–16.

Kasperson, R. E. (1992). The social amplification of risk: progress in developing an integrative framework. In: S. Krimsky & D. Golding (eds). *Social Theories of Risk*. Praeger, Westport CT, pp. 153–78.

Kasperson, R. E. & Kasperson, J. X. (1990). Hidden hazards. In: D. G. Mayo & R. Hollander (eds). *Acceptable Evidence: Science and Values in Hazard Management*. Oxford, Oxford University Press, pp. 9–28.

Kasperson, R. E. & Stallen, P. J. M. (1991). Risk communication: the evolution of attempts. In: R. E. Kasperson & P. J. M. Stallen (eds). *Communicating Risks to the Public*. Dordrecht, Kluwer, pp. 1–12.

Kasperson, R. E., Renn, O., Slovic, P. *et al.* (1988). The social amplification of risk: a conceptual framework. *Risk Analysis*, 8: 177–87.

Kingdon, J. W. (1984). *Agendas, Alternatives, and Public Policies*. Boston, Little, Brown.

Krimsky, S. & Plough, A. (1988). *Environmental Hazards: Communicating Risks as a Social Process*. Auburn, Dover, Massachussetts.

Lorenzoni, I., Pidgeon, N. F. & O'Connor, R. (2005). Dangerous climate change: the role for risk research. *Risk Analysis*, 25: 1387–98.

Lupton, D. (1999). *Risk*. London, Routledge.

Machlis, G. E. & Rosa, E. A. (1990). Desired risk: broadening the social amplification of risk framework. *Risk Analysis*, 10: 161–8.

Murdock, G., Petts, J. & Horlick-Jones, T. (2003). After amplification: rethinking the role of the media in risk communication. In N. F. Pidgeon, R. K. Kasperson & P. Slovic (eds). *The Social Amplification of Risk*. Cambridge, CUP, pp. 156–178.

Pidgeon, N. F. & Beattie, J. (1998). The psychology of risk and uncertainty. In: P. Calow *et al.* (eds). *Handbook of Environmental Risk Assessment and Management*. Oxford, Blackwell Science, pp. 289–318.

Pidgeon, N. F. & O'Leary, M. (1994). Organizational safety culture: implications for aviation practice. In: N. Johnston, N. McDonald & R. Fuller (eds). *Aviation Psychology in Practice*. Aldershot, Avebury Technical, pp. 21–43.

Pidgeon, N. F. & Rogers-Hayden, T. (2007). Opening up nanotechnology dialogue with the publics: risk communication or 'upstream engagement'? *Health, Risk and Society*, 9: 191–210.

Pidgeon, N. F., Hood, C., Jones, D., Turner, B. & Gibson, R. (1992). Risk perception, Ch. 5. *Risk: Analysis, Perception and Management. Report of a Royal Society Study Group*. London, The Royal Society, pp. 89–134.

Pidgeon, N. F., Kasperson, R. K. & Slovic, P. (2003). *The Social Amplification of Risk*. Cambridge, Cambridge University Press, p. 448.

Pidgeon, N. F., Simmons, P., Sarre, S., Henwood, K. L. & Smith, N. (2008). The ethics of socio-cultural risk research. *Health, Risk and Society*, 10: 321–9.

Renn, O. (1991). Risk communication and the social amplification of risk. In: R. E. Kasperson & P. J. M. Stallen (eds). *Communicating Risks to the Public*. Dordrecht, Kluwer, pp. 287–323.

Renn, O. (2003). Social amplification of risk in participation: two case studies. In N. F. Pidgeon, R. K. Kasperson & P. Slovic (eds). *The Social Amplification of Risk*. Cambridge, CUP, pp. 374–401.

Renn, O. & Walker, T. (2008). *Global Risk Governance: Concept and Practice Using the IRGC Framework*. Dordrecht, Springer.

Renn, O., Webler, T. & Wiedemann, P. (1995). *Fairness and Competence in Citizen Participation*. Dordrecht, Kluwer.

Rip, A. (1988). Should social amplification of risk be counteracted? *Risk Analysis*, 8: 193–7.

Rosa, E. A. (2003). The logical structure of the risk amplification framework (SARF): Metatheoretical foundations and policy implications. In: N. F. Pidgeon, R. K. Kasperson & P. Slovic (eds). *The Social Amplification of Risk*. Cambridge, CUP, pp. 47–79.

Royal Society (1992). *Risk: Analysis, Perception and Management*. London, The Royal Society.

Short, J. F. Jr. (1992). Defining, explaining, and managing risk. In: J. F. Short, Jr. & L. Clarke (eds). *Organizations, Uncertainties, and Risk*. Boulder, CO: Westview.

Slovic, P. (1998). The risk game. *Reliability Engineering and System Safety*, 59: 73–9.

Slovic, P. (2000). *The Perception of Risk*. London, Earthscan.

Turner, B. A. & Pidgeon, N. F. (1997). *Man-made Disasters*, 2nd edn. Oxford, Butterworth–Heinemann.

US National Research Council (1989). *Improving Risk Communication: National Research Council Committee*. Washington DC, National Academy Press.

US National Research Council (1996). *Understanding Risk: Informing Decisions in a Democratic Society* (eds P. C. Stern & H. V. Fineberg). Washington DC, National Academy Press.

Vaughan, D. (1997). *The Challenger Launch Decision: Risky Technology, Culture, and Deviance at NASA*. Chicago, University of Chicago Press.

## Chapter 5

# From trouble to trauma: the need for public–private health partnerships

Laurence Barton PhD (President and Professor of Management, The American College, Bryn Mawr)

Although relationships are essential in any crisis management dynamic, they potentially never have greater consequence than in the area of public health. While many are impacted by construction and industrial accidents, product recalls and financial disasters, incidents that could compromise public health are non-discriminatory: they know no boundaries, economic or geographic.

Relationships between individuals and organizations are particularly essential when the wellbeing of a community or an entire society is at stake. Consider for a moment the incredibly complex span of relationships that are embedded in the public health and emergency management disciplines:

- First responders, including police, fire, and emergency medical technicians are increasingly reliant upon technology factors outside their span, including traffic and GPS systems that allow them to navigate road and rail systems to accelerate response. These systems are often flawed and, in the case of a massive electrical or technology failure, could cause further havoc upon already taxed individuals and systems

- Doctors and nurses are increasingly reliant upon national health services and non-governmental organizations to provide early warning signs for potential pandemics and related emergencies. However, as will be explained in this article, some economies are highly sensitive to not promoting outbreaks of pandemics in their borders because of the profound economic and tourism damage that can result. Employers increasingly realize that they must have a sound relationship system in place before a public health disaster strikes. While a majority of multinational employers with more than 10 000 employees are believed to have a pandemic plan in place worldwide

◆ (Friedman, 2007), some 84% of those surveyed report that they have no updated contact names for physicians such as epidemiologists whom they may rely upon for fast response in the event of a medical disaster

◆ The medical practice to which several physicians belong is investigated for potential irregularities in billing to a government agency or insurer, causing negative headlines and questions about the integrity of the spinal specialists.

## Planning for the inevitable

Corporate planning for medical emergencies is typically assigned to one of two divisions: risk management or corporate security (Barton, 2008). In analysing corporate plans from companies in the entertainment, petroleum, and financial services industries over the past 20 years, several shared attributes emerge from these plans:

1 They typically have a 'radar screen' approach built into the notification system so that security or other managers can alert headquarters on a 24/7 basis if and when an outbreak of any medical issue occurs

2 The plans almost inevitably emphasize the limited resources available within the company to assist employees, referring the senior supervisor who may be aware of a potential problem to work directly with local public health officials

3 The planning almost always refers to the impact of a pandemic on the customers of the organization. In fact, the majority of the 'public health plan' aspect of the crisis thinking is devoted more to how to divert product from one port to another, or notify customers as to when product shipments will resume, as opposed to how to provide immediate, tangible support to employees and their families

4 A surprising number of plans, estimated by this author to be in the range of about 40% of some 300 plans reviewed over the past 11 years, only discuss pandemic-like events, ignoring internal medical issues that could emerge, including the impacts of radon, lead poisoning, mold, asbestos and water contamination, to name but a few potential threats.

There are exceptions, to be sure. Sports footwear manufacturer Nike and British Petroleum have massive planning systems in place to protect their people and brand during and after a public health disaster. Both companies have separate crisis software systems to help product managers share updated information discreetly and in real time, and both have conducted extensive simulations in their respective emergency operations centres to test both local supervisors and corporate executives on how to manage issues involving a prolonged absence of talent due to sickness. Interestingly enough, both companies routinely include their insurance companies in the planning and simulation process to ascertain whether their processes can meet or exceed best practice standards.

While no list of public health disasters is complete, any discussion of the relationship between organizational leaders and their public health counterparts should include a summary of lessons learned from major incidents over the decades. In the process of writing a new book, *Crisis Leadership Now*, over a dozen leading epidemiologists from hospitals worldwide were interviewed by the author, as well as a series of public health officials, including those associated with the European Community health agencies, as well as the Centers for Disease Control in the United States. Here is a summary of what was learned:

- The primary concern of virtually everyone interviewed was the H5N1 influenza virus. This is not only because it can mutate fast, but also because the 'creeping' period from when cases first emerge to when a community may realize that it has been overwhelmed by a deadly flu can be very short. By the time health officials realize that they are dealing with a potential pandemic, sickened residents have left their community by foot, train or plane, infecting an unknown number of unsuspecting persons

- Although there have been ten pandemics over the past three centuries—with millions of victims—physicians feel that corporations simply believe that these issues can be managed by launching 'wash your hands' campaigns to the detriment of meaningful employee education. Even when hospitals and health clinics offer to manage free educational seminars inside a company, their requests are often ignored because company executives 'don't want to create panic when a crisis doesn't exist'

- Anthrax-type cases of terrorism, admittedly difficult to orchestrate, are an inevitable part of the arsenal of weapons that a terrorist treasures. The FBI, Scotland Yard, and most other respected investigatory agencies acknowledge that the successful deployment of anthrax against public officials and broadcasters in the United States in 2001 is a precursor to future deployment. When done so in an aerosol-type environment at a business convention, for example, the impact could be catastrophic in terms of the numbers of potential victims

- Tuberculosis resurfaced in the news in 2007 when American attorney Andrew Speaker travelled to five countries in Europe on his honeymoon when he knew he was infected with TB. By the time he returned to the United States (a Canadian border agent stopped Speaker because doctors had notified the CDC immediately if he was found), the news media created near panic because hundreds of travellers had been on various flights to and from Europe with Speaker and his wife. The Speaker case reminds us that an outbreak of TB inside a manufacturing or processing plant, for example—or any closed quarters—could cause havoc not only for that employer, but for regional medical systems. The number of physicians worldwide with a career-long understanding of the nuances of TB and treatment protocol is estimated to have dropped about 84% since 1950 (Zimmerman, 2007)

• Foodborne illnesses are in the news frequently, including the massive recall of Irish lamb products in December 2008. News stories often emphasize the financial loss to farmers and processors of various meat and other food products that have been recalled. What would potentially serve the public interest far more than a business analysis is a reminder to the public of the importance of early warning signs regarding botulism, parasites, and other bacteria that can contaminate food products.

## An awakening at one multinational

In mid-2008, the author worked closely with one multinational company with a heavy manufacturing focus; the company produces and distributes a variety of products to Europe, Asia, and North America. The company has little presence in Latin America or Africa but does have one subsidiary in New Zealand. The total full-time employee population exceeds 30 000 persons. The specific challenges facing this company were reviewed in terms of the need for a comprehensive business continuity plan. Other than a modest crisis management plan (focusing primarily on the need to reallocate product if a major port were closed owing to a compliance violation), the company had little in terms of planning for any health emergency.

After meeting with the executive team and surveying over 1800 mid-level to senior supervisors worldwide (with 1278 respondents) and hosting five web-based conferences to determine levels of exposure to a variety of health-related threats, the following represents a summary of lessons learned by that organization that are appropriate for reflection by both scholars of crisis management as well as public health counterparts.

• The company determined that a health-based specialist needs to be hired in the Office of the Risk Manager to create a global framework for understanding and responding to health emergencies. That health specialist will

be responsible for ensuring that the company meets or exceeds best practice standards to alert employees to the need for prevention (e.g. HIV testing, flu shots, hand washing, diabetes education), and that the specialist
will work with internal audit to ensure that each major facility worldwide
designate a 'contact lead' for the specialist who will serve as a reference
point going forward

- A cross-functional team that included a Vice-President of operations,
human resources, environmental and safety and audit established the
health specialist position requirements. Principal qualifications include a
master's degree in public health, 10 years of experience in production,
operations or manufacturing, and preferred experience in compliance.
A Canadian whose expertise spans manufacturing and health and who
spent 8 years as a pharmacist filled the position in September 2008

- The specialist worked with the author in autumn 2008 to survey teams
worldwide on areas that they felt raised high exposure for the company.
Theme areas included natural disasters, embezzlement/extortion and
related crimes, and geopolitical and economic changes that could harm the
people, reputation, and financial condition of the company. Interestingly
enough, over 31% of respondents said that a health crisis represented the
single greatest threat to operations, second only to a fire (representing 33%
of all responses). That information was shared with the Board of Directors
of the company at their November quarterly meeting

- The specialist realized that information inside company facilities was lacking regarding how to report concerns over environmental and safety standards. While the company had established several toll-free 'whistleblower'
hotlines regarding safety infractions, those resources were rarely, if ever,
used to report concerns over the lack of internal awareness regarding sani-
tation, for instance. The specialist quickly learned about cases where
dozens of employees had become sick inside a company cafeteria owing to
suspected salmonella, for instance, and others in another country where an
employee who was cut and subsequently bled on the job had hepatitis;
workers panicked when they learned that this could potentially have compromised their health

- Web-based conference calls hosted by the health specialist proved to be a
daunting challenge. Among the challenges experienced: lack of comfort
with the native tongue of the host (French) whose attempts to host the calls
in English were frustrating for all involved. Secondly, many supervisors
worldwide were hesitant to talk about concerns of health infractions inside
their business units for fear that their executive teams would be embarrassed

and subsequently singled out by leaders. Third, the specialist felt that the global recession created considerable anxiety for those on the call and that many were afraid to identify problems in their region because they did not want anyone at corporate level to sense that they were not doing their job. In essence, a fear factor paralysed participants who did not know the specialist or trust their corporate counterparts

◆ Recognizing that the web-based calls were politely informational but largely one-way in content and delivery, the specialist secured budget approval to visit five major factories (two in Asia, two in Europe, and one in the United States) by the end of the year. Those visits allowed the specialist to build a personal rapport with members of a newly appointed Safety and Health Task Force for the company. The specialist feels that personally securing the support of contemporaries is essential for her success, and the first voluntary reports of health concerns have begun to be shared on her secure email account

◆ The law department has similarly proven to be a challenge to this specialist. Although her knowledge of health issues runs deep and her capabilities in production have been established with another multinational, the legal department has often challenged how and when the health office communicates with the business units. Lingering concerns exist that once the company is aware of a public health exposure, a lack of swift communication with local officials could be a violation of provincial or national laws. Disclosure continues to be a theme that multinationals tout in their investor and relations campaigns, but the practical dimensions of transparency in a company that is worried about headlines and sustaining its stock price makes many lawyers shutter (Barton, 2008). This specialist has learned this through several early battles in her tenure.

## Corporate planning and SARS

Corporate executives worldwide noted with great alarm the impact from the most notable outbreak of severe acute respiratory syndrome (SARS) in 2003 that migrated from Asia to Canada. The potential pandemic—medical experts continue to debate definitions—cost the Canadian economy an estimated US $800 million loss in tourism and business revenue. Traffic through Chek Lap Kok International Airport in Hong Kong dropped by 90 per cent over a 3-week period (Leung and Lan, 2004). Economists continue to debate widely the economic loss to businesses whose products were held in ports both in Asia and North America.

In the midst of the 2003 outbreak, the electronics industry claimed that over-reaction to the SARS concern could devastate trade. The trade magazine

*Silicon Strategies* (EE Times, 2003) stated that SARS was crippling 'the bottom lines of Motorola, Nokia, Qualcomm and other electronic companies'. Both that journal and at least three dozen other electronic journals and online sources complained that despite the human toll of SARS—China originally reported 6727 'probable' SARS cases and over 400 deaths—these reports did not discuss the human toll of the disaster.

Corporate planning cannot be stagnant. Nike, for example, has written and revised its pandemic plan four times over 3 years, according to Bill Turner, Corporate Director of Retail. Among the steps taken on a global scale:

- A pandemic plan is available for download on the company intranet for all business units; the plan is revised after close coordination with international health officials
- Two simulations have allowed corporate managers to test the pandemic plan in terms of its effectiveness in reaching out to employees at their homes and while on the road, and in answering questions from associates and customers
- Human resources daily track employee issues so that an outbreak of an influenza that is unusually large in a particular manufacturing or distribution plant leads to an alert that is sent to a regional office. Since that one issue could cause a drop in product distribution impacting an entire region, the early alert system is not only smart economics (since part-time replacement help can be accessed more rapidly before a flu spreads), but the regional director can also sense whether there is a 'connect the dots' situation even before some public health officials may have had the chance to look at cross-border situations.

## Private sector planning

Although formal contingency plans such as those mentioned earlier are increasingly common among multinationals, surveys by scholars in both Europe and North America find that the majority of small businesses have little or no formal planning in place in anticipation of a public health disaster. The migration and transmittal of influenza can be so rapid in any community, complicated by the ease and low cost of cross-border travel, that the daunting impact of a global pandemic has only been fully appreciated by the World Health Organization and comparable bodies; their corporate counterparts often live in denial. Many risk management executives interviewed by the author admitted that they have purchased insurance policies that will indemnify their organization against losses from a communicable disease outbreak, but they also struggled when asked these questions.

There is some good news emerging in the disaster literature. In the aftermath of the terrorist attacks of 11 September 2002, a number of communities in the United States increased the number of 'homeland security advisors' who could work with the private sector on planning for medical and other complex emergencies. As their expertise grows by visiting local employers, creating networking opportunities with public health providers, and sharing models for evaluation and response of potential outbreaks, they are also beginning to publish articles that offer sound, if not sage, counsel, to employers. One example is Adam Crowe, a health planner for Johnson County, Kansas, who also teaches at Park University. He notes:

> Every organization, regardless of the size and service provided, can be severely impacted by communicable conditions. Every employee, particularly essential personnel, should be provided education and encouragement to practise good hand washing, cough and sneeze etiquette, as well as other prevention techniques. Like all hazards, organizations must evaluate the risks of communicable conditions and other public health threats. Once this evaluation is completed, clear communication with personnel and their families will alleviate some of the fear and misunderstanding that comes with these public health threats (Crowe, 2008, p. 81).

Corporate leaders have been slow to hear such warnings, however. There is an abiding reliance upon public health officials to advise employers when a communicable disease could compromise social and business systems. Interestingly enough, however, there are few, if any, recorded standards that actually explain how and when employers are expected to advise local or provincial health officials when they see major leaps in sickness among employees, one of the first warning signs of a looming health disaster.

The following questions are intended to encourage robust dialogue between public health officials and their corporate counterparts in the environmental, health, and safety/security arenas.

## For public health officials

- Have you asked that major employers in your geographic region notify you when more than 10 employees in any one department are reporting that they are ill to their employers? What mechanism exists to track multiple reporting issues within a single geographic area?

- What kind of website information and updates can be made available when the first outbreak of a communicable disease occurs? Are these updates available in those major languages that are unique to your region?

- So as not to create panic, do you have a frequently asked question (FAQ) brochure and webpage available now in template form that can be customized to the unique public health issue that could emerge in the future?

For instance, if a Chernobyl-type industrial accident were to occur in your area that potentially compromised the health of tens of thousands because of a highly toxic cloud, how quickly could public information be shared? How long would it take for roads, rail lines, and airports to be ordered closed? What is the established process for food and water supplies to be destroyed and replenished after inspection and safety verification? How will animal deportation and slaughters be managed? What are the legal and ethical questions that public policy-makers will face in the midst of these and hundreds of other decisions?

## For corporate leaders

• Beyond existing crisis management plans, do you have a specific and separate plan in place that alerts senior management to a potential health crisis that could affect the organization? What is your business continuity plan if more than 30% of your employees were unable to work because of prolonged illness? How will you communicate with suppliers and customers during this emergency?

• When is the last time you reviewed your insurance policies with your broker in terms of how they relate to a medical emergency? Would you be indemnified for lost revenue if a major medical emergency were to compromise your sales and production for a month? For how long? Three months? What steps are required by senior management and the Board of Directors as fiduciaries in order to be reimbursed for lost revenue?

• Do you require in your sourcing contracts that headquarters is notified in real time if a key supplier finds that their manufacturing or processing has been compromised by a health disaster? If a plant or port in Hong Kong, Turkey or Vietnam shuts down for weeks or months at a time, your ability to function could be compromised. Suppliers are notoriously averse to sharing bad news. What systems do you have in place to encourage the early sharing of information?

The need for public health leaders to discuss these and related issues with corporate executives is a compelling one. In a digital world where news travels fast, we may be lulled into false comfort that 'bad news travels fast', however. Unfortunately, some of the most fragile economies in the world are also host to some of the least funded and sophisticated medical systems where detection and preventive care at large employers could identify serious risks before they blossom into a catastrophe. When these same economies are also producing foods and/or products that can contaminate a large population, we face an equation for which no model prescription of response exists. Rather than 'solving the problem on the fly', the time for synergistic planning by health officials and their corporate counterparts working in concert is now—before disaster strikes.

## References

Barton, L. (2008). *Crisis Leadership Now.* New York, McGraw-Hill.

Crowe, A. (2008). The invisible challenge: organizational continuity and public health threats. *Disaster Recovery Journal*, Spring 2008, pp. 26–29.

Friedman, A.F. (2007). *Measurement of readiness by organisational first responders* white paper for the American College program on risk management, October 2007.

Leung, G.M. and Lan, W.Y. (2004). SARS in Hong Kong: from Experience to Action. Hong Kong (SARS), China: Hong Kong Government, 2004.

Silicon Strategies column. (2003). SARS fears to impact Nokia, Motorola, Qualcomm, says report. *EE Times*, 11 May, p. 1.

Zimmerman, J. (2007). Supervisor of Medical Stockpiles, US Centers for Disease Control; interview with the author, September, 2007.

Section 2

# Public health risk communication in practice

Chapter 6

# The role of the media in public health crises: perspectives from the UK and Europe

Hugh Pennington (University of Aberdeen)

## Introduction

What is a public health crisis? Academics who study crisis management have formally defined a crisis as 'a serious threat to the basic structures or the fundamental values and norms of a system which under time pressures and highly uncertain circumstances necessitates making critical decisions' (Rosenthal *et al.*, 2001). Rightly, this is a very broad definition. A simpler way to emphasize the many different forms that a crisis can take and the difficulty in formulating a precise and concise operational definition is to draw an analogy with US Supreme Court Justice Potter Stewart's opinion of what is obscene: 'I shall not today attempt further to define the kinds of material I understand to be embraced . . . but I know it when I see it . . . ' (Jacobellis v. Ohio, 378 US184, 197 (1964)).

Nevertheless, whatever kind of definition is adopted, it is beyond dispute that for public health crises and the events that follow their initiation, the explanatory power of the Thomas theorem is very great: 'if men define situations as real, they are real in their consequences' (Thomas and Thomas, 1928); and it is also universally agreed that the media play an exceptionally important role as one of the forces that drives the theorem. In other words, 'if CNN defines a situation as a crisis, it will indeed be a crisis'. (Rosenthal *et al.*, 2001).

This account presents a series of case studies of the role of the media in public health crises. It is a personal one. As a commentator on microbiological issues (and from time to time a direct participant in crises), my involvement with the UK media has been extensive. Chairing a group that prepared a report in 1997 for the Scottish Office into a large *E. coli* O157 outbreak (Pennington Group, 1997) led to a high public profile. A readiness to respond to media inquiries (helped by residence close to two TV and two radio broadcasting stations), the regular and continuing occurrence of food poisoning outbreaks and other newsworthy events, and the operation of the Matthew effect ('For unto every one that hath shall be given, and he shall have abundance . . . ' or, to put it another way, the continued accrual of greater increments of recognition to those who already have recognition (Merton, 1968)), have further increased this public visibility. Four other factors have been important in assisting interaction with the media: being an academic gave me an almost untrammelled freedom to comment as an individual—one that is denied, for example, to a British civil servant (the UK Civil Service Code says that civil servants may not disclose official information without authority); being a Professor at an ancient Scottish university was an affiliation that endorsed a position as an expert; my career development (15 years in virology followed by 24 years in bacteriology) has allowed me to present myself as a medical microbiologist in the broad rather than as a narrow specialist; and a shortage of 'public' scientists has pushed the media in my direction. The use of the term 'public' to define someone who carries their professional work to non-academic audiences through media work and by publishing in outlets that reach non-specialists was coined by US sociologists two decades ago. It has been vigorously debated by them (Burawoy, 2005). Vaughan's vigorous defence of this kind of work is compelling (Vaughan, 2006).

The case studies that follow illustrate the interactions between the media and those involved in public health crises. The factors that determine the final media product, topic selection, and the treatment and the telling of the story (Hartley, 1982), are illustrated. The first case study, of the British necrotizing fasciitis 'outbreak' in May 1994, provides a proof for the Thomas theorem; the media was causative.

## Necrotizing fasciitis

Necrotizing fasciitis is a rapidly spreading and aggressive infection that leads to massive tissue destruction and gangrene. It was first described in 1924 by an American surgeon working in Beijing (Meleney, 1924). The causative organism in his cases was *Streptococcus pyogenes*, long known to be the cause of scarlet fever, erysipelas, and puerperal sepsis. A perception in the USA that the virulence of this organism was increasing, and the occurrence of a cluster of cases of necrotizing fasciitis and other severe infections caused by *S. pyogenes* in northern Scotland in the 1980s (Upton *et al.*, 1995) were the stimuli for my research group in Aberdeen to obtain research funding in 1992 to develop new fingerprinting methods to test the hypothesis that 'hotter' strains were in circulation in Scotland. My name was on a list held by the British Medical Association of experts willing to talk to the media, with streptococci being named as a particular interest.

Two patients from the Stroud area of Gloucestershire underwent elective surgery in the same operating theatre, one on the 4th February 1994 and one on the 7th. Both developed necrotizing fasciitis (Cartwright *et al.*, 1995). Subsequent cases of necrotizing fasciitis in west Gloucestershire presented on the 18th of February, the 7th and 15th of April, and the 11th of May. One of these patients lived in Stroud and the others lived 1, 15, and 40 km away. Two died. The cluster of cases first received media attention outside the local area at the beginning of May, when the BBC South of England health correspondent broadcast a radio item about them. The story was run by the Press Association on the 11th of May and attracted the attention of a *Daily Sport* journalist. This paper carried a report about it on the 13th of May, replacing its usual front page sex story with the headline 'BUG THAT EATS YOU ALIVE', and, in lower case, 'Killer virus scoffs three'. Two weeks later the story had spread worldwide, with items being carried on Canadian television and Australian radio. Its end was marked by leaders in the *Lancet*, the *British Medical Journal*, *Nature*, and *Science* in early June. The acute microbiology and epidemiology investigations were handled by the Public Health Laboratory Service. Its London HQ handled about 1000 enquiries during the incident and its Gloucester laboratory received 200 requests for information.

The number of media outlets (newspapers, radio programmes, and television stations) telephoning me for microbiological information between the 12th and the 28th of May is shown in Figure 6.1. Enquiries from newspapers happened in three phases. The first enquiry (*The Daily Sport*) was followed by

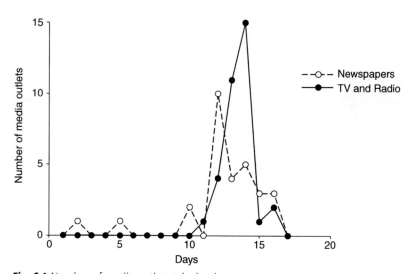

**Fig. 6.1** Number of media outlets telephoning.

another, and then by about a week of silence. The number of calls then rose rapidly, peaking on Monday the 23rd of May. A slow fall during the remainder of the week was marked by the replacement of calls from daily publications by those from Sunday papers.

Television and radio enquiries lagged behind those from the press, peaking on Wednesday the 25th of May. A graph showing the cumulative number of calls is shown in Figure 6.2. It shows an S-shaped, or logistic, curve.

It is clear that the necrotizing fasciitis media story appeared and disappeared with a dynamic not unlike the rise and fall of cases in an epidemic caused by a virus or a bacterium. It even had an incubation period. Rather than an outbreak of infection, it was an outbreak of media interest. It scored highly in the fright factors and media triggers listed in Chapter 1. For fright factors its acquisition seemed involuntary because it attacked victims at random, and its distribution was inequitable—why so many victims at Stroud, which had also had the misfortune between 1981 and 1986 to be the centre of a meningitis epidemic with more than 60 cases and two deaths? It was inescapable because risk factors appeared to be poorly defined, and it was novel because its clustering seemed to defy explanation. It caused irreversible damage through massive tissue loss, and caused death in a dreadful way—'Bug that eats you alive' (*The Daily Sport*). Its victims were identifiable. For the media triggers, it scored highly in the human interest and visual impact factors, with powerful images being conveyed by text, such as 'Thank God I'M FAT' (*Take a Break*), and 'BUG EATS HUMAN FLESH' (*Sunday Mail*).

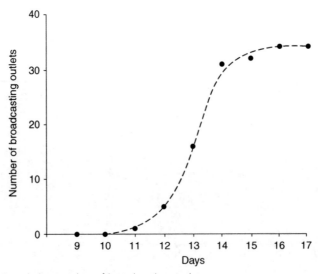

**Fig. 6.2** Cumulative number of broadcasting outlets.

It is probable that the coming together of all these features accounted for its selection by the media, its strength as a story, and, in part, its persistence. This was also aided by the discovery and description of previously unreported cases by journalists (the media were able to find a number of victims or relatives of victims willing to speak about their experiences—photographs of at least seven were published and television programmes about two were made, a significant tally considering the rarity of the disease), by the raising of uncertainties about its incidence, and by the rehearsal of arguments for and against notification. The lack of data about the incidence of the condition made it impossible to make evidence-based comments about whether it was changing, so it was not possible to curb speculation.

The dynamics of media interest in necrotizing fasciitis and the shift of interest from newspapers to broadcasting can be analysed both in terms of the bureaucratic setting which produced it and its mathematical epidemiology. Thus journalists make extensive use of media organizations other than their own in determining what is news. The influence of the early morning BBC *Today* radio programme in setting the news agenda for the rest of the day is well known. TV and radio newsrooms are always littered with newspapers. In a study of crime reporting, Fishman (1981) showed that this mutual dependence between different branches of the media is an important factor in encouraging the spread of a news theme through the community of a news organization, in his case converting a crime *theme* into a crime *wave*. There is a clear similarity between such events and the spread of necrotizing fasciitis as a news theme and its conversion thereby into an 'outbreak'. In terms of its mathematics, it is highly probable that the basic principles governing the spread of a news theme and the spread of an infective agent are the same. The course of the latter is governed by the mass action principle. This indicates that the rate of spread is proportional to the product of the density of susceptibles multiplied by the density of sources of infection. The pattern of spread following the introduction of a small nucleus of infection (the initial story) into a population of uninfected humans (journalists) and vectors (media outlets) would, if plotted, give an S-shaped curve identical in general form to that shown in Figure 6.2.

The end of the media 'outbreak' was quite sudden. It was finally killed on 28 May by a much stronger story, an attack by Prime Minister John Major on beggars. It is likely that the absence of such rival stories during the previous week had made a significant contribution to its longevity.

It is possible to read a message about risk into the Banx cartoon (Figure 6.3) published at the end of the episode—that being attacked by the flesh-eating bug and winning the lottery were equally improbable. It also indicates that by

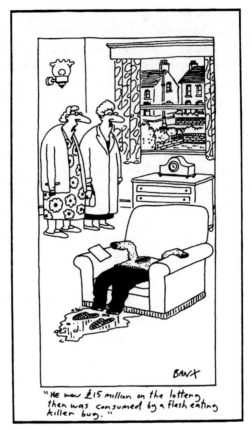

**Figure 6.3** The *Independent on Sunday*, May 1994.

this time some journalists were interpreting it not just as a health story, but as a media event and an episode meriting the application of some black humour.

## *E. coli O157* outbreaks in Scotland and Wales

No humour, black or otherwise, is associated with *E. coli* O157. Although much rarer than the usual causes of bacterial gastroenteritis, *Campylobacter* and *Salmonella*, the infections caused by it are often severe. Complications (which cannot be prevented by any specific treatment once an infection has been established) are more frequent in young children and the elderly—renal failure (which may be permanent) and brain damage are the commonest. Cardiac involvement is not uncommonly a cause of death. The incidence of human infections is higher in the UK than anywhere else in the world.

## The 1996 Central Scotland outbreak.

On the afternoon of Friday 22 November 1996, the Public Health Department of Lanarkshire Health Board became aware of several cases of infection with *E. coli* O157 in residents of Wishaw in the central belt of Scotland. By the evening, histories from confirmed or suspected cases indicated that 14 of the 15 who were ill had consumed food obtained directly or indirectly from J. Barr and Son, Butchers of Wishaw. Although outwardly a small local butcher with a bakery shop adjoining, the business was involved at the time of the outbreak in a substantial wholesale and retail trade involving the production and distribution of raw and cooked meats and bakery products from the Wishaw premises. The epidemic curve of the outbreak (Figure 6.4) shows that the number of suspected or confirmed cases increased dramatically from its onset.

Epidemiological and subsequent microbiological evidence shows that the outbreak was made up of several separate but related incidents. The largest of these were a lunch attended by more than 70 frail elderly people held in Wishaw Parish Church Hall on the 17th of November, a birthday party that took place in the Cascade Public House on the 23rd of November, and retail sales in Lanarkshire and the Forth Valley. The outbreak was declared over on Monday the 20th of January 1997, although further deaths occurred following prolonged illness. The final tally of cases was 501 (the largest ever outbreak of infection with the organism in the UK). Of these, 127 were admitted to hospital, of whom 13 required dialysis. Of those infected, 21 died; the deaths of 17 of them were caused directly by *E. coli* O157.

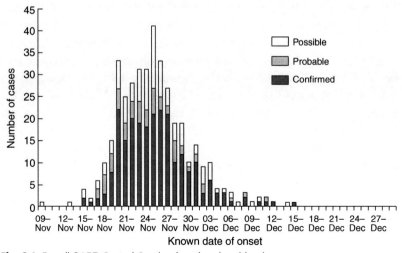

**Fig. 6.4** *E. coli* O157 Central Scotland outbreak epidemic curve.

On 28 November 1996 the Secretary of State for Scotland announced the establishment of an Expert Group with me as chairman. Our remit was 'to examine the circumstances which led to the outbreak in the central belt of Scotland and to advise on the implications for food safety and the general lessons to be learned'. In early 1997 another *E. coli* O157 outbreak occurred in a nursing home in Tayside and in its deliberations the group was asked to take account of this as well as other outbreaks that had occurred in the Borders and in Lothian. The Group convened from the beginning of December 1996 until the end of March 1997. An interim report with recommendations was submitted to the Secretary of State on Hogmanay 1996. He responded to it in the House of Commons on 15 January 1997. Our final report was submitted at the end of March and was published, with the government's response, on 8 April 1997.

In 1992 I had established the Scottish Reference Laboratory for *E. coli* O157 in Aberdeen, and so was known as a source of information about the organism. Before the Wishaw outbreak, the frequency of media enquiries in 1996 ranged from one to six per month. Eighteen of the 31 enquiries were from Scottish organizations. At the beginning of November the BBC current affairs programme *Newsnight* came to my department to film the work of a visiting Public Health Laboratory Service staff member (and *E. coli* O157 expert) as part of an item about the fiftieth anniversary of the Service, and BBC Scotland was planning with us a programme about the transmission of *E. coli* O157 to shepherds at lambing. Filming took place in the department on the 28th of November, the day when the establishment of the Expert Group was announced.

The number of telephone enquiries from the media about *E. coli* O157 during and following the outbreak is shown in Figure 6.5. Calls are plotted day by day, starting on the 25th of November 1996 (day 1) and finishing on the 16th of July 1997 (day 230). On nine occasions, enquiries peaked at 10 or more a day. The first peak, labelled (a), reflected media activity on the day of the announcement of the Expert Group. The next peak (b) coincided with the meeting at the Scottish Office at which the composition of the group was decided, and five peaks (c–f and h) occurred on the day before the meetings of the group. Media pressure was particularly sustained just before and on the day of the meeting at which the report was finalized (peak h). The largest peak of all—36 enquiries on the 6th of March 1997 (peak g)—was linked to the leaking to the press of the first draft of the Swann Report, a review by the Meat Hygiene Service of abattoir hygiene practice conducted in 1995. Highly critical of aspects of abattoir practice, the report underwent significant drafting changes and was eventually put into the public domain in a low key way in

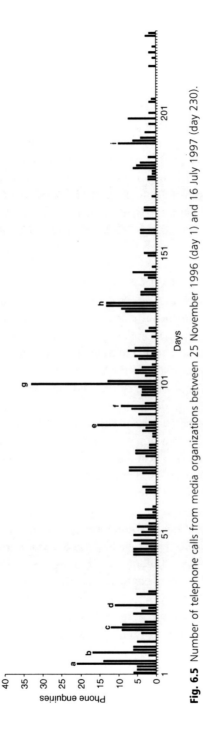

**Fig. 6.5** Number of telephone calls from media organizations between 25 November 1996 (day 1) and 16 July 1997 (day 230).

June 1996. Much of the substantial press coverage of the 6th of March, and that which followed, focused on the actions of the Meat Hygiene Service, government departments, and ministers. My involvement started with a call from the BBC radio *Today* programme at about 7.20 am asking whether I knew about the report in any of its versions. My reply was that 'I hadn't been shown any of them, and that I was not pleased'. It became part of the story. The final peak of interest on the 2nd of June (peak i) coincided with the deaths of two elderly women from *E. coli* O157 infections, one of them a victim of the Central Scotland outbreak. Of the total of 557 inquiries, 159 were from television, 126 from radio, 130 from the four Scottish broadsheets (*Press and Journal* (Aberdeen), *Courier* (Dundee), *Herald* (Glasgow), and *Scotsman* (Edinburgh)), 66 were from London broadsheets, 29 from tabloids, 20 from science journals, 12 from trade journals, 13 from press agencies, and one each from the *Lancaster Guardian* and the *West Highland Free Press*.

Fright factors for E. coli O157include its involuntary acquisition (by consuming seemingly safe but microscopically contaminated ready-to-eat cold meats, for example), its inequitable distribution (four times commoner in Scotland than in England), its ability to cause irreversible damage to kidneys and brain, particularly in small children, and its ability to cause death in a painful way (Jeremy Bray, MP: 'As the families of too many of my constituents have discovered, dying from E. coli is a horrible way to die'; Hansard, 15 January 1997). As factors determining media activity, these are almost certainly sufficient to explain the persistence of a long-term interest. But with the exception of the twentieth death, none of them seemed to play a role in determining the major fluctuations in the number of enquiries that I received after the beginning of the outbreak. These related either to the deliberations and conclusions of the Expert Group or to political events. The first five of the media triggers listed in Chapter 1 map well on to these circumstances; thus the alleged concealment of the Swann Report by the Meat Hygiene Service and the Ministry of Agriculture and the Scottish Secretary provide questions of: (1) blame, (2) cover-ups, (3) human interest, (4) links with high-profile personalities, and (5) evidence of conflict.

The Expert Group met in private. On arrival in Edinburgh from Aberdeen to chair its first meeting I was met at the railway station ticket barrier by two civil servants to shield me from reporters. At this meeting it was agreed that our discussions would be confidential. For my part, this remained the case. But there were leaks to the media. The source was never established. My interpretation of them was that they were manifestations of the battle being fought over the recommendations that the Group was developing; the representatives on the Group of London-based government departments (Agriculture and

Health) were unhappy about the radical form they were taking. The leaks were not helpful to their case. At the end of the day, although by convention not admitted, the arguments were settled by a Cabinet committee in favour of the more radical Scottish position (Pennington, 2000).

## The 2005 South Wales outbreak

The first cases of gastroenteritis presented on Wednesday 14 September 2005. By Friday the 16th it was clear that an outbreak affecting children was in progress in the Merthyr Tydfil and Rhondda Cynon Taf areas, and that micro-biological evidence was pointing to *E. coli* O157 as its cause. Within a week, 150 cases had been identified in the South Wales valleys with 42 schools affected. Following the death of 5-year-old Mason Jones on the 4th of October 2005, a police investigation was launched. By the 14th of November, 168 cases compatible with an *E. coli* O157 infection had been identified. On the 5th of October the National Assembly for Wales established a committee to consider the establishment of a public inquiry under the 2005 Inquiries Act. They recommended that one should be held and that I should chair it, with a remit 'To inquire into the circumstances that led to the outbreak of *E. coli* O157 infection in South Wales in September 2005 and into the handling of the outbreak, and to consider the implications for the future and make recom-mendations accordingly' (Pennington, 2009).

A public inquiry is inquisitorial, not adversarial. It is very different from the internal government inquiry that I chaired in 1996–97. The 2005 Act confers powers to compel the production of documents and the attendance of witnesses to give evidence. Its hearings are held in public and the evidence it gathers is published.

The hearings were held in Cardiff from the 12th of February to the 19th of March 2008. Journalists from the print and electronic media had full access. The proceedings were not televised. Transcripts went on the Inquiry website within hours. The daily newspapers that gave the most detailed coverage of the hearings were the *Western Mail* and the *South Wales Echo*. Both are published in Cardiff by the Trinity Mirror Group. The *Echo* is described as 'tabloid'. It has a circulation of about 50 000. The *Western Mail* is produced in 'compact' format and has a circulation of about 40 000. The hearings were covered mainly by two reporters. They wrote for both papers.

Three individuals had their photographs reproduced many times in both papers alongside the reports of the hearings. In the *Echo*, Mason Jones (the 5-year-old boy who died) was shown on 6 days and his mother, Sharon Mills, on 7. But William Tudor, the butcher who had supplied contaminated meat to the schools in the valleys, had his photograph in the paper on 8 days. He had pleaded guilty to six charges of supplying contaminated meat in July 2007, and in August to an additional charge of supplying contaminated meat. In September he was sentenced to 12 months in prison.

Headlines tell the story.

12 February—*Western Mail.* 'Mum wants answers from *E. coli* inquiry.' 'People need to be reminded of the human cost of *E. coli.*' 'Inquiry team has collected 36,000 pages of evidence.'

13 February—*Western Mail.* 'Councils chose "lowest cost" Tudor's meat despite scores of complaints.'

14 February—*Western Mail*, front page. '*E. coli* butcher's laid bare by inquiry.' (Double page spread inside) 'Tudor "lied to officers" about vac-packer that spread contamination to meat.' (*Echo*, front page) 'SECRETS AND LIES.' '*E. coli* butcher hid factory filth and falsified hygiene records.' (Double page spread inside) 'If it didn't smell too nice just bag it and send it out.'

15 February—*Echo*, front page. 'A TRAVESTY OF JUSTICE—Families' anger as *E. coli* butcher William Tudor is released after just three months of a year-long sentence.' (Inside) 'Mason's life was snatched away—yet Tudor's got his life back.'

16 February—*Western Mail.* 'Council officials admit falling short on checking of *E. coli* butcher's cleanliness standards.' (*Echo*) '*E. coli* butcher: How the system failed.'

19 February—*Western Mail.* 'Inspector defends her view that butchers premises were safe when she visited.'

21 February—*Western Mail.* 'Using vac-pack for dual meat role "like Russian roulette".'

28 February—*Western Mail.* 'School contracts awarded on price despite complaints.'

29 February—*Western Mail.* 'Food Standards Agency blames WAG underfunding for delaying report.'

4 March—*Western Mail.* 'One in five schools had no hot water for children to wash their hands.' *(Echo)* 'Vital hot water supplies shock.'

6 March—*Echo*, front page. 'MASON DENIED HOME VISIT "THREE TIMES".' (Inside) 'Desperately-ill Mason offered Calpol by doc.'

7 March—*Western Mail.* 'Mamma I'm dying.'

11 March—*Echo.* 'Groundhog Day for chair of *E. coli* inquiry. Hygiene failures similar to Scottish case.'

18 March—*Western Mail.* 'Tudor abattoir scored the 'lowest ever' hygiene rating.'

The way these headlines and the photographs accompanying them highlighted the events and issues being revealed at the public hearings followed the patterns found by Petts and her colleagues in their study of risk reporting in the UK (Petts *et al.*, 2001). Risk event causation was personalized to individuals. There was a powerful use of visual images. Lay experiences, initiatives, and voices figured large.

One of the reasons for setting up a public inquiry is to 'give an opportunity to all who reasonably have an interest in making representations to do so. It thus has a cathartic effect for victims, relatives and, via the media, the public in regard to distress, recriminations, speculations and rumours' (Blom-Cooper, 1992). In this inquiry the media did what was hoped—and expected—that it would do towards fulfilling this aim.

The Inquiry used a public relations specialist to advise it on media matters. So did the Outbreak Control Team. The Head of Communications at the National Public Health Service for Wales joined the team on Saturday 17 September 2005, the day after the declaration of the outbreak. It was decided that the Rhondda Cynon Taf local authority would lead on communications in general, and that a public health doctor would give broadcast interviews. In the event, because of illness, the lead for newspaper inquiries passed to the NPHS communications head. He kept a log of media inquiries and interview bids. The number of inquiries peaked at 72 on Monday the 19th of September. It remained in double figures daily until the end of the month, totalling 459. Bids (16) also peaked on the 19th; by the end of the month there had been 102. The number of enquiries rose from 6 on the 3rd of October to 58 on the 4th, when Mason Jones died. The Inquiry report was published on the 19th of March 2009. There were many media bids. My interviews were marshalled and timetabled by the Inquiry media adviser; those for the electronic media (BBC Wales, ITV Wales, ITN, Channel 4) were shorter than those given by Sharon Mills and Lisa Bray (who had given oral evidence to the Inquiry about the illnesses of herself, her daughter, and her son). On the next day, the *Western Mail* front page headline was 'We must never forget', with a picture of Mason Jones. Sharon Mills' face dominated the front page of the *South Wales Echo* with Mason's photograph in the lower corner and the headline 'Failed'.

## Foot and mouth disease in England, 2007

Memories of the draconian measures used to control the 2001 UK foot and mouth disease outbreak (which cost more than £3 billion) were still fresh when the disease was confirmed in cattle in Surrey on Friday 3 August 2007. It soon became clear that virus had escaped from nearby Pirbright, the site of the only laboratories in the UK allowed to handle it (Pennington, 2007a). The outbreak was very small, but its media impact was very great. It was the first item on the BBC 6 O'clock news on four consecutive nights. BBC News 24 (television) contacted me on the evening of the 3rd and interviewed me. I became their expert, and was interviewed by them on the 4th, 5th, 6th, 7th, 8th and 14th of August. They came back on September 12th and 13th when a second cluster of cases occurred. As well as giving interviews, the BBC reporter standing at the gate outside the Pirbright laboratory site (he was not allowed inside) telephoned me on several occasions to run past me what he was about to say on the news to check it for scientific accuracy.

I have never worked on the foot and mouth virus, although I have worked for and with ex-Pirbright virologists and was familiar with veterinary virology issues because my PhD was on Newcastle disease, an infection of birds. I guess that I was the port of call for the media (appearing on BBC News 24 and *Newsnight* on the 3rd of August was followed by interview bids from BBC *Breakfast*, BBC 5 Live, Sky and STV on the 4th) because all the real experts on foot and mouth virus in the UK were inside Pirbright and for obvious reasons were unlikely to appear at its gate to give free-ranging interviews any time soon.

## The European perspective

My personal experience of the media outside the UK is limited. Interviews at their request by Norwegian television on *E. coli* O157 and by Radio Telefis Eireann on foot and mouth disease, waterborne *Cryptosporidium* infections, and on the significance of low levels of dioxins in Irish pork gave no surprises about topic choice by journalists.

A survey in September and October 2005 of 25 642 people in the 25 Member States of the European Union commissioned by the Directorate General Health and Consumer Protection and the European Food Safety Authority (Special Eurobarometer 238, 'Risk Issues') showed that 42% of the population considered that food would damage their health (ranking fourth as a risk after environmental pollution, car accidents, and serious illness), with food poisoning coming first to mind most often (before chemicals and obesity). Top worries included new viruses such as avian influenza and the contamination of food by bacteria. Paradoxically, while 16% permanently changed their eating habits and 37% avoided food temporarily as a consequence of media coverage, only 17% regarded the media as their most trusted source of information, behind consumer groups (32%), doctors (32%), scientists (30%), and public authorities (22%).

## Conclusion

The case studies described above illustrate factors that drive media interest in public health stories. They show how they are told in newspapers and on radio and television. They also demonstrate that microbes attract the media because they have particular properties. They cause horrible diseases, like necrotizing fasciitis. *E. coli* O157 ranks high because it can kill, and because it targets children and the elderly. 'Killer viruses' initiate stories more easily if they have a high previous profile; the confirmation that the week-old corpse of a whooper swan washed up at Cellardyke on the East coast of Scotland had tested positive for H5N1 bird flu in early April 2006 caused a brief—but massive—invasion of the East Neuk of Fife by London-based correspondents. This story illustrates one of the most difficult things for a 'public' microbiologist to get right, a prediction. Is an influenza pandemic imminent? How many will it kill? Unfortunately, the randomness of evolution makes such questions *trans-scientific* (Weinberg, 1972); they can be stated in the language of science but cannot be answered by it. Evolution is at the core of many other public health stories as well. *E. coli* O157 only evolved to be a human pathogen 30 years ago. The 2008 pandemic norovirus strain only emerged in 2006 (Siebenga *et al.*, 2008). *Clostridium difficile* ribotype 027 only started to be an important pathogen in 2002 (Kuijper *et al.*, 2007), going on to be pandemic and dramatically lethal (Pennington, 2007b). So in the year that we celebrate the bicentenary of Darwin's birth and the 150th fiftieth anniversary of the publication of *The Origin of Species*, it is right and appropriate to enter evolution into the list of major causes of current media-worthy events. A safe prediction is that it will be thus for all time coming.

## References

Blom-Cooper, L. (1992). Report into the Committee of Inquiry into Complaints about Ashworth Hospital. (1992). Volume 1. London, HMSO.

Burawoy, M. (2005). For public sociology. *American Sociological Review*, 70: 4–28.

Cartwright, K., Logan, M., McNulty, C.M. *et al.* (1995). A cluster of cases of streptococcal necrotising fasciitis in Gloucester. *Epidemiology and Infection*, 115: 387–97.

Fishman, M. (1981.) Crime waves as ideology. In: S. Cohen and J. Young (ed.) *The manufacture of news: deviance, social problems and the mass media*. London, Constable, pp. 98–117.

Hartley, J. (1982). *Understanding news*. London, Methuen.

Kuijper, E. J., Coignard, B., Brazier, J. *et al.* (2007). Update of *Clostridium difficile*-associated disease due to PCR ribotype 027 in Europe. *Eurosurveillance*, 12: 163–6.

Meleney, F. L. (1924). Hemolytic *Streptococcus* gangrene. *Archives of Surgery*, 9: 317–64.

Merton, R. K. (1968). The Matthew effect in science. *Science*, 159: 56–63.

Pennington,T. H. (2000). Recent experiences in food poisoning: science and policy, science and the media. In: D.F.Smith & J. Phillips (eds). *Food, Science, Policy and Regulation in the Twentieth Century*. London, New York, Routledge, pp. 223–38.

Pennington, T. H. (2007a). Biosecurity101: Pirbright's lessons in laboratory security. *BioSocieties*, 2: 449–53.

Pennington,T. H. (2007b). Wash your hands. *London Review of Books*, 29: November 15, p. 21.

Pennington, T. H. (2009). *The Public Inquiry into the September 2005 Outbreak of E. coli O157 in South Wales*. (HMSO, also http://www.ecoliinquirywales.org).

Pennington Group Report (1997). On the circumstances leading to the 1996 outbreak of infection with *E. coli* O157 in Central Scotland, the implications for food safety and the lessons to be learned. Edinburgh, The Stationery Office.

Petts, J., Horlick-Jones, T. & Murdock, G. (2001). *Social amplification of risk: The media and the public. Contract Research Report 329/2001*. Sudbury, HSE Books.

Rosenthal, U., Boin, R. A. & Comfort, L. K. (2001). *Managing crises. Threats, dilemmas, opportunities*. Springfield, C. C. Thomas.

Siebenga, J., Kroneman, A., Vennema, H., Duizer, E. & Koopmans, M. (2008). Food-borne viruses in Europe network report: the norovirus GII.42006B (for US named Minerva-like, for Japan Kobe 034-like, for UK V6) variant now dominant in early seasonal surveillance. *Eurosurveillance*, 13(2): pii=8009.

Thomas, W. I. & Thomas D. S. (1928). *The child in America. Behavior problems and programs*. New York, A. A. Knopf.

Upton, M., Carter, P. E., Morgan, M., Edwards, G. P. & Pennington, T. H. (1995). Clonal structure of invasive *Streptococcus pyogenes* in Northern Scotland. *Epidemiology and Infection*, 115: 231–41.

Vaughan, D. (2006). NASA revisited: Theory, analogy, and public sociology. *American Journal of Sociology*, 112: 353–93.

Weinberg, A. M. (1972). Science and trans-science. *Minerva*, 10: 209–22.

Chapter 7

# Where do we go from here? The evacuation of city centres and the communication of public health risk from extreme threats

Denis Fischbacher-Smith, Moira Fischbacher-Smith, & David BaMaung (University of Glasgow)

## Introduction

> If only Hitler had known he didn't need a whole air force to paralyse London . . . just a revved-up teenager with a bottle of bleach and a bag of weedkiller—Robert Harris (2008). *The Ghost*. London, Arrow Books, p. 13.

The attacks on Tokyo, Madrid, and London's transport infrastructures illustrated the vulnerability of urban areas to terrorist attack and highlighted the problems associated with communicating risk-related and public health information to those who might be affected by the attack. The above quote illustrates inherent vulnerabilities that exist within urban spaces. Cities are double-edged entities—they are providers of health, shelter, and wellbeing, and yet crucibles within which destruction can be generated. Their interconnected nature and their underpinning critical infrastructures are a source of strength and protection and the means by which public health agencies and 'first responders' can intervene in the event of an attack. Attacking infrastructures allows terrorists to achieve a 'double hit', causing damage and mass casualties and harming the mechanisms that underpin any contingency response. This raises some important issues for public health around the redundancy of support systems for first responders, how risk is communicated before, during, and after any attack, and when to asset harden elements of the public health system and critical infrastructures.

There are many, including public health professionals, who may not consider terrorism to be an issue for public health but rather a political problem. However, several elements of terrorist attacks clearly fall within the remit of public health medicine, including mass casualties requiring treatment, information regarding hazard exposure, maintenance of medical supplies to deal with damaging agents, and the raising of awareness in the event of attack[1]. The use of chemical (Eckstein, 2008; Sauer & Keim, 2001; Stern, 1993) and biological agents (Avery, 2004; Guillemin, 2005; Hamburg, 2002; Pooransingh & Hawker, 2006), and radiological/dirty weapons (Berger *et al.*, 2006; Karam, 2005) has obvious implications for public health. Even more conventional forms of explosive have considerable public health implications, especially when combined with suicide terrorism, and in some countries they are already seen as a significant public health issue (Awofeso, 2006; Perliger & Pedahzur, 2006; Perliger *et al.*, 2005). Whilst debate remains about the nature and scale of the terrorist threat (Avery, 2004; Mueller, 2006; Neil, 2003), there has been increased interest in the relationships between these threats and the public health response (Levy & Sidel, 2003). Interest also exists around risk communication and the potential for public health practitioners to draw on their health promotion experiences in developing policy (Heldring, 2004). This chapter explores these issues, examining the relationship between the nature of the city as the 'space' within which threats occur and the population at risk lives and works, and considering types of terrorist threat and how they are shaped by the city space. We emphasize the structural elements of the city, showing that as a city's structure and pattern of interactions contributes to the threat of disease and the manner in which disease spreads amongst the population at risk, so too the interaction between the city and those who occupy it will shape the terrorist threat and determine how the threat unfolds. The city also shapes the potential for public health interventions around terrorism as it does around disease. We also consider issues in communicating risks around terrorist threats and the implications this has for multi-agency working.

## Terrorism—a problem for public management and public health

The attacks carried out by Al Qaeda on New York and Washington on 11 September 2001 marked a significant shift in the thinking amongst policymakers around the potential for harm that could be generated by terrorist groups (Baxter & Downing, 2001; Burns, 2001; Flynn, 2004; 2007; Lehman & Sicherman, 2002; Walker, 2002). They also highlighted how terrorists could

---

[1] Creating the UK's Health Protection Agency with a remit to consider the response to biological and chemical agents, brings terrorism directly onto the public health agenda (Nicoll & Murray, 2002).

expose the inherent vulnerability and the potential for escalation within many core 'systems' in urban areas (Boin & Smith, 2006; Cameron & Pate, 2001; Flynn, 2004). Such asymmetrical approaches by terrorists are a hallmark of 'new' forms of terrorism and the techniques developed in Iraq and Afghanistan—methods that continue to be refined and disseminated to new generations of recruits. The issue of terrorist threats and their implications for public management is a real and present danger for policy-makers, security agencies, and public health officials. There is little agreement, however, over the nature of that threat and the necessary policy response (Avery, 2004; Crutchley *et al.*, 2007; Emanuel, 2002; Giacomello, 2004; Laffey & Weldes, 2004; May, 2005; Neil, 2003; Quillen, 2001). The attacks of 9/11, 7/7, and, more recently, Mumbai, along with other (foiled) plots, illustrated the potential public health problems that arise from terrorism in large urban centres and the potential for mass casualties. Unsurprisingly, since 2001, the vulnerability of urban areas has received considerable academic and political attention, both in the UK and the USA (Azar & Ruiz, 2003; Boin & Smith, 2006; Coaffee & Wood, 2006; Flynn, 2002). The attacks on Glasgow airport in 2007 and Mumbai in 2008 also illustrated the particular vulnerability of 'port cities' and the creativity of terrorist groups. Collectively, these attacks illustrate the processes through which networks—both terrorist and agency—are central to generating and dealing with risk (Enders & Su, 2007; Jones, 2005; Strom & Eyerman, 2007).

Terrorism has been accepted as one of a range of threats that the state seeks to deal with as part of its civil contingency programme and is therefore a key issue for public management. A common element of many threats is the importance of the city and how its physical, social, and economic characteristics combine to shape the potential damage pathways and to determine the effectiveness of any contingency response. As such, we need to consider the nature of the city as a key element in our understanding of the challenges that face public health strategies around dealing with the impacts of terrorist attacks.

## The city as 'risky space'

> The city is everywhere and in everything. If the urbanized world now is a chain of metropolitan areas connected by places/corridors or communication (airports and airways, stations and railways, parking lots and motorways, teleports and information highways) . . . then what is not the urban? . . . The traditional divide between the city and the countryside has been perforated— (Amin & Thrift, 2002), p. 1.

Cities are complex entities in that they are dynamic sociotechnical systems with a high potential for emergent properties, i.e. conditions that arise out of the interactions between the various elements of the cityscape. For those who live within the confines of cities, their interconnected nature generates the services and functions that are essential to the maintenance of what we have come to expect as 'normal'. Any disruption to these services can create considerable problems for those who 'manage' the various elements of the city and those who rely on those services for their existence. As the above quote suggests, they are also highly connected entities and, as such, are vulnerable to an attack, with the consequences 'migrating' throughout the 'system'.

Cities, and the varied districts within them, are also the frameworks within which elements of the population are 'structured' together. Every city has its own complex set of districts, many of which are home to particular ethnic groups. In certain circumstances, these districts may create an environment in which potential terrorist recruits are identified, radicalized, and even trained. They may also provide highly concentrated areas in which potential target populations congregate. Many cities have a 'quarter' in which particular ethnic groups are to be found, where the sites of their worship are located, and their children are educated. For groups who see any such ethnic group as a potential target, the fact that they occupy such a well defined space makes targeting them all the more straightforward. Conversely, the target group can pay particular attention to how they can defend themselves as they 'own' the space that they need to defend. Cities therefore provide the landscape in which such 'predator–prey' interactions are carried out.

The nature of urban space is also important when exploring issues relating to risk communication and evacuation. There are, however, difficulties associated with raising awareness of the nature and degree of terrorist threats, problems of creating and communicating evacuation plans to often transient populations, and particular difficulties managing in the aftermath of an attack.

Public health responses and risk communication in relation to terrorist attacks need to take account of the motives of terrorist attacks, as this sheds light on the type of approaches that may be taken and the nature of the associated risk. Also important is the 'attractiveness' of cities as a target, owing to the particular ways in which they are configured and their potential as a means of political and ideological gain for terrorists. Thus, before considering risk communication we must first understand the approach of the terrorists and the particular vulnerability around cities.

## Motives, strategies, and targets for terrorist attack

Attempts to explore the targeting preferences of terrorists have highlighted a number of issues. In a study for the US Department of Homeland Security, for example, the RAND Corporation identified four hypotheses that served to explain the motivation of terrorists (Libicki *et al.*, 2007), set within the wider context of Al Qaeda's assumed ultimate goals of creating an 'Islamic caliphate, which would eventually govern the umma' (p. xiii) and removing 'western influences' from this caliphate. Within this framework, Libicki *et al.* suggest that attacks may be primarily intended:

1 To achieve *coercion* potential—forcing the western countries out of the Muslim world by making any 'occupation' of Muslim lands too expensive a process. This coercion strategy could be employed within western countries but need not be spatially bounded: the majority of attacks may be aimed at western interests in Islamic states. Direct attacks on western nations may also have the presumed aim of mobilizing political and social opinion against the continued 'occupation' of Muslim lands.

2 To inflict *damage* on the abilities to continue 'meddling' in the interests of the Muslim world. As with the coercion hypotheses, this would interpret the targeting of economic, social, and military interests as a means of increasing the 'costs' of continued western action at home and abroad.

3 To *rally* support for the terrorists' cause via a process of radicalization. Here, the focus of attacks would be chosen as a means of fuelling that radicalization process and garnering support for the 'cause'.

4 To allow Al Qaeda to draw upon a number of 'affiliated jihadist groups' (p. xiv) in order to maximize its resource base. This is referred to as the *franchise* hypothesis.

The RAND team argue that the four hypotheses may overlap and are less likely to serve in an explanatory manner when considered in isolation. If attacks are 'centrally determined' by the Al Qaeda leadership then they will involve *coercion* and *damage* as the core strategies and that resource constraints on the group might prompt them to consider the use of suicide bombers. Similarly, suicide bombing might be the preferred choice of the 'franchised' terrorist, as illustrated by the attacks on the London Underground. Suicide bombing is an effective way of inflicting a great deal of damage with relatively minimal resource utilization that creates the maximum amount of fear and unease amongst the general public.

If, as has been suggested, there is a greater likelihood of terrorist attacks being made by suicide bombers (Perliger *et al.*, 2005; Perliger and Pedahzur, 2006), then further issues may arise around defending against those events, and responding to the threat (Awofeso, 2006). These issues were brought into sharp focus when the Metropolitan Police mistook the Brazilian, Jean Charles de Menezes, for a suicide terrorist and shot him. The argument often articulated by security personnel is that the only viable response to a suicide bomber is to shoot them before they can trigger their device. Individuals determined to die for their cause are likely to detonate their devices if apprehended—even if they are not at their chosen target. Such a strategy is notoriously difficult to defend against without incurring loss of life.

## Cities as 'attractive' targets

In addition to terrorist motivations, it is necessary to consider how the city itself might exacerbate these problems. Amin & Graham (1999), for example, identify several issues that are important. The first is that institutional, economic, and social relationships underpinning supply and value chains have become 'stretched across space' (Amin & Graham, 1999, p. 8). Cities, and the activities that take place within them, are now connected in ways that were virtually impossible in the past. This provides both the opportunity for terrorists to strike at global interests in several city locations and the means by which knowledge about mounting such an attack can be disseminated. The population of a city may also be a source of potential terrorists, intelligence, and support networks.

The 'place' of attack against corporate interests is no longer constrained to the country of origin of a particular company (Steen *et al.*, 2006) but stretches out across space within the urban mosaic. This provides terrorists with the opportunity to be dynamic in terms of the specific locations they seek to harm, whilst maintaining their strategy of attacking particular interests. It also means that cities are connected through the corporate networks that transcend them. The interests of 'company x' in London, Milan, Paris, and New York may all prove to be potential targets of equal merit, and the damage caused by attacking any of them has the global impact that terrorist groups now seem to crave.

Amin & Graham also argue that the interconnections between places and cities have become intensified through globalization. This intensification allows the rapid transmission of damage between places within a network, and potentially generates further vulnerability elsewhere, especially when elements of the critical national infrastructure are attacked (Boin & Smith, 2006). The attacks on New York on September 11th had a global impact on other cities that were connected to companies operating in the World Trade Centre.

A further issue concerns the permeability of cities:

> Cities juxtapose cultures, people and flows within more or less concentrated material spaces through which they become proximate. Because of this it is not possible—if indeed it ever was—to ascribe to any city a singular purpose or fixed coherence. Dig deep enough and you will find diverse social worlds even in cities which at first sight seem apparently homogeneous—Amin & Graham (1999), p. 9.

This permeability has generated policy problems for governments trying to prevent terrorist cells from planning and mounting attacks. That potential terrorists can operate unnoticed within communities is compounded by the flexibility of electronic forms of communication that allow cells to remain socially proximate yet physically separated. The result is a city environment that is 'interactively complex' and 'tightly coupled' (Perrow, 1984). In other words, the city and the communities that occupy its space are linked together in myriad ways and in such a manner that the flows between those nodal elements can impact in a short space of time.

Also of relevance here are three further distinguishing features of the 'urban'. Firstly, cities are 'sites of proximity and co-presence' (Amin and Graham, 1999), i.e. they have multiple functions and land uses juxtaposed against each other, bringing together several potential targets in a well defined geographical area. This might include several targets whose destruction would fall within the stated aims of Al Qaeda and its affiliates. A shopping area, for example, may be located near to a busy business district and transport hubs. The interactive nature of many targets adds a further layer of complexity to the issues of target hardening and public health responses given the size and density of the population present in the area, the chaos arising from disrupting transport hubs/links, and the likely ensuing population movement through self-evacuation in the event of an attack. Each provides significant difficulties in terms of reaching those in need of emergency help or indeed reaching and diagnosing the nature of any chemical, biological, radiological, and nuclear (CBRN) attack.

Secondly, cities mix together space and time in a variety of ways. The move towards a 24-hour society means that certain parts of the city may have quite different 'populations at risk' at different times of the day and night. The abortive car bomb attacks in London in 2007 were allegedly targeting nightclubs and their patrons. The same 'target' locations during the day would have exposed a different population to the hazard. Similarly, the transport infrastructure that exists within and between cities ensures that terrorists can travel over considerable distances in a short space of time. This means that there are considerable numbers of potential targets located within well defined spaces. Risk communication will need to vary for these locations depending on the time of day or indeed particular point in the year (e.g. when religious festivals or public events may be taking place).

Finally, cities serve as 'meeting places' (Amin & Graham, 1999)(p. 10). Obvious examples include high profile government-organized events, annual general meetings of high profile companies, and sporting events. The forthcoming London Olympics coincide with, amongst others, the Notting Hill Carnival and Wimbledon, thus concentrating the density of meetings in one place and increasing pressure on support and emergency services. In addition, the transience of many populations means terrorists can meet inconspicuously.

Table 7.1 illustrates the impact that these various elements of the city have in terms of a number of terrorist attacks. In the context of risk communication, the issues create some important challenges. Firstly, the notion of 'proximity and co-presence' (Amin & Graham, 1999) brings with it the problem of the interactive nature of hazards. Shopping centres and transport systems are a particular problem in terms of asset hardening. They invariably have multiple occupants, multiple points of access and egress, often draw a diverse and transient population, and may be constructed of materials that compound the impacts of any explosive overpressure. Additionally, they are often co-located symbiotically—attacking one site will impact upon others. It is difficult, however, for the 'owners' of the site to ensure effective communication of what to do in the event of any attack or accident given the transience of the population. It is clearly problematic to brief every member of the public who visits the site in the actions that they should take in an emergency. Even if that were possible, there are issues around the training that these people would be given in order to allow an evacuation to progress smoothly. Moreover, those who use the site may also be physically impaired or not fluent in the local language, therefore making it difficult for shopping centre staff to communicate effectively. Sports venues bring additional problems of 'volume' whilst hospitals face the problems of evacuating people with poor mobility or who are in intensive care, which generates another layer of complexity, as does the potential for hospitals to become targets themselves. Each of these events brings with it specific demands for risk communication.

## With evil intent: evacuations associated with terrorist threats

It was obvious the moment I got outside that another bomb had gone off. At Tottenham Court Road, people were surging up above ground from all four exits of the tube station like storm water from a blocked drain. A loudspeaker said something about 'an incident at Oxford Circus'. . . I carried on up the road, unsure of how I would get home—taxis, like false friends, tending always to vanish at the first sign of trouble.

—Robert Harris (2008). *The Ghost*. London, Arrow Books, p. 12.

In the opening chapters of his novel, Robert Harris highlights the fear and confusion that follows a terrorist attack and the difficulties that can ensue for the authorities in communicating the exact nature and source of any risk. The events of 9/11, the attacks on the train networks in Tokyo, Madrid, and London, the attacks on a local school at Beslan, and the bombings of tourist areas have all illustrated the fear and confusion that invariably accompanies

**Table 7.1** Terrorist attacks and their implications for elements of the city

| Elements of the urban | New York [9/11] | Tokyo (Sarin Gas Attack) | London (7th July) |
|---|---|---|---|
| Proximity and co-presence | ◆ the World Trade Centre co-located many major financial and commercial organisations in a well defined space<br>◆ New York's emergency management centre was located close to WTC I and 2<br>◆ Lower Manhattan contained many potential targets in addition to the WTC. The disruption had wider economic impacts. | ◆ attacks were targeted at various underground trains in the Tokyo Underground<br>◆ the underground system was attacked in a way that impacted on the government district | ◆ attacks made against the London Underground and Bus networks (the latter was a contingent response from one of the terrorists and may not have been the initial target)<br>◆ the manner in which the attacks occurred brought key parts of the city to a standstill. |
| Critical National Infrastructure elements | ◆ the attacks, and the use of aircraft, led to the grounding of all flights and heightened security at airports that impacted upon the US transport network<br>◆ New York's subway network was severely compromised<br>◆ the New York telephone network was disrupted<br>◆ healthcare organisations were on alert but the lack of survivors means that early estimates of task demand were not met | ◆ the attacks were designed to disrupt the Tokyo underground and cause disruption to the business and government districts<br>◆ impact on connecting elements of the transport system<br>◆ hospitals were affected as the casualties were dealt with | ◆ attacks made on the transport system in London. Could be seen as an attempt to attack the political and financial elements of the country by creating fear within the City of London. The aborted follow-up attacks two weeks later would have compounded this fear.<br>◆ the number of injured created considerable task demands for local hospitals |

**Table 7.1** (continued) Terrorist attacks and their implications for elements of the city

| Elements of the urban | New York [9/11] | Tokyo (Sarin Gas Attack) | London (7th July) |
|---|---|---|---|
| Mixing of Space and Time | ◆ timing of the attack was designed to maximise casualties over space<br><br>◆ the attacks unfolded through various stages from the hijacking through to the attacks on the buildings<br><br>◆ recovery and rehabilitation processes were carried out over a long time period<br><br>◆ casualties drawn from both East and West coasts of the USA thereby heightening the 'political' impact | ◆ timing of the attack was designed to maximise casualties<br><br>◆ timing of the attack was designed to cause maximum disruption to the workings of the city | |
| Meeting places and permeable spaces | ◆ initial vulnerability exposed in the security of the airports and subsequently the aircraft itself (security permeable)<br><br>◆ WTC buildings were permeable and served as meeting spaces<br><br>◆ terrorists able to avoid detection prior to the attack | ◆ the Tokyo underground is the busiest in the world with a large transient population<br><br>◆ disruption to the underground impacted on the daily life of the city | ◆ disruption to the underground impacted on the daily life of the city<br><br>◆ terrorists able to avoid detection prior to the attack |

such attacks. These attacks have taken place within cities and have generated considerable public health issues around casualties. Of course, the significant threat in public health terms is the risk of a dirty bomb—the use of CBRN materials with conventional explosives—as this would have both acute and chronic healthcare implications.

Earlier terrorist threats in the UK were marked largely by the tendency of the Provisional IRA (PIRA) to provide warnings of a bomb's presence[2]. This allowed for the evacuation of an area and minimal casualties. Suicide terrorism, in contrast, is marked by the lack of an early warning and the intention to cause mass casualties. As such, it brings a new set of problems around risk communication, city centre evacuation, and the restoration of order within the urban space. The so-called 'new' forms of terrorism (largely suicide-based) generate considerable problems for the emergency services and how risk-based information can be communicated. There are several reasons for this.

Firstly, the current wave of terrorist threats carried out by fundamentalist extremists is based on the strategy of striking without warning. As such, there is little scope for evacuation prior to the 'attack' and any evacuation after the event is likely to be shaped by fear and uncertainty. Suicide terrorism is notoriously difficult to defend against when the intelligence-led approach breaks down. The paradox seems to be that arguably the only effective way of dealing with a suicide bomber is to kill them before they can detonate their weapon. Invariably, this leads to accusations of a 'shoot to kill' policy and goes against the principles of justice that prevail in most western countries. How these issues are communicated is a major challenge to the security services enforcing the policy. Secondly, the current wave of terrorist attacks is concerned with inflicting mass casualties as a core aim. Unlike previous waves of terrorism, the targets chosen are not political, military or commercial targets per se, but are members of society of all creeds and nationalities who happen to be travelling on public transport or occupying 'public' space. These two factors mean that more of our cities are now open to potential attack, and this generates challenges for how we protect the various potential targets and develop effective communications strategies to warn and inform the public of any potential hazards.

---

[2]  There were some obvious exceptions where no warning was given or where the warning was miscommunicated.

## Communicating with the population at risk

Cities provide a complicated setting for risk communication. The population is heterogeneous, made up of different ethnic and social groupings with multiple, often competing, interests and different languages. An effective communications strategy for one group may not prove successful with another. In certain cities, there will be a need to ensure that the messages about risk are communicated in multiple languages and that the message is constant across languages. The transience of large populations—especially in central business and shopping areas—means messages relating to risk will also be required to take account of the potential lack of familiarity within the geography of the area. These difficulties are compounded by the fact that any terrorist attack will create confusion and chaos.

In the midst of the event itself, effective communication will be difficult and many of the messages received by those at risk may be confusing. In this context, the trust that the receivers have in the source of the message will be important. Much of the information that needs to be provided, especially in the case of attacks with complex health effects, may have to be simplified in order to ensure that the various groups within the city can make sense of it but, at the same time, that information needs to provide the basis for effective action in both the short and the medium term. It is therefore important to separate the signal from the noise in the messages. Ideally, a single, trusted source of communication should be provided, although in practical terms this will be problematic. The mechanisms by which we channel the information will also be important. There is currently no all-encompassing communications technology within the UK that allows all members of the public within a city to receive risk information. It is therefore crucial that multi-channel forms of communication are available to ensure that the same message is reinforced by a number of delivery mechanisms such as television, radio, SMS text messaging, email or even via loud hailer messages.

These issues illustrate the complexity associated with communicating risks to the public and that the diverse nature of our cities will ensure that no single strategy is appropriate across them all. Each city will need to develop a tailored approach that recognizes the complexities outlined above. Against this background, it is possible to identify a number of key elements of a potential communications strategy set out within the key stages of a major incident involving terrorism. Some of these issues are shown in Table 7.2 where a health promotion approach (Naidoo & Wills, 2000) illustrates potential avenues for dealing with terrorist threats. It should be noted, however, that this approach can also be used for multiple forms of risk within a civil contingencies perspective rather than simply terrorist threats. The focus here is on two of the main

**Table 7.2** A health promotion approach to dealing with terrorist threats. Adapted from Naidoo & Wills (2000)

| APPROACH | Sub-themes | Worker/Client relationship | Potential strategies to be considered |
|---|---|---|---|
| Medical or Preventative (based upon the use of medical data around the potential for harm) | Primary Prevention | Expert driven between doctors, first responders and professional societies such as health and social workers, teachers to raise awareness of the risks associated with potential terrorist threats<br><br>Role of first responders and civil contingency professionals in identifying potential areas of vulnerability and likely threat scenarios<br><br>Process of 'target hardening' key vulnerable sites | ◆ Based on a risk analytical approach to Identifying potential vulnerable sites and the main failure modes and effects of any attack<br>◆ Assessment of capacities to prevent and respond to such threats - involving acute care but also assessment of 'walk-In' centre capability for dealing with casualties<br>◆ provision of information around the strategies to be taken in the event of any terrorist attack<br>◆ raising awareness within primary care about the likely effects of terrorist attacks, particularly involving CBRN (due to the likelihood of self presentation by potential victims)<br>◆ targeted strategy of informing local businesses, especially in city centres, of tie main issues around terrorist attacks with a view to developing a network around early warning.<br>◆ Identification of key issues around communication in terms of evacuation strategies and advice for victims exposed to CBRN agents |
| | Secondary Prevention | Expert driven by making potential attacks increasingly difficult in business and commercial situations<br><br>Identification of training needs for first responder organisations | ◆ Identification of potential vulnerabilities *within the first responder community* through awareness raising and early intervention around potential scenarios for attacks<br>◆ key skills audits around acute care<br>◆ awareness raising around the early warnings of terrorist behaviours within the communities at risk |

**Table 7.2** (continued) A health promotion approach to dealing with terrorist threats. Adapted from Naidoo & Wills (2000)

| APPROACH | Sub-themes | Worker/Client relationship | Potential strategies to be considered |
|---|---|---|---|
| | Tertiary Prevention (Direct Response) | Expert driven and involving a collaboration with a number of agencies. The main emphasis here will be on first responder organizations and acute care. It could also involve elements of primary care provision. | ◆ Communication strategies for evacuation<br>◆ Health protection advice about response needs for CBRN agents (information packs)<br>◆ Decontamination areas and strategies for dealing with self presenters in acute and primary care (risk of secondary contamination of treatment centres)<br>◆ strategies for dealing with victims of attacks across the range of potential weapon options open to terrorists<br>◆ joint exercising of plans key agencies |
| Educational | Cognitive (Information and Understanding) | Likely to be driven by expert groups but may involve local parental/faith/school-based groups via police and health promotion worker. Success may be dependent on the ability of the programme of change to address the specific needs of the client groups and to do so in a language that is accessible to that group. | ◆ awareness raising programmes within the local business community about incident prevention and response<br>◆ ensuring that the threat is seen in its context and that the response is proportionate (avoiding scaremongering) |
| | Affective (Attitudes and Feelings) | | ◆ prevention of initial process of radicalization by effective programmes within those areas with a high percentage of groups known to have an 'affinity' with the particular terrorist cause.<br>◆ anti-radicalisation campaigns offered in local schools |
| | Behavioural (Skills) | | ◆ communications training for key personnel (both within the first responder community but also within businesses in the areas 'at risk')<br>◆ table-top and other exercises for potential target areas (eg, nightclubs, shopping centres, business parks, educational establishments etc) |

approaches to health promotion as these are seen as the most relevant to the risks associated with terrorist threats. Each has a focus on different aspects of the problem. The medical or preventative approach is largely focused on the provision of effective strategies and associated infrastructures for dealing with the task demands associated with a terrorist attack. It is mainly organization-ally focused and is concerned with pre-attack planning and provision. The educational approach is wider in its scope and seeks to build upon the provi-sion of capabilities around preventing and responding to terrorist attacks by developing effective awareness-raising strategies for responding to events. Many of these strategies will require multi-agency working and will not simply be within the domain of the public health professional.

## Conclusions

Perhaps more than ever before, there is a recognition that cities are vulnerable to attack. When terrorists can manufacture powerful explosives in a bathtub and then deploy them via back-pack bombs with devastating effects, then it is clear that attacks need not be of the so-called 'spectacular' form to be damag-ing. Attacks on several transport infrastructures also illustrate the vulnerability of urban areas to terrorist attack and highlight the problems associated with the communication of risk and public health information to those who might be affected by the attack. The interconnected nature of cities and the critical infrastructures that support them are potential targets for terrorist-related attacks. Thus, by attacking the infrastructure, terrorists achieve the 'double hit' of both causing damage and mass casualties and harming the mechanisms that underpin any contingency response. For public health, this raises some impor-tant issues around how risk is communicated before, during, and after any attack, and the means by which it is possible to asset harden key elements of the public health system.

There are implications for public health and acute care with any terrorist attack, especially in a CBRN attack. Questions remain as to whether there are sufficient police officers, fire, and paramedic staff trained to deal with a CBRN attack and who would be available to manage any such event at any target within the UK. In addition, there would be a requirement for sufficient equip-ment to be made available to the emergency services in terms of dealing with multiple attacks of this nature. The communication aspects of dealing with CBRN attacks also generate a new set of task requirements for public health and first responders. It is argued here that the skills currently available to pub-lic health organizations have an important role to play in dealing not just with the aftermath of any attack but also with the issues of radicalization and 'warning and informing' the public prior to any attack. For this potential to be realized, public health organizations will need to work more closely with other agencies to ensure that these skills are utilized.

## References

Amin, A. & Graham, S. (1999). Cities of connection and disconnection. In: J. Allen, D. Massey & M. Pryke (eds). *Unsettling cities.* London, Routledge, pp. 7–48.

Amin, A. & Thrift, N. (2002). *Cities. Reimagining the urban.* Cambridge, Polity Press.

Avery, G. (2004). Bioterrorism, fear and public health reform: Matching a policy solution to the wrong window. *Public Administration Review*, 64(3): 275–88.

Awofeso, N. (2006). Suicidal terrorism and public health. *Public Money & Management*, 26(5): 287–94.

Azar, C. F. & Ruiz, Y. (2003). 'We are All Public Health': September 11 and its aftermath through the eyes of public health educators at ground zero. *Health Promotion Practice*, 4(4): 362–6.

Baxter, J. & Downing, M. (eds) (2001). *The day that shook the world. Understanding September 11th.* London, BBC Worldwide Ltd.

Berger, M. E., Christensen, D. M., Lowry, P. C., Jones, O. W. & Wiley, A. L. (2006). Medical management of radiation injuries: current approaches. *Occupational Medicine*, 56(3): 162–72.

Boin, A. & Smith, D. (2006). Terrorism and critical infrastructures: implications for public–private crisis management. *Public Money and Management*, 26(5): 295–304.

Burns, J. F. (2001). A day of terror: The Militant; America the vulnerable meets a ruthless enemy. *The New York Times*, September 12th 2001(Accessed online 7th January 2008 at http://query.nytimes.com/gst/fullpage.html?res=9904E0DC1238F931A2575AC0A9679 C8B63&sec=&spon=&pagewanted=all).

Cameron, G. & Pate, J. (2001). Covert biological weapons attacks against agricultural targets: assessing the impact against US agriculture. *Terrorism and Political Violence*, 13: 61–82.

Coaffee, J. & Wood, D. M. (2006). Security is coming home: rethinking scale and constructing resilience in the global urban response to terrorist risk. *International Relations*, 20(4): 503–17.

Crutchley, T. M., Rodgers, J. B., Whiteside, H. P., Vanier, M. & Terndrup, T. E. (2007). Agroterrorism: where are we in the ongoing war on terrorism? *Journal of Food Protection*, 70(3): 791–804.

Eckstein, M. (2008). Enhancing public health preparedness for a terrorist attack involving cyanide. *Journal of Emergency Medicine*, 35(1): 59–65.

Emanuel, G. (2002). Self-defense against terrorism—what does it mean? The Israeli perspective. *Journal of Military Ethics*, 1(2): 91–108.

Enders, W. & Su, X. (2007). Rational terrorists and optimal network structure. *Journal of Conflict Resolution*, 51(1): 33–57.

Flynn, S. (2004). *America the vulnerable. How our government is failing to protect us from terrorism.* New York, Harper Collins Publishers.

Flynn, S. (2007). A manageable risk: assessing the security implications of liquefied natural gas and recommendations for the way forward. *Written Testimony before the House*

*Subcommittee on Coast Guard and Maritime Transportation of the Committee on Transportation and Infrastructure*, May 7, 2007: http://www.cfr.org/publication/13287/manageable_risk.html?breadcrumb=%13282Fbios%13282F13301%13282Fstephen_e_flynn (Accessed online January 2008).

Flynn, S. E. (2002). America the vulnerable. *Foreign Affairs*, 81: 60–74.

Giacomello, G. (2004). Bangs for the buck: a cost–benefit analysis of cyberterrorism. *Studies in Conflict and Terrorism*, 27(5): 387–408.

Guillemin, J. (2005). *Biological weapons. From the invention of state-sponsored programs to contemporary bioterrorism*. New York, Columbia University Press.

Hamburg, M. A. (2002). Bioterrorism: responding to an emerging threat. *Trends in Biotechnology*, 20(7): 296–8.

Heldring, M. (2004). Talking to the public about terrorism: promoting health and resilience. *Families, Systems & Health*, 22(1): 67–71.

Jones, D. (2005). Structures of bio-terrorism preparedness in the UK and the US: Responses to 9/11 and the anthrax attacks. *The British Journal of Politics & International Relations*, 7(3): 340–52.

Karam, P. (2005). Radiological terrorism. *Human and Ecological Risk Assessment*, 11(3): 501–23.

Laffey, M. & Weldes, J. (2004). US foreign policy, public memory, and autism: representing September 11 and May 4. *Cambridge Review of International Affairs*, 17(2): 355–75.

Lehman, J. F. & Sicherman, H. (eds) (2002). *America the vulnerable. Our military problems and how to fix them*. Philadelphia, Foreign Policy Research Institute (Available online at http://www.fpri.org/americavulnerable/BookAmericatheVulnerable.pdf).

Levy, B. S. & Sidel, V. W. (eds) (2003). *Terrorism and public health: A balanced approach to strengthening systems and protecting people*. New York, Oxford University Press.

Libicki, M. C., Chalk, P. & Sisson, M. (2007). *Exploring terrorist targeting preferences*. Santa Monica, RAND Corporation.

May, T. (2005). Funding agendas: has bioterror defense been over-prioritized? *American Journal of Bioethics*, 5(4): 34–44.

Mueller, J. (2006). Is there still a terrorist threat? The myth of the omnipresent enemy. *Foreign Affairs*, 85(5): 2–8.

Naidoo, J. & Wills, J. (2000). *Health promotion. Foundations for practice,* 2nd edn. Edinburgh, Bailliere Tindall/Royal College of Nursing.

Neil, A. (2003). Terrorist use of weapons of mass destruction: how serious is the threat? *Australian Journal of International Affairs*, 57: 99–112.

Nicoll, A. & Murray, V. (2002). Health protection—a strategy and a national agency. *Public Health*, 116(3): 129–37.

Perliger, A. & Pedahzur, A. (2006). Coping with suicide attacks: Lessons from Israel. *Public Money & Management*, 26(5): 281–6.

Perliger, A., Pedahzur, A. & Zalmanovitch, Y. (2005). The defensive dimension of the battle against terrorism—an analysis of management of terror incidents in Jerusalem. *Journal of Contingencies and Crisis Management*, 13(2): 79–91.

Perrow, C. (1984). *Normal Accidents*. New York, Basic Books.

Pooransingh, S. & Hawker, J. (2006). Are we prepared for a deliberate release of a biological agent? *Public Health*, 120(7): 613–17.

Quillen, C. (2001). Terrorism with weapons of mass destruction: the congressional response. *Terrorism and Political Violence*, 13: 47–65.

Sauer, S. W. & Keim, M. E. (2001). Hydroxycobalamin: Improved public health readiness for cyanide disasters. *Annals of Emergency Medicine*, 37(6): 635–641.

Steen, J., Liesch, P. W., Knight, G. A. & Czinkota, M. R. (2006). The contagion of international terrorism and its effects on the firm in an interconnected world. *Public Money & Management*, 26(5): 305–12.

Stern, J. E. (1993). Will terrorists turn to poison? *Orbis*, 37(3): 393–410.

Strom, K. J. & Eyerman, J. (2007). Interagency coordination in response to terrorism: promising practices and barriers identified in four countries. *Criminal Justice Studies*, 20(2): 131–47.

Walker, D. M. (2002). 9/11: the implications for public-sector management. *Public Administration Review*, 62(Special Issue): 94–7.

Chapter 8

# Radiation in London: managing risk communication in the Litvinenko affair

Pat Troop (former Chief Executive, Health Protection Agency) & Anton Dittner (Emerging Health Threats Forum)

## The context

On 23 November 2006, Alexander Litvinenko died from a massive dose of Polonium-210 (Po-210). Many organizations became involved, but the primary responsibility for managing and communicating the public health risk fell to the Health Protection Agency (HPA). The Agency had been established in 2003 to bring together a range of skills and knowledge in infectious diseases, chemical and radiation hazards and emergency response, and included specialist centres and a national network of frontline staff. A prime motive in setting up the Agency was the specialist management of public health emergencies, and the Po-210 incident became its most significant in its short history. At the time of this incident, one of the authors (PT) was the Chief Executive of the Health Protection Agency, taking overall lead for the response and communication.

Mr Litvinenko had been admitted to hospital on November 1st and, following his death, the police found radiation contamination in two locations he had visited that day. These findings triggered a police investigation into an unexplained death, later classified as a murder. For the HPA and its partners, it was a public health problem, for the government a potential diplomatic incident, and for the media, all of these plus a 'spy story'. It attracted the attention of the world media and was a major news story for many weeks. One way of describing the situation was a 'non-explosive dispersed contamination incident', and, as more contaminated premises were found, it affected an increasing number of people, and raised concern amongst the general public.

The HPA had emergency plans in place, but not surprisingly did not have a 'polonium plan' and fell back onto basic principles in its response.

## Radiation and public perception

Ionizing radiation cannot usually be seen, heard or immediately felt. Unlike in science fiction films a source does not helpfully glow green, and someone who has been exposed to harmful radiation will usually be unaware of the fact until some time later. The harmful effects of various types of radiation can range from infertility and cancer, to the painful and lingering death experienced by Alexander Litvinenko, images of which were published in all forms of visual media in Britain and beyond. This is enough to generate a great deal of public fear, a state exacerbated by a generalized lack of knowledge and understanding. The term 'radiation' is a vague one, which simply describes the manner in which energy is emitted. It can refer to electromagnetic energy such as visible light, X-rays, gamma rays, and radio waves, or to particles such as alpha and beta radiation. It is unlikely that the average person on the street has a working knowledge of how a microwave oven works, or how light and other electro-magnetic radiation travels across the vastness of empty space. Millar (1994) describes research in which a representative sample of 16-year-olds was given a written test on their understanding of radiation. The results were disappoint-ing if not unexpected.

This lack of understanding extends to some degree to professionals, some of whom work with radiation. Research has been carried out into whether or not doctors (Shiralkar *et al.*, 2003; APSA, 2007) and nurses (Stanbridge *et al.*, 2007), who administer radiation treatments, have a full appreciation of the doses received by their patients. The conclusion drawn was that there is a mixed level of understanding, and that some professionals 'have no idea as to the amount of radiation received by patients undergoing commonly requested investigations, despite them all having undertaken the radiation protection course' (Shiralkar *et al.*, 2003).

Harmful ionizing radiation can be found in a number of forms, which have different properties. The type emitted by polonium-210 is alpha radiation. An alpha particle is a positively charged helium nucleus, composed of two neutrons and two protons, which is emitted from the radioactive nucleus of a large element such as uranium or, in this case, polonium-210. Alpha particles are highly ionizing, but have a low penetration; they will only travel about 10 cm through air at one atmosphere and can be blocked by a single sheet of paper. Alpha sources are difficult to identify, as they cannot be detected using certain types of Geiger counter. Because of the low penetration of alpha radiation, occasional external contact with a small amount of it is unlikely to be harmful.

To be significantly injurious the source must be absorbed internally, for example, through ingestion or inhalation.

An added confusion is that radiation is measured in different ways depending on the context. The amount of radiation emitted by a source is measured in Becquerels (Bq)[1] or milli-Becquerels (mBq). The 'dose' of radiation is measured in Grays (Gy)[2], whereas when a person has been contaminated the dose they have received is measured in sieverts (Sv)[3] or milli-sieverts (mSv). Dose levels, as relevant to this case, are discussed more fully later in the chapter.

## The beginning

As with most other emergencies, the information at the beginning was sparse, leading to risk assessment and communication in an 'information-free zone'. The HPA knew that Mr Litvinenko had died in hospital from Po-210, and that alpha-emitting radiation sources had been found in a restaurant and a hotel bar. This led to three key objectives:

- Identify and support those potentially at risk
- Prevent further risks to public health
- Reassure the general public.

Although the full implications of the contamination were not known at the beginning, HPA staff were familiar with Po-210, a naturally occurring material, albeit their experience was usually with small doses. As an alpha emitter, they knew that its effect was very localized, that it could not pass through simple barriers, and that at low doses its harm was limited. Therefore, unless someone had been in direct contact with the material, they were very unlikely to come to harm. This formed the basis of their first risk assessment and communication. At this early stage, the HPA acted in a very precautionary way. They did not know if there were others who had suffered high exposure, nor the full public health implications of the contamination found.

Information was given out first through a press conference held on 24 November, and NHS Direct, the UK Health Information helpline, which responded to people with concerns. Advice was also placed on the NHS Direct

---

[1] A Becquerel (Bq) is an SI-derived unit for the measurement of radiation. One Bq is equal to one nuclear decay or other nuclear transformation per second.

[2] A gray (Gy) is the SI-derived unit of absorbed dose, equal to the amount of ionizing radiation absorbed when the energy imparted to matter is 1 J/kg.

[3] A sievert (Sv) is the SI-derived unit of ionizing radiation for measuring an absorbed dose. It is calculated as a product of the absorbed dose measure in grays and a dimensionless factor (Q), stipulated by the International Commission on Radiological Protection, and indicating the biological effectiveness of the radiation.

and HPA websites. The press conference was held less than 24 hours after the death of Mr Litvinenko, but was attended by the world's media. It was agreed that the emphasis would be on public health and was led by the Chief Executive of the HPA, herself a doctor, and the Director of the HPA's specialist centre for Chemical, Radiation, and Environmental Hazards, a specialist in radiation.

The key messages at this early stage and maintained throughout were that Po-210 was only harmful if ingested, inhaled or taken in through broken skin; the risk to the general public was very low; and if more information was needed, people could contact NHS Direct. During the press conference, to illustrate this, the Director held a glass of water and explained that if it contained Po-210 it would not harm him. Over the following period, whilst some of the HPA specialists provided expert briefing, it was agreed that to maintain continuity and build confidence, the key presenter on broadcast media would be the Chief Executive, and there were many media interviews.

Over its first 3 years of existence, the HPA had worked to demonstrate its independence, which it thought vital if the public were to regard it as an objective and authoritative, recognized factor in effective communication. Nevertheless, because of the multiple agendas, the HPA worked with all other relevant organizations, especially the police, to ensure that inappropriate information was not given out. With a criminal investigation being conducted in parallel, there was a potential for conflict between the usual open approach taken in public health emergencies and the need to maintain confidentiality of information that might jeopardize that investigation and any future prosecution. The government and police were clear that the first priority was public health, but the HPA worked with them to ensure that they did not compromise these other objectives whilst still giving sufficient public health information. Because of this, some commentators complained that the HPA was not giving the full picture. One reason may have been that they were the only organization giving out daily information. Not releasing information that would compromise the police case, whilst protecting public health, was a fine balance to maintain and represented a new challenge for many health staff used to a less restrictive approach. In a stressful and fast-moving situation, some tensions inevitably arose, but were generally well managed. These negotiations took considerable resources from all of these agencies to ensure common messages and understanding.

For the general public, the broadcast and written media were the most useful forms of communication. For those potentially at risk, the situation was more difficult. Relevant staff in hospitals where Mr Litvinenko had been treated and in locations where contamination was found were identified through rotas. They were met with in groups or individually and offered a test to assess whether or not they had been in contact with Po-210. Whilst not completely straightforward, this was relatively easy compared with finding those who had been customers in the restaurant and bar. Up to that stage, NHS Direct had been used in its usual way, for maintaining up-to-date information and as a call centre for advice. For the customers, an additional system was set up. Through the media, they were asked to contact NHS Direct, who confirmed their attendance at the relevant time, and passed their names and contact details to the HPA. Clinical staff from the HPA followed up the contacts, and administered a simple questionnaire. If there were any symptoms potentially associated with radiation, the individuals were referred to a clinic: all others were asked to remain on a register. In fact, only 29 people were found to have relevant symptoms, and none to have health problems related to radiation. However, this follow-up process met with considerable difficulty. Many customers did not hear the messages; some were from overseas and had moved on; others had left telephone details but did not answer when called. Many required a number of calls, and it was agreed that if there was no response, a letter would be sent, although this was not regarded as ideal. Not surprisingly, many who did respond needed considerable reassurance that their risk was low, making the process very time-consuming. This approach to contact tracing was new for the HPA and NHS Direct, but useful lessons were identified should the need arise in future situations.

## Explaining the results

Explanation of the results of testing and the level of risk was a further problem. Po-210 is found in the bloodstream of many people, especially smokers, but at 'trace' levels. It is also used in industry, where there are health and safety regulations on the level of exposure of workers to radiation. There was no agreed safe level for the public in this situation, so a new algorithm was devised to assess the risk to individuals. The test required a 24-hour urine collection, from which a measure of radiation output could be calculated, expressed in Becquerels (Bq) or milli-Becquerels (mBq) per day. This data was entered into an established biokinetic model to calculate the intake in Becquerels and hence the dose. The dose is expressed in milli-sieverts (mSv) and is a measure of long-term risk. One milli-sievert adds an additional lifetime cancer risk of 0.0005%, against a current risk of 23%, and therefore 100 mSv around a 0.5% additional lifetime risk.

To establish the risk to an individual, 30 mBq excretion per day was taken as the starting point, being considered above the level due to background radiation, including smoking. If the level was above that, a more detailed calculation was carried out to determine the dose using the biokinetic model. The next cut-off point was a dose of 1 mSv, which was equivalent to the annual dose limit for members of the public for forward planning purposes, and about half the typical UK natural background. The third point was 6 mSv, which is a level of occupational exposure, above which ongoing medical surveillance would be introduced. Those with outputs less than 30 mBq were told the result was 'below reporting levels'. Because of the complicated nature of this message, it was initially decided that those with above 30 mBq per day output but with a dose less than 1 mSv would be reported as 'below 1 mSv,' those with doses between 1 and 6 mSv would be told that the risk was 'slightly raised but of no concern'; and only those with levels above 6 mSv would be given a more detailed picture. However, it soon became clear that many who showed evidence of low exposure (though above 30 mBq output per day) wished to know their actual figure. They were subsequently given this information.

There was no precedent for what was carried out—or the levels chosen, which were calculated using a pragmatic risk assessment. Explanation of the figures was clearly not straightforward. There were often requests for the number testing 'positive' or 'negative', which required explanation that there was a continuum, with relevant 'cut-off points'. To enable better understanding, the HPA held a press technical briefing to explain the approach taken and its rationale. To put the figures in context, the briefing used some comparable doses, e.g. one CT head scan results in a dose of 2 mSv, whilst a pelvic scan is almost 10, and 2 weeks on a space station gives a dose of around 7 mSv. It also pointed out that, whilst the UK annual average background radiation dose is 2 mSv, there is wide variation, with levels of 8 mSv in some parts of SW England. Most people who received their results acknowledged that the risk was negligible, but a few required considerable reassurance, even amongst those whose levels were below 1 mSv.

## The unfolding situation

The situation developed rapidly, with new features occurring daily. The police identified more locations showing contamination, including offices, hotels, aeroplanes, and the Emirates Stadium. For each of these, the HPA tested the public areas to check their safety, carried out a risk assessment based on the levels found, and either carried out remedial work or advised the Local Authority to close the area. This was followed by a risk assessment for people considered to have been at most risk of exposure, who were traced and offered testing. Because of the novel nature of the incident, the HPA had also been required to set safe levels for locations, which they did on a precautionary basis. However, as experience grew, they were able to match the human results against the levels in the locations and modify their risk assessment and hence communication with individuals in those locations.

Information was given in a daily press release, often backed up by media interviews. The press release was in a standard format, giving updates on locations tested, the number of people who had contacted NHS Direct, the number tested, and a summary of the results. The core messages were repeated each time about the low risk to the public. As no other agency was giving out daily information, these updates were a key source for journalists, and there was strong pressure to issue the press releases before the evening news deadlines. New events triggered more media interest, as did statements in Parliament, each with requirements for more explanation of the risks to individuals and the public. At one stage, there was concern about a potential second person being affected. In the event, this was not the case, but this led to another round of speculation and major international interest.

This incident was different from many emergency incidents in a number of ways. It was neither a 'big bang', not a developing infectious disease epidemic. Rather it was a rapidly emerging situation, with new features daily in the first 2–3 weeks, followed by a sustained level of response over many weeks. The 'tail' of the incident continued for many months, well after the media interest had died down.

## New results

After 2 weeks, test results for staff in the hotel bar showed that a number had doses above 6 mSv, albeit still at levels which did not give rise to any significant long-term risk. These people were counselled individually, and any other potential staff sought out. In view of these results, all those who had contacted NHS Direct reporting they had been in the hotel bar were contacted and offered testing, and a further call went out via the media to ask anyone else who had not yet contacted them to do so. In the first week, there had been several hundred calls per day to NHS Direct, but this new call generated little interest, and the press response was much less, although the results were fully reported. Press releases continued daily, but were often not commented on, and after 6 weeks they became weekly.

The final results showed that the HPA had carried out 78 tests on healthcare workers. Ten had been exposed to Po-210, but none had received a dose above 6 mSv and only one in the 1–6 mSv range. Of the 675 non-healthcare workers tested, 86 had above 30 mBq per day output but a dose of less than 1 mSv, 36 had received 1–6 mSv, and 17 above 6 mSv, giving a total of 129 (19%) who had been exposed. The total number of people found to be exposed was thus 139, probably an underestimate because of the difficulty of tracing individuals.

Some critics argued that the level of response from the HPA was unnecessary but, equally, there were many who expressed surprise at the number of people identified as having been exposed and the potential public health risk that had been found.

## The international dimension

From an early stage, it was evident there were international implications. The bar and restaurant were in Mayfair, with many overseas customers, and aeroplanes were included in the investigation. Also, the potential second case was from Italy. There were two key aspects. First, both the international media involvement and the internet meant that the story was widely shared across the world from the beginning. One of the authors received a number of calls and emails from colleagues overseas saying they had seen the press conference and follow-up media. The HPA worked closely with the UK media, and the press briefings, regular updates, and a willingness to answer questions and do interviews meant that the relationship was largely positive. This in turn meant the reporting was accurate and often helpful in communicating difficult ideas, such as the nature of alpha-emitting radiation sources. It was more difficult with media in other countries, and the HPA received examples of sensational reporting—sometimes suggesting that London was contaminated. One country sent senior representatives for written confirmation that this was not the case, as they reported that their citizens were unwilling to come to London for fear of exposure. This episode was before the introduction of the new International Health Regulations[4], although the HPA did inform the World Health Organization (WHO) about the situation. The new arrangements might have made it easier to share the information with public health and radiation specialists in a more systematic way to help with their local media, although the information was fed back through radiation networks and public health contacts.

The second aspect was following up overseas contacts. NHS Direct is operated on a free phone basis, but this cannot be accessed outside the UK. Information was placed on websites, and a dedicated email address and helpline were set up to respond to concerns, both from individuals and agencies. Over time, the international team grew quite considerably to cope with the work, often operating across time zones and different languages, with all the inherent difficulties in expressing risk. On occasions, the HPA was asked to

---

[4] International Health Regulations (2005) require countries to report to WHO disease outbreaks or public health events of international significance. They were adopted by the World Health Assembly in 2005, but had not been fully implemented by 2007.

brief representatives from embassies and consulates. This was organized by the Foreign and Commonwealth Office (FCO), who became another significant partner. The FCO also arranged for the names of potential contacts to be passed to other countries' embassies and on to public health authorities. They also produced packs of information on the approach, testing, and risk assessment methods they had used, so that other countries could adopt these if they wished. It was left to each country, with its own arrangements for public health, to act in a way that was appropriate for them, although the feedback was that the information was helpful. By the time the packs were sent out, the emerging picture was of an extremely small risk (if any) to most people casually involved in the incident. Some countries took the view that it was therefore a low priority. Many others did carry out testing but, despite many requests, the feedback on the results was disappointing.

A smaller dimension of the international work was 'mutual help', with a number of countries offering assistance. A number of other agencies were drawn in to test locations, but this need could be met within the UK. For the urine testing, other laboratories were used, although this meant dummy testing and setting up quality control. Overseas laboratories were included in this setting up of systems, but in the event were not needed.

## Evaluation

As previously mentioned, the HPA set out three objectives at an early stage:

- Identify and support those potentially at risk
- Prevent further risks to public health
- Reassure the general public.

All three required communication in a variety of ways, often putting forward difficult concepts for those with little science knowledge. The calls to NHS Direct over this incident reached a peak of around 900 after 6 days, in response to the media asking people to call if they had been in certain locations at key times. This number is very small compared with NHS Direct's overall workload of over 20 000 calls per day, suggesting that people not directly involved did not see the need to call. There was informal feedback, which was broadly positive. Two more formal surveys were carried out.

The first (Rubin *et al.*, 2007) was led by the Department of Psychology in King's College London's Institute of Psychiatry, but with some input from the HPA. Their objectives were to identify public perceptions of the risk to health after the poisoning of Alexander Litvinenko and to assess the impact of public health communications. They carried out a cross-sectional telephone survey of the general public, and a qualitative study of some of those more directly involved.

The cross-sectional survey was carried out between 8 and 11 December, around 2 weeks after the death of Mr Litvinenko, and just after the second call to those who had been in the hotel bar on 2 November. The survey involved around 1000 adults, chosen to reflect the make-up of London's population. On the primary outcome measure, 11.7% of participants perceived their health to be at risk as a result of the incident. Recognition of the HPA's messages varied from 15% (polonium-210 can be removed from clothes using a washing machine) to 58% (polonium-210 is only dangerous when it enters the body. However, 71% recognized the statement about there being no risk to health if someone had not been in a contaminated area—one of the key points being put across to reassure the public about their safety. Most also thought that the HPA's response had been about right (80%). There were differences between different sections of the population, with non-white ethnicity, an income below £30 000 per annum, living in rented accommodation and travelling into London less than once a week being associated with a higher number perceiving risk. Those who thought the incident related to terrorism or a threat to public health were more likely to believe their health was at risk than those who reported the incident as related to crime or espionage. Similarly, those who thought the incident was aimed at the wider public were more likely to perceive that personal health was at risk than those who believed it was targeted at one person. With radiation being one of the most feared environmental hazards, the authors were surprised that only 11.7% of people expressed concern about their health. They considered that two factors helped to limit the presumption of risk. The first was that the HPA message about the restricted nature of the risk was successful and the second was the perception of the incident being related to espionage or targeted at one person.

The other part of the survey was based on interviews with people who had been contacted by the HPA after reporting that they were in the restaurant or bar, some of whom had not responded to the HPA or had declined testing. Whilst many were reassured by the information they received, there was particular concern amongst some of those tested about the lack of detailed information. Some reported that they found terms such as 'of no concern' too vague to be reassuring. More detailed information had not been given initially owing to concern about its complexity, at a time when the staff would not have been able to spend time explaining the results to large numbers of people. However, the HPA also received this feedback and sent out individual results. In retrospect, writing a short leaflet to go with the results at an early stage would have been better. There was also a desire for up-to-date information and, whilst some people praised the daily updates on the HPA website, some were unaware of these, suggesting that the written communications that were sent out could have brought these to everyone's attention.

Few participants reported that the incident had any major impact on their life and any heightened anxiety was temporary for most. However, following the publication of this paper, a case study was reported about a healthcare worker suffering alopecia areata, who presented 7 months after the incident (Macbeth *et al.*, 2007). She wrongly thought the condition to be due to radiation, even though the level of exposure had been less than 30 mBq per day, and whilst it could have been coincidental, it was attributed by the clinicians to psychological stress. The healthcare workers had been given priority for testing. However, setting the test up had taken a little longer than anticipated, so that results were returned 5–7 days after being sent, rather than the 3 days initially expected. Some people reported that they found the general reassurance unhelpful, and this delay heightened the anxiety of some staff.

The second survey, commissioned by Westminster City Council and supported by the HPA, was based on 500 interviews with London residents who had heard of the radioactive contamination[5]. It was carried out by an independent polling company, the sample weighted to reflect the known profile of London. In all, 72% reported knowing a 'great deal' or 'fair amount' about the incident, with television being the most significant source of information, followed by national newspapers and radio. A smaller number used websites, with less than 1% reporting the use of the HPA or NHS Direct website. Of those who knew about the incident, 72% had heard that the health risk to the general public was low, and 70% agreed with the statement that the health risk to the population is likely to be very low, suggesting that the message had been received. In addition, 69% said they agreed with the statement that if people are concerned, they should contact NHS Direct.

Nearly half of those who had heard about the incident thought that central government was responsible for keeping them informed, and 35% that they were responsible for cleaning up, with smaller numbers identifying other agencies. However, only 27% said they were satisfied with the central government response, compared with 40% dissatisfied. Sir Ian Blair and the Metropolitan Police received 40% satisfaction with 26% dissatisfied, while 25% were satisfied with the HPA and 19% dissatisfied. The important measure of public perception for each organization is the ratio of satisfied to dissatisfied, as opposed to the magnitude of the actual percentages.

Only 20% of those who heard about the incident said they were worried. This was dependent on a number of factors, with women more than men, and black and minority ethnic groups more worried than white groups. Those living outside London and those less informed were also more worried.

---

[5]  Wholey N, Compton J. (2007). Litvinenko Survey, communications evaluation. City of Westminster. Personal communication.

These findings are similar to the other study. Both studies compared their results with surveys after the London bombings, but found less demonstrable anxiety, which may be for the factors cited above.

These findings confirmed that the key messages were received, and that there was general reassurance, with small numbers showing concern. Although this survey was aimed at public health, it was also a criminal investigation, which probably underlines the satisfaction with the police. There was less clarity about the public health aspects and where the messages were coming from. For example, in the question on trust, 9% and 10% reported 'don't know' for government and the police, whereas for the local council, NHS Direct, and the HPA it was 25%, 20%, and 28%, respectively. At this stage, the HPA was 3 years old, and not known to many in the population, which might explain this figure.

## Conclusions

This was a complex, fast-moving situation involving many agencies, with international dimensions and involving radiation contamination. Although government and all agencies put public health concerns as the top priority, the criminal, potentially political, and 'spy' connotations added to the complexity. There were features similar to any emergency, such as lack of early information, the need to update the risk assessment continually, working across agencies, and the need to allay public concern. It demonstrated the value of a team of professional communications staff, and the resource-intensive nature of this type of situation. There have also been other instances where the media have been used to encourage people to contact a helpline, but the use of NHS Direct asking customers to report in was novel. There were other new features. There was no precedent for a radiation incident involving an alpha-emitting substance, and there was a rapidly evolving set of circumstances in which the death of one man changed to a situation including many locations and contact with over 50 countries. In terms of evaluation, it is unusual for a survey to be carried out early during an incident, although this had been done during the London bombings the year before.

For the public, the process of giving out early and regular information, based on repeated simple messages, appeared to be successful, as was the close working with the media, who generally repeated those messages. Similarly, feedback from stakeholders was generally positive. There was less understanding of the origin of the messages and there were mixed reactions over who was trusted. It also demonstrated that the media, especially broadcast media, remain the key source of information, and that the internet, despite its wide use, is not the prime source for most people. Both studies showed similar characteristics of groups reporting more concern than others, which should be pointers for future communication.

The method of identifying potentially contaminated people appeared successful, with the numbers reporting being reasonable for the expected number of customers. Nevertheless, the problem of dispersal of customers, including those overseas, meant that inevitably some were missed. Some who were contacted declined testing, citing the low perceived risk, and there may have been others who did not call for the same reason. Communicating complex messages with these people was difficult, and whilst many were happy with the information they received, the need for detailed personalized information became clear. This is difficult in a high pressure situation and can be resource-intensive when the same staff are responding to the incident. But forward planning on a 'generic' arrangement that could be tailored would be worthwhile, for example, identifying the most likely hazards to be encountered and producing text for each of these. The HPA had learnt this from a major chemical incident, and as a result had drawn up a 'compendium of chemicals' on its website that could be used in this way. It also has graphic presentations on understanding radiation that could be similarly used. Individuals could have been directed to the website, but information sent with letters might have been helpful.

Another lesson identified was the difficulty in communicating the risk internationally. This included the same two aspects as the domestic situation—the need to reach individuals and the need to allay pubic concern. The former was very time-consuming, and hopefully will be simpler following the introduction of the new International Health Regulations and the coordinating role of the WHO. The latter was important, as seen by the concern over visiting London. Tourism is a major industry for the UK, and, by comparison, an estimated £425 million was lost as a result of the 2001 foot and mouth epidemic (Thompson *et al.*, 2002). At the other end of the scale, after the incident, some staff within the HPA reported that they had felt uninformed. Although staff members were drawn in from across the country, and there were daily press releases, not everyone understood the need for the scale of the response. This was partly because of a lack of understanding of the numbers of contaminated premises found and tests carried out, and some had not experienced working in such a high profile situation with all that entails. Others reported that it had raised the profile of the HPA and made it easier to describe their own work. However, it highlighted the need for consistent internal communication to ensure that those not directly involved have better understanding.

In this incident, it was agreed by government and other agencies that the HPA should be the central source of communication on public health.

Many new lessons were identified, but the approach of clear, simple repeated messages appears to have been successful in allaying public anxiety.

## References

APSA Education Committee, ETATS-UNIS. (2007). Peer assessment of paediatric surgeons for potential risks of radiation exposure from computed tomography scans. *Journal of Paediatric Surgery*, 42(7): 1157–64.

Macbeth A. E., Levell, N. *et al.* (2007). Alopecia areata following polonium-210 exposure: a psychological trigger? *BMJ Communications*, 6 December.

Millar, R. (1994). *Public Understanding of Science*, 3(1): 53–70.

Rubin G. J., Page L., Morgan O. *et al.* (2007). Public information needs after the poisoning of Alexander Litvinenko with polonium-210 in London: cross sectional telephone survey and qualitative analysis. *British Medical Journal* doi: 10.1136/bmj.39367.455243.BE.

Shiralkar, S., Rennie, A., Snow, M. *et al.* (2003). Doctors' knowledge of radiation exposure: questionnaire study. *BMJ Communications*, 16 Aug 2003.

Stanbridge, K., Latus, K., Robinson, C. *et al.* (2007). Radiation dose from cardiac investigations: A survey of cardiac nurses' knowledge. *British Journal of Cardiac Nursing*, 2(3): 143–9.

Thompson, D., Muriel, P., Russell, D. *et al.* (2002). Economic costs of the foot and mouth disease outbreak in the UK in 2001. *Review of Science and Technology*, 21: 675–87.

Chapter 9

# Risk communication in the British pertussis and MMR vaccine controversies

Rachel Casiday (University of Wales Lampeter)

## Introduction

Vaccination is heralded as 'the most important public health intervention in history, after safe drinking water. It has saved millions of lives over the years and prevented hundreds of millions of cases of disease' (Centers for Disease Control and Prevention, 2007, p. 9). However, because vaccination involves the introduction of foreign antigens into a healthy body, advocates have always worked against fears about the risk that vaccination might entail. Since the introduction of the first vaccine for smallpox, public debates about vaccination have expressed contested notions of risk and tensions between public health and individual liberty (Streefland, 2001).

This paper examines and compares two vaccination controversies from recent decades—about the safety of whole-cell pertussis vaccine in the 1970s and 1980s and the more recent controversy about the measles, mumps, and rubella (MMR) vaccine from 1997 onwards. Both of these controversies emerged in Britain with the publication of case reports of alleged paediatric neurological damage following immunization. Both were propelled by parental advocacy groups and legal actions on behalf of the affected children. And both resulted in diminished confidence in the vaccine in question and, more generally, in the state-sponsored public health system. This final aspect prompted widespread public health concern in both cases about under-immunization in the population and ways to improve risk communication and public confidence. A critical evaluation of the points of convergence and divergence between these two controversies is necessary to improve our understanding of why controversies about particular vaccines emerge even when the bulk of scientific evidence points to their safety and utility, and will help develop effective risk communication strategies for the vaccine controversies that will surely arise in the future.

## Chronology of the pertussis vaccine controversy

The 1970s saw a global controversy about the safety of the pertussis, or whooping cough, vaccine that has been called 'the most significant setback for the cause of immunization since the smallpox vaccine debates of the previous century' (Baker, 2003, p. 4003). Although the debate originally emerged in Britain, it ultimately spread to Japan, the United States, the Soviet Union, and Australia, leading to sharp declines in pertussis vaccination followed by a series of whooping cough epidemics (Gangarosa et al., 1998).

Whooping cough is a highly infectious bacterial disease characterized by an irritating cough, sometimes resulting in severe complications and death for infants less than 6 months of age. Before a vaccine for the disease was introduced in England and Wales in the 1950s, over 100 000 cases were reported annually (Salisbury and Begg, 1996). In the early 1960s the pertussis vaccine was combined with vaccines for diphtheria and tetanus in the formulation known as DTP (Anonymous, 1961). With the new vaccine, notifications and deaths from whooping cough decreased dramatically. With the exception of some concerns that the pertussis vaccine was not particularly effective at protecting against new strains of the disease-causing bacteria (Anonymous, 1966; 1969), the combined DTP vaccine was widely accepted and attracted little negative attention until 1974, when the controversy about its safety erupted.

The controversy emerged with the publication of an article describing 36 children who had suffered severe neurological complications following DTP immunization (Kulenkampff et al., 1974). Because the pertussis component of the triple vaccine used at the time contained whole bacterial cells and was more reactogenic than the other antigens in the DTP vaccine, this component was assumed to be the culprit in reactions following immunization with DTP (Department of Health and Social Security, 1977, pp. 20–21).

The medical community initially appeared to be sharply divided over this issue. Early newspaper reports contained expert admonitions that the vaccine was 'worthwhile and safe' and that 'lives could be lost' if public fears forced the vaccine to be withdrawn (Anonymous, 1974). The Joint Committee on Vaccination and Immunization (JCVI) met immediately following this newspaper coverage and expressed support for the vaccine (Anonymous, 1975), but the government did not take any further action to restore public confidence in the vaccine. Meanwhile, several prominent physicians, including one of the authors of the article that had raised the initial concern and one member of the JCVI, publicly criticized the JCVI's decision to continue to endorse the vaccine. At the same time, general practitioners and health visitors were following much more liberal interpretations of the contraindications to vaccination than the government, withholding it for reasons such as being 'jittery' or having a family history of allergies (Baker, 2003; Hull, 1981). In February 1978, the British government launched a £150,000 campaign to promote vaccines for polio, diphtheria, tetanus, and pertussis, emphasizing that serious reactions were uncommon but stopping short of urging parents to vaccinate their children (Anonymous, 1978).

A parents' advocacy group, the Association of Parents of Vaccine-Damaged Children, was formed to provide support for parents and to focus public attention on the issue. In addition to ensuring a prominent media profile and campaigning to place pertussis vaccine high on the nation's political agenda, the Association of Parents of Vaccine-Damaged Children also requested that cases of children with neurological damage, allegedly caused by the pertussis vaccine, be investigated. As a result, in 1979 the government passed the Vaccine Damage Payments Act, resulting in a lump sum payment to each of 638 people allegedly harmed by whooping cough vaccination (Healy, 1978; 1980).

In 1977, the government launched a series of investigations into the vaccine's safety (Baker, 2003; Department of Health and Social Security, 1977). Two advisory panels reviewed individual cases, including those submitted by the Association of Parents of Vaccine-Damaged Children. In addition, a very large case–control study, the National Childhood Encephalopathy Study (NCES), examined the possibility of immunization as a risk factor for acute neurological illness. While the advisory panels reviewing individual cases concluded that they could neither prove nor disprove whether the vaccine caused encephalopathy, the NCES authors reported in 1981 that the risk of acute neurological illness from pertussis vaccine was very small, and that the risk of permanent neurological damage was even smaller (Baker, 2003; Department of Health and Social Security, 1981). At this point, the government launched another major education and media campaign to increase vaccination uptake. Most physicians seemed to feel the debate had been resolved by this study, but the controversy continued in the legal battle of the parents who believed their children had been damaged by the vaccine. The final legal case ended in 1988, when the Wellcome Foundation undertook to clear the vaccine's reputation through a detailed critical analysis of the few cases that had led the NCES to the conclusion that pertussis vaccine might cause neurological damage (Griffith, 1989). The key finding revealed in this hearing was 'that permanent brain damage did not occur within 48 hours of DTP vaccination [as previously alleged to explain the putative link between neurological damage and DTP vaccination] in any child in England, Scotland, and Wales from mid-1976 to mid-1979 when 2 million doses of vaccine were used' (Griffith, 1989, p. 199).

## Chronology of the MMR controversy

In 1968, a vaccine for measles was introduced in the UK; prior to that the UK saw 160 000–800 000 cases of measles per year, possibly killing over 100 children annually (Boseley, 2002). The combined measles, mumps, and rubella vaccine (hereafter referred to as MMR) was introduced in 1988 in the UK, though the MMR had already been in use in the United States since 1975.

Following its introduction in the UK, the MMR vaccine received little special attention until August 1997, when newspapers reported an as yet unpublished study conducted by researchers at the Royal Free Hospital in London suggesting a link between the MMR vaccine, autism, and bowel disorder (Anonymous, 1997a). The following month, parents from the group JABS (Justice, Awareness and Basic Support, providing support for parents who believe their children have been damaged by vaccines) publicly requested that the MMR vaccine be withdrawn after gathering details of 1000 cases of alleged adverse reactions (Anonymous, 1997b).

In February 1998 the Royal Free researchers, led by Dr Andrew Wakefield, published the results of their study in *The Lancet* (Wakefield *et al.*, 1998). The paper described a small group of children suffering from developmental regression and gastrointestinal problems, and anecdotally mentioned that the parents of eight of the 12 children had first noted these problems following MMR vaccination (Wakefield *et al.*, 1998). The research team held a press conference in which Andrew Wakefield unexpectedly stated that he felt enough doubt had been cast on the MMR to avoid giving it to his own children, and suggested that administering the three vaccines separately might be safer (Laurance, 1998b). A group of 37 scientific experts was assembled to evaluate the evidence on MMR and concluded that the vaccine was safe (Laurance, 1998a). However, the director of JABS publicly expressed concern that the issue was not given sufficient time for debate.

In December 2000, another widely publicized paper by Wakefield in *Adverse Drug Reactions & Toxicology Review* questioned the adequacy of the pre-release safety testing of MMR (Wakefield, 2001). By this time, 500 parents were planning to sue the Department of Health, claiming the vaccine had damaged their children (Hall, 2001b). By the start of 2001, Department of Health officials launched a £3 million advertising campaign to promote MMR (Hall, 2001a). In December 2001, Wakefield resigned under pressure from the Royal Free Hospital in London (Meikle, 2001).

The controversy continued in the preparation of legal cases, parliamentary debates, further Department of Health promotional materials and scientific publications, and demand for separate measles, mumps, and rubella vaccines rose dramatically. In March 2003, Desumo Information and Health Care was ordered to stop offering single vaccines until the company was registered with the National Care Standards Commission, leaving 5000 families uncertain about how their children's vaccination courses would be completed (Fraser, 2003).

Debate about the acceptability of private clinics offering single vaccines— and of the NHS's refusal to administer separate vaccines to those who wanted them—reached a peak in July 2003, when two clinics offering separate vaccines were shut down for improperly administering them (Hawkes, 2003). Additionally, limited supplies of single mumps vaccines left many children whose parents had refused the MMR unimmunized for mumps (Ebron, 2003). In September, annual immunization uptake figures were released, showing MMR uptake to be at a record low (79%) since the vaccine was introduced (Boseley, 2003). Simon Murch, a co-author of the original *Lancet* paper (Wakefield *et al.*, 1998), warned that measles epidemics were likely to occur in the coming winter if MMR uptake did not increase (Murch, 2003; Derbyshire, 2003).

In October 2003, the parents (by now, more than 1500) who were suing the vaccine manufacturers over alleged damage to their children lost their legal aid funding for the case (Martin, 2003). In February 2004, a High Court judge rejected an application for judicial review of this withdrawal (Taylor, 2004; Hawkes, 2004). MMR litigation costs had so far run to £15 million.

By 2004 there was some optimism among health officials that the contro- versy over MMR was waning. The Health Protection Agency reported the first rise in MMR uptake since April 2002, increasing by 0.9% over the previous quarter to 79.8% of all 2-year-olds (Frith, 2004). That this small increase was cause for special comment and pride demonstrates how deep the concern about MMR uptake had been.

The controversy was re-ignited in February 2004 with new allegations of ethical misconduct and undisclosed conflict of interest levelled against Dr Wakefield (Horton, 2004; Deer, 2004b). Richard Horton, the editor of *The Lancet,* proclaimed that he would not have published the 1998 paper had he known about this conflict of interest (Meikle, 2004a; Wright *et al.*, 2004). Wakefield was ultimately cleared of this charge (Horton, 2004), but his profes- sional reputation was seriously compromised by the allegations.

By March, most of Wakefield's former collaborators retracted their support for the hypothesis linking MMR with autism.

John O'Leary said his findings 'did not support the MMR/autism hypothesis' and that he was 'shocked' to learn of Wakefield's 'misconduct' (Deer, 2004a). Of the 12 co-authors of the original paper, 10 retracted their 'interpretation' of the data that MMR might lead to autism, in a statement published by the *Lancet* (Meikle, 2004b; Rogers and Deer, 2004). However, the MP Ian Gibson (Chairman of the Science and Technology Select Committee) expressed outrage that the paper was not retracted completely (Coates, 2004). Wakefield continued to defend his concern, saying that he had always advised that children be vaccinated, and blamed the government for failing to offer separate vaccinations as an alternative to the MMR.

## 'Bad science'

The apparent similarities between these two vaccine controversies have led to many comparisons, with authors concluding that both illustrate 'bad science' leading to unfounded, irrational fears with serious public health consequences (Goldacre, 2008; Elliman and Bedford, 2001). In both cases, fears were initially based on anecdotal reports of small numbers of children allegedly harmed by the vaccine, which were none the less published in respected medical journals and widely publicized. At the same time that panels of medical experts were being convened to review the statistical evidence, increasing numbers of 'vaccine-damaged' children were featured in the media and lawsuits. Competing statistical and narrative paradigms were invoked, with both sides claiming to be supported by medical experts. A review in the *BMJ* by prominent medical advocates of the MMR demonstrates the frustration of many in the medical community with what they saw as the public's willingness to listen to unfounded, unscientific scare tactics, specifically comparing the MMR scare to the pertussis vaccine scare that preceded it:

> Wakefield and Montgomery's review provides no justification for offering the single antigens. But this is not the media's interpretation. However weak the scientific evidence which triggers vaccine safety scares, they provoke anxiety among parents and health professionals which can lead to a decline in vaccine uptake. The pertussis vaccine scare in the 1970s was based on similarly flawed research and resulted in unnecessary suffering and deaths. We need urgently to identify and use the most effective methods for training and updating health professionals so that they can respond promptly and appropriately to parents' concerns (Elliman and Bedford, 2001, p. 184).

The 'rapid responses' to the online version of this editorial were particularly revealing of the competing paradigms for demonstrating risk. Specifically, those whose firsthand experience led them to believe in a causal link between vaccination and adverse effects wanted those concerns to be taken seriously on their own merits, and were not persuaded by statistical reasoning to the contrary. The first of these responses, for instance, begins:

> My personal experience is with the DTP triple antigen vaccine. The concerns about this vaccine were also decried by many in the medical profession as well as of course those in the pharmaceutical industry. History can repeat itself and it behoves all who see the honest concerns of some parents and professionals as 'idiosyncratic' to have the sackcloth and ashes ready in case they are wrong (Challoner, 2001).

Public health advocates in the midst of the MMR controversy sought to apply lessons from the earlier pertussis experience (NHS Health Promotion England, 2001). A firm, consistent approach was needed, they said, to avoid the confusion and public health disaster brought about by the pertussis vaccine scare. However, as I argue below, this approach fails to take into account the different forms of narrative and reasoning about risk that were at work in many parents' decision-making.

## Impacts of pertussis and MMR vaccine scares

Over the decade and a half of the pertussis vaccine controversy, the public health impact was dramatic. By 1977, pertussis immunization uptake had fallen to just 33% (Swansea Research Unit of the Royal College of General Practitioners, 1981). At least four significant outbreaks of whooping cough occurred during the course of the vaccine scare. The first of these, in 1979, had 102 500 reported cases throughout the UK and an estimated 36 deaths. By comparison, the impact of the MMR controversy on immunization rates was much more modest, with an uptake rate of 82% at the height of the controversy in 2002 (Swansea Research Unit of the Royal College of General Practitioners, 1981; Department of Health, 2004). Although there were some isolated outbreaks of measles and mumps, no epidemics of measles, mumps or rubella occurred on the scale of the 1970s pertussis outbreaks.

It might be argued that the consistent response from the Department of Health to the MMR controversy was responsible for lessening the impact of this controversy on immunization uptake, relative to the pertussis vaccine scare. However, there were other important differences that have been largely overlooked in comparisons of the two controversies. There was a crucial difference in the purported culprit for the damage: in the first controversy, one component (pertussis) of the combined DTP vaccine was held to be responsible, while in the second it was the combination per se of measles, mumps, and rubella vaccines that was thought to cause problems. Thus, in the MMR controversy an alternative form of immunization, through a series of separate, single antigen injections, was proposed. The Department of Health's firm stance on MMR was in part based on the argument that separating the components of the DTP had resulted in unacceptably low uptake of pertussis vaccine. But whereas parents in the 1970s had come to fear the pertussis component of the DTP vaccine in particular, many parents in the latter controversy wanted their children to be vaccinated against all three diseases but feared the combined MMR formulation. By this reasoning, it makes sense that when diphtheria, pertussis, and tetanus vaccines were offered separately, uptake of the pertussis component would remain very low; however, the same logic does not necessarily apply in the case of MMR, when the value and safety of each component was generally recognized but objections to combining the three into a single dose had been raised. The policy of allowing only the combined MMR vaccine, rather than separated single antigen vaccines for the three diseases, came to be viewed by many as undermining children's and parents' right to choice for safe vaccinations in favour of other financial and political interests, and may have contributed to a difference in impacts of the controversies noted by Michael Fitzpatrick (2004, p. 27): whereas the pertussis scare resulted in a much greater reduction in vaccine uptake, the MMR scare seems to have had a greater political impact (see below).

An additional difference between the two controversies concerns which groups of children were being vaccinated and which groups were meant to benefit from immunity. At the time of the pertussis vaccine scare, DTP was administered to children over 6 months of age, which was after the age at which whooping cough was considered to be a particularly dangerous disease. Parents were being asked to vaccinate their children to prevent the spread of the disease in the population and thus to protect children who were then deemed too young to be vaccinated themselves—a worthy objective, but not one that was necessarily compelling for parents who were concerned that the vaccine itself might cause irreversible harm to their own children, who were not the primary intended beneficiaries. As Rogers and Pilgrim (1995) have noted, the success of mass childhood immunization campaigns means that the relative risk of vaccine-preventable diseases diminishes while the potential risks of vaccines increase in importance, presenting a conundrum for public health promoters. In the MMR controversy, measles (and, to a lesser extent, mumps) infection was a lively concern for parents of children at the age of MMR immunization (12–15 months). However, many parents understood the purpose of childhood rubella vaccination to be more about promoting herd immunity to protect unborn children from congenital rubella exposure than with an imminent threat to their own children, and parents varied as to whether they considered this to be sufficient grounds for subjecting their children to the vaccine (Casiday, 2007).

One of the most significant consequences of the MMR controversy in the UK is a loss of trust in the government's role in health service provision and protection from risk. In this light, the MMR controversy follows in the path of such crises in public trust as the bovine spongiform encephalopathy (BSE) epidemic, in which government scientific advisors lost credibility by reversing their assurances to the public that BSE posed no health threat to humans (Bellaby, 2003; Caplan, 2000; Murphy-Lawless, 2003; Rowell, 2003). The breakdown in trust occurring as a result of controversies like those surrounding the safety of MMR and human risks from BSE (discussed in Chapter 11) may spill over to other aspects of healthcare provision, fundamentally damaging the trust that is necessary for the implementation of effective public health measures and the provision of medical care. Recent data suggest that while trust in government and—to a lesser extent—in the medical profession may have suffered during the MMR debate, trust in individual practitioners remained good as long as parental and professional responsibilities for promoting children's health were mutually recognized and respected (Casiday et al., 2006; Smith et al., 2007).

## Risk communication and trust

The worrying reports that sparked both of these vaccine controversies and the public health responses to them clearly framed vaccination as a 'risk' issue. To handle risk, government and medical authorities create policies and distribute 'expert' knowledge to the public. However, in the case of both the pertussis and MMR vaccine controversies, this top-down communication approach was at odds with many parents' experiences and concerns.

Mary Douglas's cultural theory of risk (Douglas, 1985; 1992; Douglas and Wildavsky, 1982) posited that societies have deep, possibly irreconcilable, disagreements about risk because members of different social groups have competing notions about what sort of outcomes would be undesirable. Risk is invoked to hold individuals, corporations, and governments accountable for harm when they do not comply with accepted ways of behaving. This line of analysis also supports the claim made by other, psychometric, risk researchers (Fischhoff et al., 1993; Freudenberg, 1988; Slovic, 2000; Kasperson et al., 1998; Pidgeon, 1999) that technical risk experts and lay members of the public may well be focused on different considerations when making their evaluations and comparisons of risks. Understanding these differences is key to formulating strategies of risk communication that take into account both 'expert' knowledge and the needs and priorities of 'lay' audiences. As found by Poltorak and colleagues, 'MMR talk' did not take place in isolation, but rather was situated among many other social issues, including personal and family histories, feelings of control, personal assessments of children's health and vulnerabilities, engagement with the health services and social networks and conversations (Poltorak *et al.*, 2005).

Douglas (1992, pp. 46–47) has suggested a set of four topics of inquiry to understand risk in a particular cultural context: the bearing and extent of a particular risk on individual perceivers' purposes; the role of the community in individuals' purposes relating to risk perception; individual versus collective good; and community support for authority, commitment, boundaries, and structure. The importance of Douglas's cultural factors for risk perception is amply demonstrated for the MMR vaccine controversy by several recent studies on parental perceptions and decision-making (Brownlie and Howson, 2005; Casiday, 2006; 2007; Hobson-West, 2007; Poltorak *et al.*, 2005). In the vaccine debates presented here, parents varied in the extent to which they perceived risks of vaccinating (e.g. brain damage or autism) and of not vaccinating (principally, developing communicable and life-threatening diseases), though all overwhelmingly shared the the chief purpose of protecting their own children from harm. However, other purposes also played an important part in shaping what factors parents thought would harm their children. Parental resistance to pharmaceutical corporations' monetary interests or to government control over medical choice disposed some to give a credence to the suggested link with autism, while for others, the communitarian argument that protecting all children from disease depends on immunizing as many children as possible was more salient (Casiday, 2007; 2008). Just as parents differed in their purposes related to risk perception and their emphases on individual and communal welfare, so too did they vary in their support for authority and structured social boundaries. First and foremost, they demanded support for parents to act in the interest of their children's health. For some, the unique relationship between parents and children meant that other social authorities should have little scope for intervention. According to this view, parents must be believed when they report changes in their children's behaviour, and other parents must be free to choose whether, when, and how (i.e. by means of MMR or separate vaccines) to immunize their children, because they understand their own children's needs and vulnerabilities best. At the other end of the spectrum were parents who saw their role as part of a social order with space for many others to contribute to their children's upbringing and health. Such parents welcomed the involvement of a central authority to fund and interpret medical research, administer a complex national health service, and support families coping with difficult conditions like autism or complications arising from measles.

For many parents, medical decisions on behalf of children, such as immunization, symbolize what it means to be a good parent (cf. Alderson, 1990; Casiday, 2007; 2008). Vaccine decision-making is an important way of exercising parental responsibility. It is important for parents to feel that their responsibilities, and their good intentions to fulfil these responsibilities, are recognized by other parents, by health professionals, and by government officials. Such recognition is vital to foster trust between parents and the professionals offering advice or delivering policy about vaccination, and may ultimately be the most important lesson for improving risk communication about this issue.

The risks invoked in both vaccines reviewed here were at once intensely personal and intensely political. Parents' chief concern was to protect their own children from harm, but uncertainty about the nature and likelihood of different harms meant that parents had to turn to other sources for information and interpretations. Therefore, trust—in information sources, in government, and in medical authority—was a key component of parental decisions. The fundamental role of parents in protecting their children from risk made trust especially important. This trust was determined by and contributed to the wider social and political concerns of the parents. Events resulting in the erosion of trust between parents and healthcare professionals have detrimental effects on the effectiveness of medical intervention (Safran *et al.*, 1998), invite micromanagement of healthcare (Mechanic, 1998), and 'could lead to disharmony and discord' (Calman, 2002, p. 168) that undermine public participation in the democratic political process.

In modern societies, trust is necessary to reduce complexity to manageable proportions, allowing us to abdicate responsibility for day-to-day operations to expert systems (Giddens, 1990; 1994; Luhmann, 1979). In matters of public health, decisions must be made at the level of public policy, because they affect the population collectively. Furthermore, they typically involve technical evaluations that are beyond the everyday knowledge of most individuals who will be affected by the policy-makers' decisions. Members of the public could certainly learn the relevant concepts to take part in this decision-making, but it is not feasible for every person to learn all the details of all the situations necessitating public policy decisions in our society. Trust is then crucial, both to legitimize the decisions taken by representative bodies and to avoid the sense of paralysis arising from lack of trust in institutions (Giddens, 1990, p. 100).

In the pertussis and MMR vaccine controversies, trust appears to have broken down in many respects. Many parents felt that they could not accept professional and government interpretations of the evidence on the basis of trust, and indeed saw contradictory messages emanating from different professionals.

Perhaps even more importantly, parents often felt that trust was not reciprocated when policy-makers and health practitioners did not communicate respect for parents' good intentions to protect their children's health and rationale for challenging official reassurances about the vaccine's safety (Casiday, 2006; 2007).

Earle and Cvetkovich (1995) have argued the need for a 'cosmopolitan social trust,' relying on flexibility, communication across social boundaries, and imagination to find common values *across* different social groups and to develop solutions to problems that were previously beset by inter-group divisions. In the case of public health disputes, cosmopolitan social trust could provide a platform for agreed norms of dialogue and decision-making, as advocated by Beck (1994, pp. 29–30). This scenario would not eliminate dissent, but dissent would be more tolerable if all parties recognized the fairness of the process by which decisions were made. It would also provide a mechanism for incorporating diverse concerns into decision-making and communication strategies. For example, parents may be more comfortable giving their children a controversial vaccine if they understand that the claims of parents alleging damage to their children have been taken seriously and investigated clinically, rather than relying on broad epidemiological studies alone to demonstrate vaccine safety.

This form of robust social trust is, naturally, very difficult to bring about and maintain. Earle and Cvetkovich (1995) suggested that a key tool for fostering this form of trust is narrative. Recognizing the power of parents' narrative anecdotal accounts will go a long way toward making them feel listened to and empowered by the medical establishment, and in turn more likely to trust the considered judgements of experts who take their concerns into account alongside the accumulated evidence from epidemiology and clinical studies. Indeed, Hobson-West (2003) has argued that the focus on 'risk' and the attendant emphasis on statistical evidence are inconsistent with parents' basic conceptions of health and disease; she proposed that a more appropriate set of concepts for presenting public health messages about vaccination may be uncertainty and necessity. Powerful narrative accounts about the importance of parental responsibility, recognizing the difficulty of the decisions but also the importance of vaccination to protect children, could be developed by focusing on these categories. Some good examples of this sort of narrative did emerge from the MMR controversy, including Michael Fitzpatrick's moving account of how he navigated his own roles as GP and parent of an autistic child in making the decision to give his son the MMR vaccine (Fitzpatrick, 2004 p. vii–viii), and personalized newspaper stories of children affected by whooping cough or measles subsequent to diminished vaccine uptake as a result of these controversies.

## Conclusion

This paper has demonstrated points of similarity between the pertussis and MMR vaccine controversies, including their basis in medical papers reporting small numbers of children believed to have suffered damage following immunization, the roles of parent advocacy groups in highlighting the concern and making, and diminished confidence in the vaccine in question and the public health system. However, the impact on immunization uptake was far less for the MMR than for the pertussis controversy, while the MMR controversy arguably had a greater political impact (cf. Fitzpatrick, 2004). A variety of factors may account for these differences, including the perceived benefits of the vaccines (and particularly their intended beneficiaries, as pertussis vaccine was given at the time to infants older than those most at risk of the disease), and official public health responses. Department of Health doctors cited the experience of the pertussis vaccine scare as justification for the current policy of not providing separate vaccines for measles, mumps, and rubella (NHS Health Promotion England, 2001), but this chapter has presented reasons why that logic may have been unpersuasive to many parents and may indeed have resulted in diminished trust and confidence in the vaccine and its proponents.

These incidents are not the first time that vaccination has provoked public controversy (Greenough, 1995; Leask and McIntyre, 2003; Nichter, 1995; Streefland, 2001; Streefland et al., 1999), and there will certainly be more vaccine debates in the future. We need to have public health strategies in place that will protect children both from diseases and harmful vaccine side effects, rebuild trust, and thus cope successfully with similar controversies in the future. To this end, it is important to find ways to involve the public more fully in framing the research agenda about health risks. Richard Horton, in his book on the MMR controversy (Horton, 2004, pp. 154–7), praised several innovations around the UK that aim to make science more publicly accessible. These include the Science Media Centre, an organization for promoting scientific voices to the news media; Café Scientifique, a forum for scientists to hold informal talks with members of the public; and the very successful Cheltenham Festival of Science. Another platform, not mentioned by Horton, is the Science Museum in London. From October 2002, the Science Museum hosted an exhibit on the MMR controversy (Science Museum, 2002), including a series of drop-in events for members of the public to meet experts, an evening discussion and debate about controversial vaccines, and a website on which people could post questions and opinions about the MMR vaccine (http://www.sciencemuseum.org.uk/antenna/mmr). Clearly, these endeavours represent a positive step toward developing the interface between science and society. But for the most part, the focus of all of these initiatives is on presenting science *to* the public. What we still lack, and urgently need, are similar platforms for presenting public concerns to scientific funding bodies and policy-makers.

In addition, sound relationships based on trust between patients and healthcare practitioners should be fostered as one of the chief strengths of the National Health Service. There is some evidence from cross-country comparisons that vaccine policies involving compulsion foster distrust and are less effective, in the long run, than those involving encouragement and education (Greco, 1997; Greenough, 1995). In addition, 'top-down' vaccine promotion can be detrimental to parental confidence if it comes from a little-trusted source. For the most part, though, parents did express satisfaction and trust in individual healthcare practitioners, with whom they had developed interpersonal relationships (Casiday, 2007; Casiday *et al.*, 2006). These relationships should be fostered and should be the primary basis for further communication about health risks. Putting trust and multidirectional communication at the heart of public health risk communication strategies may be fostered through the innovative use of narrative to complement the epidemiological, statistical evidence that has traditionally informed public health policy and communication.

## References

Alderson, P. (1990). *Choosing for Children: Parents' Consent to Surgery*. Oxford, Oxford University Press.

Anonymous (1961). Fewer injections for children. London, *The Times*.

Anonymous (1966). Protecting your child. London, *The Times*.

Anonymous (1969). Poor cough protection. London, *The Times*.

Anonymous (1974). Peril in 'undue anxiety' over whooping cough vaccine. London, *Times*.

Anonymous (1975). Science report whooping cough: Verdict on vaccine. London, *The Times*.

Anonymous (1978). New vaccination campaign will take softer line. London, *The Times*.

Anonymous (1997a). Health: The truth about the MMR jab; Childhood illnesses may be on the wane, but are vaccines damaging our children's immune systems? London, *The Independent*.

Anonymous (1997b). Parents seek jabs bar. London, *The Independent on Sunday*.

Baker, J. P. (2003). The pertussis vaccine controversy in Great Britain, 1974–1986. *Vaccine*, 21: 4003–10.

Beck, U. (1994). The reinvention of politics: towards a theory of reflexive modernization. In: Beck, U., Giddens, A. & Lash, S. (eds). *Reflexive Modernization: Politics, Tradition and Aesthetics in the Modern Social Order*. Cambridge, Polity Press.

Bellaby, P. (2003). Communication and miscommunication about risk: understanding UK parents' attitudes to combined MMR vaccination. *BMJ*, 327: 725–8.

Boseley, S. (2002). A shot in the arm: There are likely to be outbreaks of measles because the MMR scare means fewer children are being vaccinated. But does that really matter? London, *The Guardian*.

Boseley, S. (2003). MMR jab rates hit record low. London, *The Guardian*.

Brownlie, J. & Howson, A. (2005). 'Leaps of faith' and MMR: An empirical study of trust. *Sociology–the Journal of the British Sociological Association*, 39: 221–39.

Calman, K. C. (2002). Communication of risk: choice, consent, and trust. *Lancet*, 360: 166–8.

Caplan, P. (2000). Eating british beef with confidence: a consideration of consumers' responses to BSE in Britain. In: Caplan, P. (ed.). *Risk Revisited*. London, Pluto Press.

Casiday, R. (2006). Uncertainty, decision-making and trust: lessons from the MMR controversy. *Community Practitioner*, 79: 354–7.

Casiday, R. (2007). Children's health and the social theory of risk: insights from the British MMR controversy. *Social Science & Medicine*, 65: 1059–70.

Casiday, R. (2008). Making decisions about vaccines: interactions between parents and 'experts'. In: Nathanson, J. & Tulley, L. (eds). *Mother Knows Best: Talking Back to the Babycare Experts*. Toronto, Demeter Press.

Casiday, R., Cresswell, T., Panter-Brick, C. & Wilson, D. (2006). A survey of UK parental attitudes to the MMR vaccine and trust in medical authority. *Vaccine*, 24: 177–84.

Centers for Disease Control and Prevention (2007). *Parents' guide to childhood immunizations*. Atlanta, United States Government Printing Office.

Challoner, A. (2001). Peculiar to persons: rapid response to Elliman and Bedford, 2001, 'MMR vaccine: the continuing saga'. *BMJ*, 322: 183–4.

Coates, S. (2004). MPs call for full retraction of study linking MMR to autism. London, *The Times*.

Deer, B. (2004a). MMR doctor's Irish ally rejects link to autism. London, *Sunday Times*.

Deer, B. (2004b). MMR: The truth behind the crisis. London, *Sunday Times*.

Department of Health. (2004). *Statistical Bulletin: NHS Immunisation Statistics 2003–04*. London, Department of Health.

Department of Health and Social Security. (1977). *Whooping Cough Vaccination: Review of the Evidence on Whooping Cough Vaccination by the Joint Committee on Vaccination and Immunization*. London, HMSO.

Department of Health and Social Security. (1981). *Whooping Cough: Reports from the Committee on Safety of Medicines and the Joint Committee on Vaccination and Immunisation*. London, HMSO.

Derbyshire, D. (2003). MMR scare scientist warns of impending measles epidemic. London, *Daily Telegraph*.

Douglas, M. (1985). *Risk Acceptability According to the Social Sciences*. London, Routledge & Kegan Paul.

Douglas, M. (1992). *Risk and Blame: Essays in Cultural Theory*. London, Routledge.

Douglas, M. & Wildavsky, A. (1982). *Risk and Culture: An Essay on the Selection of Technical and Environmental Dangers*. Berkeley, CA, University of California Press.

Earle, T. C. & Cvetkovitch, G. T. (1995). *Social Trust: Toward a Cosmopolitan Society*. Westport, Praeger.

Ebron, S. (2003). No mumps vaccine left. London, *The Times.*

Elliman, D. & Bedford, H. (2001). MMR vaccine: The continuing saga. *British Medical Journal,* 322: 183–4.

Fischhoff, B., Bostrom, A. & Quadrel, M. J. (1993). Risk perception and communication. *Annual Review of Public Health,* 14: 183–203.

Fitzpatrick, M. (2004). *MMR and autism: What parents need to know.* London, Routledge.

Fraser, L. (2003). Red tape shuts down parents' single jabs clinic; Children left without immunisation as officials refuse families the right to opt out of MMR vaccine. London, *Sunday Telegraph.*

Freudenberg, W. R. (1988). Perceived risk, real risk: Social science and the art of probabilistic risk assessment. *Science,* 242: 44–9.

Frith, M. (2004). MMR jab uptake rises for the first time in a year. London, *The Independent.*

Gangarosa, E., Galazka, A., Wolfe, C. *et al.* (1998). Impact of anti-vaccine movements on pertussis control: the untold story. *The Lancet,* 351: 356–61.

Giddens, A. (1990). *The Consequences of Modernity.* Cambridge, Polity Press.

Giddens, A. (1994). Risk, trust, reflexivity. In: Beck, U., Giddens, A. & Lash, S. (eds). *Reflexive Modernization: Politics, Tradition and Aesthetics in the Modern Social Order.* Cambridge, Polity Press.

Goldacre, B. (2008). The media's MMR hoax. London, *The Guardian.*

Greco, D. (1997). Vaccination: Legal obligation vs. education. *Biologicals,* 25: 319–21.

Greenough, P. (1995). Intimidation, coercion and resistance in the final stages of the South Asian smallpox eradication campaign, 1973–1975. *Social Science and Medicine,* 41: 633–45.

Griffith, A. H. (1989). Permanent brain damage and pertussis vaccination: is the end of the saga in sight? *Vaccine,* 7: 199–210.

Hall, C. (2001a). Campaign to persuade parents that the MMR jab is safe. London, *Daily Telegraph.*

Hall, C. (2001b). Mother of five children with autism to sue over MMR jabs. London, *Daily Telegraph.*

Hawkes, N. (2003). Clinics in measles jab scare withhold children's names. London, *The Times.*

Hawkes, N. (2004). MMR case parents lose legal aid fight. London, *The Times.*

Healy, P. (1978). Bill to help victims of vaccine damage. London, *The Times.*

Healy, P. (1980). New campaign to win state help for vaccine-damaged. London, *The Times.*

Hobson-West, P. (2003). Understanding vaccination resistance: moving beyond risk. *Health Risk & Society,* 5: 273–83.

Hobson-West, P. (2007). 'Trusting blindly can be the biggest risk of all': organised resistance to childhood vaccination in the UK. *Sociology of Health and Illness,* 29: 198–215.

Horton, R. (2004). *MMR: Science and Fiction.* London, Granta Books.

Hull, D. (1981). Interpretation of the contraindications to whooping cough vaccination. *British Medical Journal,* 283: 1231–3.

Kasperson, R., Renn, O., Slovic, P. *et al.* (1998). The social amplification of risk: A conceptual framework. In: Löfstedt, R. E. & Frewer, L. (eds). *The Earthscan Reader in Risk and Modern Society.* London, Earthscan Publications, Ltd.

Kulenkampff, M., Schwartzman, J. S. & Wilson, J. (1974). Neurological complications of pertussis inoculation. *Archives of Disease in Childhood*, 49: 46–9.

Laurance, J. (1998a). Children's vaccine is safe, say experts. London, *The Independent*.

Laurance, J. (1998b). From MMR to autism: Case study. London, *The Independent*.

Leask, J. & McIntyre, P. (2003). Public opponents of vaccination: a case study. *Vaccine*, 21: 4700–3.

Luhmann, N. (1979). *Trust and Power*. Chichester, John Wiley and Sons.

Martin, N. (2003). Parents seeking MMR compensation lose legal aid for court fight. London, *Daily Telegraph*.

Mechanic, D. (1998). The functions and limitations of trust in the provision of medical care. *Journal of Health Politics, Policy and Law*, 23: 661–86.

Meikle, J. (2001). Doctor who linked jab to autism quits. London, *The Guardian*.

Meikle, J. (2004a). Lancet regrets MMR report: Paper that questioned vaccine might never have been published. London, *The Guardian*.

Meikle, J. (2004b). National roundup: Health: Retraction from MMR authors. London, *The Guardian*.

Murch, S. (2003). Separating inflammation from speculation in autism. *The Lancet*, 362: 1498.

Murphy-Lawless, J. (2003). Risk, ethics, and the public space: The impact of BSE and foot-and-mouth disease on public thinking. In: Hawthorn, B. H. & Oaks, L. (eds). *Risk, Culture, and Health Inequality: Shifting Perceptions of Danger and Blame*. Westport, CT, Praeger.

NHS Health Promotion England. (2001). MMR: What parents want to know. London.

Nichter, M. (1995). Vaccinations in the Third World: A consideration of community demand. *Social Science and Medicine*, 41: 617–32.

Pidgeon, N. (1999). Risk communication and the social amplification of risk: theory, evidence, and policy implications. *Risk Decision and Policy*, 4: 1–15.

Poltorak, M., Leach, M., Fairhead, J. & Cassell, J. (2005). 'MMR talk' and vaccination choices: An ethnographic study in Brighton. *Social Science & Medicine*, 61: 609–19.

Rogers, A. & Pilgrim, D. (1995): The risk of resistance: perspectives on the mass childhood immunisation programme. In: Gabe, J. (ed.). *Medicine, Health and Risk: Sociological Approaches*. Oxford, Blackwell.

Rogers, L. & Deer, B. (2004). Scientists desert MMR maverick. London, *The Times*.

Rowell, A. (2003). *Don't Worry, It's Safe to Eat: The true story of GM food, BSE and foot and mouth*. London, Earthscan.

Safran, D. G., Taira, D. A., Rogers, W. H., Kosinski, M. M., Ware, J. E. & Tarlov, A. R. (1998). Linking primary care performance to outcomes of care. *Journal of Family Practice*, 47: 213–20.

Salisbury, D. & Begg, N. (eds). (1996). *Immunisation against Infectious Disease*. London, HMSO.

Science Museum. (2002). Antenna: The MMR Files.

Slovic, P. (2000). *The Perception of Risk*. London, Earthscan.

Smith, A., Yarwood, J. & Salisbury, D. M. (2007). Tracking mothers' attitudes to MMR immunisation 1996–2006. *Vaccine*, 25: 3996–4002.

Streefland, P. H. (2001). Public doubts about vaccination safety and resistance against vaccination. *Health Policy*, 55: 159–72.

Streefland, P. H., Chowdhury, A. M. R. & Ramos-Jimenez, P. (1999). Patterns of vaccination acceptance. *Social Science and Medicine*, 49: 1705–16.

Swansea Research Unit of the Royal College of General Practitioners. (1981). Effect of a low pertussis vaccination uptake on a large community. *British Medical Journal*, 282: 23–6.

Taylor, M. (2004). Judge confirms legal aid refusal in MMR litigation. London, *The Guardian*.

Wakefield, A. (2001). Measles, mumps, rubella vaccine: through a glass, darkly. *Adverse Drug Reactions & Toxicological Reviews*, 19: 265–83.

Wakefield, A., Murch, S., Anthony, A. *et al.* (1998). Ileal-lymphoid-nodular hyperplasia, non-specific colitis, and pervasive developmental disorder in children. *The Lancet*, 351: 637–41.

Wright, O., Hawkes, N. & Lister, S. (2004). Lancet criticises MMR scientist who raised alarm. London, *The Times*.

Chapter 10

# Risk communication and pandemic influenza

Judith Petts, Heather Draper, Jonathan Ives,
& Sarah Damery (University of Birmingham)

## Introduction

This chapter (written before the 2009 'Swine Flu' pandemic) examines a risk
scenario that could form one of the most significant communication challenges both nationally and globally—an influenza pandemic. The threat of
pandemic influenza has attracted significant international attention. A pandemic occurs when a new influenza strain emerges and spreads rapidly because
people have no natural resistance to it (Department of Health, 2007). The
most notable influenza pandemic of the last century occurred in 1918–19, the
so-called 'Spanish flu', which caused an estimated 20–40 million deaths worldwide (250 000 of these in the UK). Two significant but less serious (in terms of
deaths) pandemics occurred in 1957–58 (Asian flu) and 1968–69 (Hong Kong
flu). Pandemic influenza is much more serious than a seasonal flu outbreak—a
point to which we will return.

There has been scientific agreement for some years (e.g. Morse *et al.*, 2006)
that another pandemic is not only possible but probable, yet the risk has been
difficult to predict. The UK National Risk Register (Cabinet Office, 2008)
assessed an influenza pandemic as having the highest potential impact relative
to all high consequence risks (from terrorist attack to flooding to major chemical or transport accidents). A pandemic could be catastrophic in terms of
morbidity and mortality; the Department of Health (DH) estimated that up to
half of the UK population could become infected; 25% of the workforce may
be absent from work through illness, and there may be up to 750 000 deaths
under the reasonable worst case scenario (Department of Health, 2007). In the
United States, disaster planning scenarios estimate potentially 2.25 million
deaths (Paek *et al.*, 2008). Disasters such as pandemics that take a heavy toll on
human life are inherently characterized by rapid social change, high levels of
uncertainty, and interactive complexity (Reynolds & Quinn, 2008). In all

countries, normal life could face severe economic and social disruption, which could last weeks to months (a pandemic 'wave' is expected to last up to 15 weeks but may recur 2–3 times).

The World Health Organization (WHO, 2005) defines six phases of an influenza pandemic, including phase 3, the pandemic alert period and phase 6 in which there is sustained human-to-human transmission. An influenza virus (H5N1) circulating among birds in Africa, Asia, and Europe has demonstrated the ability to cross the species barrier to humans, but is currently not spread easily from person to person. WHO has warned of a potential pandemic should the H5N1 strain mutate and become more easily transmitted, as happened in the case of severe acute respiratory syndrome (SARS).

In such dire circumstances, effective risk communication will be essential not only to provide advice, information, and reassurance, but to encourage individuals to take personal preventative actions (e.g. isolation of sick people, voluntary home quarantine of non-ill family members, working from home) and to encourage support for necessary national response and contingency measures. The latter may raise difficult ethical issues and choices (for example, about who should be treated), and might require unpopular measures with differential social impact such as travel restrictions, refusal of visas for travellers from affected countries, and bans on public gatherings (Garoon & Duggan, 2008). Public support for such action cannot be taken for granted.

Retrospective analysis of the 1918–19 pandemic identified social vulnerability (e.g. nutritional status, household size, economic capacity to rest and recuperate) as a key determinant of morbidity and mortality (Mamelund, 2006; Garoon & Duggan, 2008). Vulnerable individuals are more likely to be at risk during a pandemic (exposure), may be less able to cope with the effects (resistance), and may be least able to recover afterwards (resilience) (Bankoff, 2001). In general, socially excluded individuals who are already considered 'hard to reach' are under-represented in national planning (Lee et al., 2008), yet will inevitably be hardest hit by any pandemic. Social unrest is a possibility that planners must anticipate as well as seek to avoid by communication and consultation.

Over the past 20 years, significant advice and guidelines on risk communication have developed. Focus is now on understanding and analysing risk-related decisions and behaviour in society so as to mediate at the public–expert interface (Leiss, 1996; Wynne, 1996; Lofstedt & Renn, 1997; Yearley, 2000). In any crisis, an open and empathetic style of communication that can engender public trust is essential, since distrust is known to heighten public concerns and disrupt responses to risk messages (Kasperson et al., 1992; Flynn et al., 1993; Lofstedt & Horlick-Jones, 1999; Petts et al., 2001).

The UK National Framework for Responding to an Influenza Pandemic (Cabinet Office and Department of Health, 2007) stressed the need for communication before, during, and after a pandemic. But prior to the 2009 'Swine Flu' outbreak, public engagement had been limited. Most of the public probably had only relatively little understanding of the link between novel viruses and pandemic influenza, and had yet to engage with the potential personal implications of a pandemic. There had been comparatively little attempt to gauge public understanding and likely response, in comparison with the increase in international surveys conducted over the last few years (Blendon *et al.*, 2006; Elledge *et al.*, 2008; Freimuth *et al.*, 2008).

Responses to major events such as a pandemic depend on perceptions of responsibility. However, the notion of responsibility, and to whom—oneself, one's family, or society—is complex and can vary significantly between different types of health risk (Petts, 2005). We can expect people to seek information actively when they have to make important decisions (in the event of a pandemic), but this raises questions about the impact of risk communication prior to this. Importantly, when risks are unpredictable and complex, people tend to base their response as much on what friends and neighbours do as on what officials say should be done (Neuwirth & Frederick, 2004). People do not need information for information's sake, but as a means of taking responsibility for personal choices, improving their own or their family's wellbeing, or supporting their role in society (Moore, 2002). Health risk communication has to be responsive to developing (and potentially highly differentiated) social representations of risk (Petts, 2005).

This chapter draws upon one of the first and most comprehensive UK surveys of healthcare workers' willingness to work and other potential responses to pandemic influenza (Draper *et al.*, 2008; Ives *et al.*, 2009). Healthcare workers will be fundamental to the emergency response in a pandemic, but will also be in the frontline of exposure to infection with potentially far-reaching personal and family impacts. The limited data on factors influencing willingness to work highlight a sense of professional obligation, estimated risk to oneself and one's family, and inclusion in preparedness planning (Tzeng & Yin, 2006; Young & Persell, 2005; Shaw *et al.*, 2006; Ehrenstein *et al.*, 2006; Qureshi *et al.*, 2005). But our discussion here is not focused on the potential implications of the findings for the health service and the emergency response. Rather, we use the evidence gathered from healthcare workers—who might plausibly have an enhanced understanding of the potential risks—to consider how information and knowledge might be exchanged amongst the wider public. This should help in understanding how risk communication efforts might most effectively engage with people, before (as well as during) an outbreak. Before outlining this evidence, the next section summarizes the characteristics of pandemic influenza that may impact on people's understanding, information needs, and response.

## Pandemic risk signature

Different risk issues possess different risk 'signatures' (Petts et al., 2001), or 'images', in terms of their capacity to engender certain patterns of public understanding. At a basic level, there is no simple correlation between scientific accounts of any risk issue and how an individual finds meaning in that issue. Rather, people draw upon individual and collective resources derived from direct and mediated experience to interpret any risk, whether real or potential.

In the context of pandemic influenza, this 'meaning' will develop with time, firstly as evidence of viral spread elsewhere in the world[1] becomes evident, and then as the potential risk becomes increasingly real to an individual and their family and friends, and as normal life is increasingly disrupted. Most importantly, it can be expected that these meanings will vary between and within communities, reflecting ethnic and socioeconomic diversity, and how sociocultural variables and past experience shape the exchange of ideas and information (Vaughan, 1995). This presents a potential dilemma for authorities focused on large scale risk communication and on national emergency planning as opposed to the strengthening and enabling of *local* public health infrastructure and *local* 'interpersonal bonds and social discourse' (Middaugh, 2008).

Risk 'signatures' comprise at least four dimensions (Petts et al., 2001), relating to: (1) the nature and specificity of the effects or harm; (2) the potential for harm to others, especially to family and friends; (3) the extent to which the authorities responsible for management are trusted; and (4) moral considerations, including questions about where responsibility for action lies.

Pandemic influenza will be unpredictable—in terms both of timing of outbreak and speed of spread. Evidence is likely to be confused at the outset. Once a pandemic has taken hold, there could be widespread and rapidly increasing mortality and morbidity. Everyone could be at risk, but those with pre-existing vulnerabilities are particularly likely to be affected (e.g. those with chronic heart and bronchial disease, the very young and the old). As the number of people affected escalates, normal access to health services may have to be

---

[1] It was anticipated that the virus would mutate in Asia and that if efforts to contain it in the country of origin fail, it will reach in UK within 2–4 weeks (Cabinet Office & Department of Health, 2007). Certainly, Swine Flu spread rapidly from Mexico.

restricted, provoking strong reactions as people are denied health services they have come to depend upon in normal times, and urgently need during the pandemic. As increasing numbers of people are absent from work, and deaths increase, all services and economic and social activity will be affected. This complexity of impact is significant; this is not just an issue of *health* risk communication.

Evidence of viral spread will raise anxiety about infection risk to the elderly or otherwise vulnerable individuals and to parents with young children. As the pandemic takes hold, adult carers will be under increasing (personal and social) pressure to look after the sick within the home rather than going to work. Socially and economically disadvantaged families may be unable to provide adequate care and may have to continue working despite the risks. Even amongst local communities and those who are not ill, tensions and concern may rise as services become increasingly disrupted or shut through absenteeism or to prevent spread of disease. Fear of contagion may lead to suspicion of others' behaviour and whether individuals are behaving 'responsibly'. Traditional neighbourhood solidarity and social cohesion around local institutions may be called into question.

In a pandemic, people need to have confidence in effective preparedness and response. This has implications for those charged with providing the response—which will not be limited to the health services. Confidence will be challenged by any identifiable lack of consensus amongst experts and authorities about the arrival and spread of the disease, and the actions required. A critical objective of any communication strategy will be to convince people to comply with recommended control measures, but people need to have confidence in this strategy and trust in those managing the risk. Evidence from other health crises, such as the controversy over the MMR vaccine in the UK, suggests that local general practitioners (GPs) may be the most trusted to provide personal health information and advice (Petts & Niemeyer, 2004). However, people with influenza symptoms are encouraged not to go to their GP, but to use the 'flu line'—a telephone service—for self-diagnosis and prescription of antiviral drugs (Department of Health, 2007, Para 9.8.1). This will isolate them from their traditional source of trusted information. Trust will be required if the government is to achieve its objective of 'business as usual' as far as possible. But if people become fearful of interacting with each other, if panic buying affects supply chains, or if public order begins to break down as services are restricted or withdrawn, then both interpersonal and political trust will be severely tested.

Perceived responsibility for dealing with the crisis is likely to be central to people's concerns—whether it be the responsibility of healthcare workers to continue to deliver an effective health service; that of transport and other infrastructure operators to maintain normal levels of service, or that of individual members of the public to take responsible measures to minimize spread of the virus, including voluntary isolation. The UK National Framework has a strong sense of 'expectation' of responsibilities being accepted. But we need to understand whether people will even recognize these responsibilities, let alone act on them.

## Public response to pandemic influenza

Public attitudes towards the threat of pandemic influenza are relatively poorly understood, as is the likely public response during or after the event. Evidence by the Academy of Medical Sciences (2005) to the UK House of Lords Science and Technology Select Committee Inquiry into Pandemic Influenza stressed that improved public understanding of the disease and its potential implications is crucial. In 2006, a questionnaire survey of the UK public reported that 50% of respondents ($n = 216$) could correctly identify the characteristics of a pandemic. While only 25% understood the likely socioeconomic impacts, 61% would consider staying away from work as a means of protecting themselves. Most (97%) said they would be prepared to wash their hands regularly if asked to do so, and 86% said they would be willing to stay away from public gatherings (Gupta et al., 2006). Similar findings were reported by one US poll (Blendon et al., 2006). An Australian telephone survey also reported willingness to undertake increased hand washing if recommended, though 10% stated they would not keep their children home from school even if this was recommended by the government (Jones & Iverson, 2008). Finally, another US study surveying both healthcare professionals ($n = 39$) and members of the public ($n = 97$) found a generally low understanding of the term 'pandemic' with some conflation with seasonal flu. Although respondents were interested in learning about protective measures, there was less interest in taking preventative action 'when a pandemic was neither present nor imminent' (Janssen et al., 2006).

These limited studies provide a sketchy picture of a public that is relatively ill-informed about pandemic influenza, but possibly willing to engage in protective behaviours if recommended by a relevant authority. However, surveys have limitations in terms of understanding what underpins these views. Unless we can begin to understand how and why people are motivated to act before, during or after a pandemic, we can have little hope of building an effective risk communication strategy.

In this context, healthcare workers are an interesting group to consider. The National Health Service (NHS) is Europe's biggest employer, with 1.3 million people on the payroll (NHS Information Centre, 2008). The NHS workforce is diverse, from highly paid medical professionals and managers (typical of those outside the health service); to semi-skilled or unskilled workers, working for the minimum wage or just above. Just under half of the NHS workforce are non-professional workers. It might be expected that many of those working in the NHS would be better informed than the general public about the risks of pandemic influenza given their frontline role and the vast resources being spent in the UK on pandemic planning. At the same time, because of this role, fears about risks are likely to be more acute and the need to communicate more urgent to maintain this essential service during any pandemic.

## The concerns of healthcare workers

Our survey work examining healthcare workers' attitudes to working during pandemic influenza was completed in 2008 and had two phases. In the first, qualitative phase, we conducted focus groups amongst healthcare workers of different types (e.g. hospital doctors, ancillary staff, professions allied to medicine, nurses, managers, GPs, community nurses, etc.). The findings were then used to inform a survey, completed by about 150 members for each category of worker. Participants were drawn from both rural and inner city areas. Here, we draw largely on the qualitative work to identify the ways in which they discussed and interpreted the risks of working during pandemic influenza.

As DH planning documents (NHS Employers and Department of Health, 2008) suggest, there is a perception of an NHS culture of dedication to patients, reinforced by a professional duty to care under even the most difficult of circumstances. Our participants confirmed this, referring to professionalism, public service, the 'Dunkirk/Blitz' spirit, and a more general work ethic as motivators for working during an influenza pandemic despite the risks (Ives et al., 2009).

Given the significant challenges that will face the UK if up to 25% of the workforce is affected by influenza, the willingness of unaffected workers to work is clearly going to be vital if chaos in the NHS is to be avoided. Estimates of likely NHS absenteeism during a pandemic range up to 50% (NHS Employers and Department of Health, 2008), in line with that suggested by Balicer et al. (2006) in the USA and also Qureshi et al. (2005) in relation to SARS. Many absentees will themselves have influenza; others with young children may be affected by local school closures; and some will wish to take time from work to care for family members and friends who are ill. We found, however, that some workers may be absent because of their own assessment of the acceptability of the risks of working, either to themselves or to their family members. Few participants recognized that not all healthcare workers would be exposed to influenza patients (so working during a pandemic may pose no greater risk than usual), nor that 'pandemic' meant that the virus was rife in the community in which they spent their non-working time (i.e. there would be exposure to risks even if they did not work).

When considering motivators *for* working, some participants did attempt to assess whether an influenza pandemic would pose any greater risk to them than other infections to which they were routinely exposed at work—like *Clostridium difficile* or MRSA. Both absolute and relative risks feature in attempts to determine whether healthcare professionals have an obligation to work during epidemics (see, for instance, Reid, 2005; Huber and Wynia, 2004). The NHS Employers and DH Human Resources guidance (2008) advises that: 'The employment contracts of staff will oblige them to treat patients and refusal to do so may put them in breach of their contracts' (Section 3.10). In our study, many NHS workers expressed concern that they might face legal action post-pandemic for damages resulting from decisions they made during the pandemic or whilst working in extended roles. This concern about litigation did not appear sufficient to deter individuals from working. But it seemed to add to a cumulative case for not working that also included low morale and lack of trust in reciprocity—the (societal) expectation that if healthcare workers are expected to work despite high personal risk, they should in turn be adequately supported and protected, and their efforts acknowledged (Barr *et al.*, 2008). For example, there were concerns as to whether personal protective equipment would be forthcoming (and adequate) as well as fears for personal and family welfare.

One clear limitation of our work is that we asked participants to imagine how they might feel about a pandemic about which, it emerged, they felt inadequately informed, and about which it was difficult to provide information owing to a general uncertainty about the precise nature of a virus yet to emerge. National planning has been made according to assumptions based on the 1918–19 pandemic—when British society was very different, not least because the country had been at war.

Our research suggests that many healthcare workers did not feel (and were not) well informed about pandemic influenza (as measured by current DH planning assumptions). They wanted more information, but it is unclear what form this should take. Some participants were aware that information must exist, and that it could probably be found on their work websites, but felt that it would take too long to find and read. Some of the GPs said that they would prefer to wait until the pandemic started, as they would then be provided with the information they needed and told what to do. At the time their focus group ran in February 2008, only one GP (out of ten) had actually considered making any pandemic plans—though this would have changed once guidance for primary care trusts and professionals was finalized (Department of Health, 2008). Very few of our participants had been involved in any planning and none had received any form of pandemic training other than completing online tutorials. Whilst there was a large amount of information readily available on the DH website, this did not appear to be reaching healthcare workers other than those directly involved in planning.

## Lessons for public risk communication

The evidence set out here suggests some tentative hypotheses about how best to communicate effectively about pandemic risk with the public.

If there is little general understanding of what an influenza pandemic is, what its effects may be, and how it differs from ordinary seasonal flu, people are likely to draw on ideas about communicable disease that are already familiar to them (making analogies with seasonal flu, MRSA, etc.). Importantly, their understanding will draw not only on official medical and scientific information but also upon personal experience, familial and social traditions, socio-economic factors, and cultural health beliefs (Helman, 2007). We can hypothesize that people will be inclined to take protective measures and lifestyle changes if advised to by a trusted source, in a manner that they understand and which speaks to their current understanding rather than the understanding experts would like them to have. Even then, the links between understanding and behaviour are far from straightforward. Whether understanding has a material impact on subsequent behaviour to reduce risk to self or others is determined by a number of context-specific factors (Blake, 1999). Like our healthcare workers, we can expect that familial concerns and responsibilities will strongly affect people's willingness to continue working and to maintain their normal daily routines unless they are reassured of their own protection.

Giving a clear and consistent message is difficult when the facts (health, economic, social, etc.) are uncertain. Uncertainty often breeds fear and may lead to 'worst case' or overly precautionary assessments of risks and panic. Some of the managers and public health doctors in our focus groups displayed 'expert caution' in stating that they were unwilling to give out information that might later turn out to be wrong. This correlates with UK planning as public information dissemination only commences in WHO phase 6, UK 6.1 (i.e. no confirmed cases in the UK but sustained human-to-human transmission evident in other countries). However, it was intended that several seasonal flu campaigns would be run prior to any pandemic in an effort to improve general standards of respiratory and hand hygiene in the population. It was hoped that this would pay dividends in terms of lessening transmission of infection during pandemic influenza. In addition, advice to adopt particular behaviours during a pandemic may find a more receptive audience if these behaviours have already been assimilated into everyday practice.

However, whether these campaigns can adequately reflect the likely dramatic and complex risk signature of a pandemic is highly debatable. There was some consensus in our GP focus group that they would simply cope with pandemic influenza just as they routinely cope with seasonal influenza. This seems unrealistic. There are obvious similarities between pandemic influenza and seasonal flu, and the promotion of a 'business as usual' message is facilitated by likening one to the other. However, conflating the two may leave the public unprepared for the likely severity of the personal, societal, and economic impacts of pandemic influenza. For this reason, we favour writing/speaking about pandemic *influenza*, which maintains some similarity but avoids total conflation of the two conditions.

User-centred risk communication (Petts & Niemeyer 2004) will be essential, not only informed by an understanding of information needs, but also responding to rapid changes in these needs, not least as media (including internet) reporting cascades new information into people's homes and as experiential knowledge takes hold. This is particularly important, as information transmission via multiple pathways has the potential to lead to public confusion if mixed or conflicting risk messages come from different sources (Bennett, 1999). As suggested by its risk signature, a pandemic is likely to produce heightened local and social communication and awareness as well as potentially tragic and alarming media stories as the death rate increases. While communication strategies will have to be able to respond to this stage of a pandemic, it seemed essential to at least start to prepare the public for the likelihood of a pandemic and to generate a public discussion of how to limit its effects. Our healthcare workers were concerned to have information on the planning already being undertaken. We think that the same could apply to the general public.

While the seasonal flu campaign seems to be attempting to generate a general health responsibility and awareness, it seems relevant to reflect that in the MMR case, prior general messages about childhood immunization and even embedded parental practice were severely challenged when an actual concern arose and became a national issue (see Chapter 9). The sudden change in the risk signature of MMR—from a beneficial and common vaccination to a perceived threat to children's health through a media story making a link (falsely) with autism—prompted heightened communication amongst parents that served to undermine expert communication as well as prior personal parental experience (Petts & Niemeyer, 2004). The MMR 'crisis' severely challenged notions of personal (in this case parental) versus societal responsibility (casiday, Chapter 9, this volume). Although this is a very different health issue, we suggest that experience of seasonal flu is not likely to provide a sufficiently robust basis for promoting the type of social response and individual responsibility required in an influenza pandemic.

Once it is clear that there is imminent danger of a pandemic (WHO phase 5), it is likely that there will be an additional demand for information about where the outbreaks are occurring, what impact the influenza is having, and what people can do to protect and treat themselves. Experience suggests this will require communication by trusted sources, including GPs, although it is likely that trusted experts and possibly celebrities may also be essential communicators. Planning should ensure advanced identification of potentially effective and empathetic communicators—a key dimension underlying trust (Renn & Levine, 1991; Fischhoff, 1995; Reynolds & Quinn, 2008). We can expect differential ability to access information amongst those from lower socioeconomic groups. Yet, these will be the very people potentially most at risk during a pandemic and least able to take personal protective measures (including time for recuperation from illness). Careful attention will be needed to communication in different forms and languages as well as opportunities for people to listen to messages, not just read them.

There will be intricacies of messages that may be difficult to predict in terms of public response once a pandemic has taken hold. Consistency of information is essential as people become confused and concerned when they are exposed to different interpretations of what should happen, e.g. over whether or not face masks are useful protection against exposure to the virus[2]. However, confusion will also arise from different social interpretations of what is 'best'. For example, staying away from mass gatherings such as football matches might be regarded differently to staying away from places of worship, particularly as people have tended to migrate towards communal worship at times of hardship, uncertainty, and danger (Ano & Vasconcelles, 2005; Siegel et al., 2001). If people are persuaded of the potential risks of mass gatherings, they may become fearful of using crowded public transportation (like the London underground) or of working in open plan offices with central air conditioning units. If this leads to people staying away from work, this will serve to heighten

---

[2] Simple face masks, frequently changed, are more likely to be effective if used by infected persons than by uninfected persons because the particles leaving the infected person are large enough to be contained with the mask. This means that face masks are likely to be more effective in protecting others rather than those wearing them. However, people may feel reassured if they are wearing a mask.

economic and service disruption further. Willingness to avoid some sorts of mass gatherings but not others will depend upon people having a shared understanding of necessary and unnecessary risk-taking, and of the relationships between collective and individual good.

A key message from our study of healthcare workers is that a willingness to pull together in a crisis will inevitably be tempered by the desire to protect oneself and one's family. We can expect parents or carers to feel a burden of responsibility to make the 'right' decision to protect those they care about. People may have difficulty balancing perceived risks against the potential personal blame for making the wrong decision. Of central significance, therefore, will be careful explanation of the utilitarian calculation that the best means of protecting individuals is by protecting the majority, and the best means of protecting the majority is by mutual cooperation rather than the anarchy of self-interest (Harris, 1992). It follows that early attention to the motivation behind the planning may be more significant to risk communication in the pre-pandemic stage. In other words, it will be just as important to communicate the reasoning behind the planning as it is to communicate the plans themselves. This is an important prerequisite if communications are to be trusted and believed. For example, a communication strategy relating to banning some gatherings that emphasizes the risk of spreading the virus in the community may encourage compliance in some people. For others, compliance may be improved by a communication strategy that emphasizes the risks of catching the virus oneself and spreading it to one's family. The former strategy may have little effect on a person who cares little about social cohesion, and the latter may have no effect on a person with no family.

An alternative to the current strategy may be to bring forward public information about pandemic influenza to lessen its sensational impact. The dangers of 'pandemic fatigue' and possible misinformation (resulting from unavoidably imprecise predictions) may be outweighed by the normalizing of the information.

In conclusion, pandemic influenza may represent one of the most catastrophic risks to public health. Effective response will depend on public support for required actions and individual willingness to take on responsibilities with wider social benefit. This will have to be achieved amidst significant levels of public concern, anxiety, and uncertainty. The risk signature for pandemic influenza has yet to be defined robustly, both for the current Swine Flu outbreak, and more generally. Social discourse around the full potential of a pandemic remains limited, and national plans are largely divorced from the engagement of the very people upon whom their success will depend. While fear of communicating risks associated with significant uncertainties is evident amongst professionals, this might underestimate the potential of members of the public to engage with the key health, social, and individual issues that a pandemic raises.

The social responses required by members of the public during a pandemic are far more complex than those associated with responses to other health issues—including the seasonal flu virus. This raises challenges that must not be ignored.

## Acknowledgements

This chapter draws on independent research undertaken as part of the study "Healthcare workers' attitudes towards working during pandemic influenza", commissioned by the UK National Institute for Health Research (NIHR). We acknowledge the important contributions of other members of the research team to this work – Dr Sheila Greenfield, Dr Christine Gratus, Professor Jayne Parry, Professor Sue Wilson and Professor Tom Sorell. The views expressed in the chapter are those of the authors and not necessarily those of the NHS, the NIHR or the Department of Health.

## References

Academy of Medical Sciences. (2005). *Pandemic Influenza* (a submission to the House of Lords Science and Technology Select Committee inquiry into 'pandemic influenza'). London, Academy of Medical Sciences. Available online: http://www.acmedsci.ac.uk/p48prid33.html. Accessed 21 January 2009.

Ano G. G. & Vasconcelles E. B. (2005). Religious coping and psychological adjustment to stress: a meta-analysis. *Journal of Clinical Psychology*, 61(4): 461–80.

Balicer R. D., Omer, S. B., Barnett, D. J. & Everly G. S. Jr. (2006). Local public health workers' perceptions toward responding to an influenza pandemic. *BMC Public Health*, 6: 99–9.

Bankoff, G. (2001). Rendering the world unsafe: 'vulnerability' as Western discourse. *Disasters*, 25(1): 19–35.

Barr, H. L., Macfarlane, J. T., Macgregor, O., Foxwell, R., Buswell, V. & Lim, W. S. (2008). Ethical planning for an influenza pandemic. *Clinical Medicine*, 8(1): 49–52.

Bennett, P. (1999). Understanding responses to risk: some basic findings. In: Bennett, P. & Calman, K. (eds). *Risk Communication and Public Health*. New York, Oxford University Press, pp. 3–19.

Blake, J. (1999). Overcoming the 'value-action gap' in environmental policy: tensions between national policy and local experience. *Local Environment*, 4(3): 259–78.

Blendon, R. J., Benson, J. M., DesRoches, C. M., Weldon, K. & Herrmann, M. J. (2006). Working Papers Project on the Public and Biological Security Harvard School of Public Health 19. Avian Flu Survey. Available online: http://www.hsph.harvard.edu/research/horp/files/WP19AvianFlu.pdf. Accessed 6 January 2009.

Cabinet Office. (2008). *National Risk Register*. London, Cabinet Office.

Cabinet Office and Department of Health. (2007). *A National Framework for Responding to an Influenza Pandemic*. London, Department of Health.

Department of Health (2007) *Pandemic Flu: A national framework for responding to an influenza pandemic*. London, Department of Health. Available online: http://www.dh.gov.uk/en/Publicationsandstatistics/Publications/PublicationsPolicyAndGuidance/DH_080734. Accessed 21 January 2009.

Department of Health. (2008). *Pandemic influenza: Guidance for primary care trusts and primary care professionals on the provision of health care in the community in England*. London, Department of Health. Available online: http://www.dh.gov.uk/en/Publicationsandstatistics/Publications/PublicationsPolicyAndGuidance/DH_091993. Accessed 8 January 2009.

Draper, H., Wilson, S., Ives, J. *et al.* (2008). Healthcare workers' attitudes to working during pandemic influenza: a multi-method study. *BMC Public Health*, 8: 192–8.

Ehrenstein, B. P., Hanses, F. & Salzberger, B. (2006). Influenza pandemic and professional duty: family or patients' first? A qualitative survey of hospital employees. *BMC Public Health*, 6: 311–13.

Elledge, B. L., Brand, M., Regens, J. L. & Boatright, D. T. (2008). Implications of public understanding of avian influenza for fostering effective risk communication. *Health Promotion Practice*, 9(4): 54S–9S.

Fischhoff, B. (1995). Risk perception and communication unplugged: twenty years of progress. *Risk Analysis*, 15: 137–45.

Flynn, J., Slovic, P. & Metz, C. K. (1993). The Nevada initiative—a risk communication fiasco. *Risk Analysis*, 13(6): 643–8.

Freimuth, V. S., Hilyard, K. M., Barge, K. & Sokler, L. (2008). Action, not talk: a simulation of risk communication during the first hours of a pandemic. *Health Promotion Practice*, 9(4): 35S–44S.

Garoon, J.P. & Duggan, P. S. (2008). Discourses of disease, discourses of disadvantage: a critical analysis of National Pandemic Influenza Preparedness Plans. *Social Science & Medicine*, 67: 1133–42.

Gupta, R. K., Toby, M., Bandopadhyay, G., Cooke, M., Gelb, D. & Nguyen-Van-Tam, J. (2006). Public understanding of pandemic influenza. *Emerging Infectious Diseases*, 12(10): 1620–1.

Harris, J. (1992). *The value of life: An introduction to medical ethics*. London, Routledge.

Helman, C. G. (2007). *Culture, Health and Illness*, 5th edn. London, Hodder and Arnold.

Huber, S. J. & Wynia, M. K. (2004). When pestilence prevails...Physician responses in epidemics. *The American Journal of Bioethics*, 4(1): W5–W11.

Ives, J., Greenfield, S., Parry, J. *et al.* (2009). Healthcare workers' attitudes to working during pandemic influenza: a qualitative study. *BMC Public Health*, 9: 56.

Janssen, A. P., Tardiff, R. R., Landry, S. R. & Warner, J. E. (2006). "Why tell me now?" The public and healthcare providers weigh in on pandemic influenza messages. *Journal of Public Health Management and Practice*, 12(4): 388–94.

Jones, S. C. & Iverson, D. (2008). What Australians know and believe about Bird Flu: results of a population telephone survey. *Health Promotion Practice*, 9(4): 73S–82S.

Kasperson, R. E., Golding, D. & Tuler, S. T. (1992). Social distrust as a factor in siting hazardous facilities and communicating risks. *Journal of Social Issues*, 48(4): 161–87.

Lee, C., Roger W. A. & Braunack-Mayer, A. (2008). Social justice and pandemic influenza planning: the role of communication strategies. *Public Health Ethics,* 1(3):223–34.

Leiss, W. (1996). Three phases in the evolution of risk communication practice. *Annals of the American Academy of Political and Social Science,* 545: 85–94.

Lofstedt, R. E. & Horlick-Jones, T. (1999). Environmental regulation in the UK: politics, institutional change and public trust. In: Cvetkovich, G. & Lofstedt, R. E. (eds). *Social Trust and the Management of Risk.* London, Earthscan, pp. 73–88.

Lofstedt, R.E. & Renn, O. (1997). The Brent Spar controversy: an example of risk communication gone wrong. *Risk Analysis,* 17: 131–6.

Mamelund, S.-E. (2006). A socially neutral disease? Individual social class, household wealth and mortality from Spanish Influenza in two socially contrasting parishes in Kristiania, 1918–19. *Social Science & Medicine,* 62: 923–40.

Middaugh, J. P. (2008). Pandemic influenza preparedness and community resiliency. *Journal of American Medical Association,* 299: 566–8.

Moore, N. (2002). A model of social information need. *Journal of Information Science,* 28(4): 297–303.

Morse, S. S., Garwin, R. L. & Olsiewski, P.J. (2006). Next flu pandemic: what to do until the vaccine arrives, *Science,* 314(5801): 929.

National Health Service Information Centre. (2008). *NHS Staff 1997–2007.* Available online: http://www.ic.nhs.uk/webfiles/publications/nhsstaff2007/Staff%20in%20 the%20NHS%20leaflet.pdf. Accessed 31 December 2008.

NHS Employers and Department of Health. (2008). *Pandemic Influenza: a Human Resources Guide for the NHS.* London, COI for Department of Health. Available online: http://www.dh.gov.uk/en/Publicationsandstatistics/Publications/ PublicationsPolicyAndGuidance/DH_086833. Accessed 31 December 2008.

Neuwirth, K. & Frederick, E. (2004). Peer and social influence on opinion expression: combining the theories of planned behaviour and the spiral of silence. *Communication Research,* 31(6): 669–703.

Paek, H.-J., Hilyard, K., Freimuth, V. S., Barge, K. & Mindlin, M. (2008). Public support for government actions during a flu pandemic: lessons learned from a statewide survey. *Health Promotion Practice,* 9(4): 60S–71S.

Petts, J. & Niemeyer, S. (2004). Health risk communication and amplification: learning from the MMR vaccination controversy. *Health, Risk and Society,* 6(1): 7–23.

Petts, J. (2005). Health, responsibility and choice: contrasting negotiations of air pollution and immunisation information. *Environment and Planning A,* 37: 791–804.

Petts, J., Horlick-Jones, T. & Murdock, G. (2001). *Social Amplification of Risk: The Media and the Public.* Contract Research Report 329/2001. Sudbury, HSE Books.

Qureshi, K., Gershon, R. R., Sherman M. F. *et al.* (2005). Health care workers ability and willingness to report to duty during catastrophic disasters. *Journal of Urban Health,* 82: 378–88.

Reid, L. (2005). Diminishing returns? Risk and the duty to care in the SARS epidemic. *Bioethics,* 19(4): 215–361.

Renn, O. & Levine, D. (1991). Credibility and trust in risk communication. In: R. E. Kasperson & P. M.Stallen (eds). *Communicating Risks to the Public: International Perspectives.* Dordrecht, Kluwer.

Reynolds, B. & Quinn, S. C. (2008). Effective communication during an influenza pandemic: the value of using a crisis and emergency risk communication framework. *Health Promotion Practice*, 9(4): 13S–17S.

Shaw, K.A., Chilcott, A., Hanson, E. & Winzenberg, T. W. (2006). The GPs' response to pandemic influenza: a qualitative study. *Family Practice*, 23: 267–72.

Siegel, K., Anderman, S. & Schrimshaw, E. W. (2001). Religion and coping with health-related stress. *Psychology & Health*, 16(6): 631–53.

Tzeng, H.-M. & Yin, C.-Y. (2006). Nurses' fears and professional obligations concerning possible human-to-human avian flu. *Nursing Ethics*, 13(5): 455–70.

Vaughan, E. (1995). The significance of socioeconomic and ethnic diversity for the risk communication process. *Risk Analysis*, 15(2): 169–80.

World Health Organization. (2005). Outbreak Communications Guidelines. Available online: http://www.who.int/infectious-disease-news/IDdocs/whocds200528/whocds200528en.pdf. Accessed 31 December 2008.

Wynne, B. (1996). May the sheep safely graze? A reflexive view of the expert-lay knowledge divide. In: Lash, S., Szerszynski, B. & Wynne, B. (eds). *Risk Environment and Modernity: Towards a new ecology*, Chapter 2 , London, Sage, pp. 44–83.

Yearley, S. (2000). Making systematic sense of public discontents with expert knowledge: two analytical approaches and a case study. *Public Understanding of Science*, 9: 105–22.

Young, C. & Persell, D. (2005). Biological, chemical and nuclear terrorism readiness: major concerns and preparedness of future nurses. *Disaster Management and Response*, 2(4): 109–14.

Chapter 11

# CJD: risk communication in a healthcare setting

David Pryer (Chair CJD Incidents Panel) &
Patricia Hewitt (NHS Blood & Transplant)

Creutzfeldt–Jakob disease (CJD) is an incurable and ultimately fatal degenerative neurological disease. Sporadic (or 'classical') CJD appears across the globe, though fortunately it is very rare. In March 1996, researchers in the UK first reported a variant of the disease, vCJD (Will *et al.*, 1996). Unlike sporadic CJD, younger people were affected, and the research suggested that infection had resulted from exposure to bovine spongiform encephalopathy—BSE, or 'mad cow disease'—in cattle (Bruce *et al.*, 1997). This discovery followed repeated and fervent denials by government that BSE posed any conceivable risk to human health. Not surprisingly, vCJD has created a new theatre of interest in risk communication. To understand why this is so, a short historical summary may be helpful. We then move on to consider the role of the CJD Incidents Panel in helping to manage the consequences of vCJD, and in communicating both to individuals and to wider audiences.

## Background: vCJD and the 'BSE crisis'

BSE had first been identified in 1986. Both BSE and CJD are diseases known as transmissible spongiform encephalopathies (TSEs), associated with abnormal forms of protein particles (prions). One key feature of TSEs is that they can have very long incubation periods prior to any symptoms appearing. In reality, the question of whether BSE was transmissible to humans could thus not be answered with any certainty for many years. In 1988, the government set up a working party on BSE chaired by Sir Thomas Southwood (Department of Health and Ministry of Agriculture, Fisheries and Food, 1989). It concluded that if BSE were to be transmitted to humans, it would be likely to resemble CJD and suggested that surveillance be put in place to identify atypical cases or changing patterns of the disease. This task was entrusted to the CJD Surveillance Unit, funded jointly by Department of Health (DH) and the Scottish Office

Home and Health Department, leading to the prompt detection of vCJD when it did emerge in 1996. A committee to consider research needs was chaired by Dr David Tyrrell, who then became the first Chair of the Spongiform Encephalopathy Advisory Committee (SEAC), which has remained the principal source of scientific advice in the UK ever since.

Despite this activity, the official view presented to the public until 1996 was that BSE posed no risk—or at least negligible risk—to human health. This view was promulgated by leading politicians and officials with a confidence that proved to be entirely mistaken (Maxwell, 1997). Undoubtedly, politicians were concerned to avoid a 'food scare'. However, they were also essentially following the prevailing scientific orthodoxy. In some instances, scientific advice came with caveats that were overlooked or downplayed. Nevertheless, scientists too were sometimes prepared to give assurances that—with the benefit of hindsight—can be seen as far too categorical.

Thus, the Southwood Report, published jointly by DH and the Ministry for Agriculture, Fisheries and Food (MAFF) in February 1989, concluded that 'it was most unlikely that BSE would have any implications for human health'. This was based on the view that:

- BSE was probably derived from scrapie (a long-established TSE affecting sheep) and could be expected to behave like scrapie. Scrapie had not been transmitted to humans in over 200 years and so BSE was not likely to transmit either

- So far as occupational and medicinal risks were concerned, the authorities which had been notified about these could be relied upon to take appropriate measures.

The Report did comment that, if the assessment was incorrect, the implications would be extremely serious. However, this warning was lost from sight. The Southwood Report was repeatedly cited as showing that no precautionary measures were needed other than those recommended by the Working Party. In response to public concerns about the safety of beef, Dr Tyrrell wrote publicly to the Chief Medical Officer in July 1990 that 'any risk as a result of eating beef or beef products is minute. Thus we believe that there is no scientific reason for not eating British beef and that it can be eaten by everyone.' Many similar statements were given.

Nevertheless, the balance of evidence shifted—especially as cats and other species were found to be suffering from 'scrapie-like' disorders. In 1994, SEAC still evaluated the risk of transmissibility to humans as remote—but only on the assumption that precautionary measures had been put in place. Well thought out measures had indeed been designed to eradicate BSE—notably by banning the use of ruminant-derived meat and bone meal (MBM) in cattle feed—and to prevent cattle affected by BSE from entering the human food chain. But it later became clear that the very message that human health was not at stake had undermined their rigorous implementation. Increasing knowledge about BSE gradually threw doubt on the theory that it would behave like scrapie. This was not actively concealed, but the impression was still given that BSE was not transmissible to humans. This exacerbated the public feeling of betrayal following the March 1996 announcement.

One casualty of the resulting crisis was that MAFF, whose dual role in promoting both food safety and the farming and food supply industries, now appeared untenable. The guardianship of food safety was transferred to a new Food Standards Agency, charged with protecting consumer interests. Critically, it is entitled (and expected) to make public its advice to government ministers. This means that the Agency can be seen to act openly and independently (Food Standards Agency, 2008).

The new government also set up the Phillips Inquiry:

> To establish and review the history of the emergence and identification of BSE and new variant CJD in the United Kingdom, and of the action taken in response to it up to 20 March 1996; to reach conclusions on the adequacy of that response, taking into account the state of knowledge at the time; and to report on these matters . . .

Amongst the report's extensive conclusions (Phillips, BSE Inquiry Report Volume 1, 2000), the following extracts, from the Executive Summary, are particularly relevant.

- BSE developed into an epidemic as a consequence of an intensive farming practice—the recycling of animal protein in ruminant feed. This practice, unchallenged over decades, proved a recipe for disaster

- At the heart of the BSE story lie questions of how to handle hazard—a known hazard to cattle and an unknown hazard to humans. The government took measures to address both hazards. They were sensible measures, but were not always timely nor adequately implemented and enforced

- The rigour with which policy measures were implemented for the protection of human health was affected by the belief of many prior to early 1996 that BSE was not a potential threat to human life

- The government introduced measures to guard against the risk that BSE might be a matter of life and death not merely for cattle but also for humans, but the possibility of a risk to humans was not communicated to the public or to those whose job it was to implement and enforce the precautionary measures

◆ The government did not lie to the public about BSE. It believed that the risks posed by BSE to humans were remote. The government was preoccupied with preventing an alarmist over-reaction to BSE because it believed that the risk was remote. It is now clear that this campaign of reassurance was a mistake . . . Confidence in government pronouncements about risk was a further casualty of BSE.

The transmission of BSE to humans had been considered most unlikely, but had nevertheless happened: an unknown number of people had been infected. In the few years from 1996 onward, new vCJD cases rose year on year, while projections for the eventual number of cases ranged from small numbers to many millions. International repercussions multiplied as other nations attempted to minimize their own exposure to both BSE and vCJD—for example, by preventing anyone who had visited the UK for significant periods from donating blood.

Fortunately, the 'worst case' scenarios have not materialized—albeit for reasons that remain unclear. The number of new vCJD cases peaked in 2000 and has consistently declined since, with the cumulative UK total of confirmed and probable cases now standing at 168. However, this is not necessarily a good indicator of the number infected, which remains highly uncertain even now. A survey of stored tissue (Hilton et al., 2004) found evidence of abnormal prion protein in three samples in roughly 12 000 appendix samples, indicating a prevalence of the order of 1 in 4000, albeit with very wide confidence intervals.

While some believe that the current, and thankfully low, number of new cases of vCJD indicate the outbreak is tailing off, others would argue that this is only 'the end of the beginning' of the problem and further waves of cases will still manifest. This argument is based in part on the fact that all the definite and probable clinical cases of variant CJD who have been tested come from one genetic group (MM homozygotes at codon 129 on the prion protein gene), comprising just under 40% of the population. Evidence both from animal models and from the human TSE kuru suggest that all genotypes (MM, MV, and VV) may be susceptible to infection, but with MM homozygotes developing symptoms first. This differential has to be considered when attempting to understand the current prevalence of infection and possible future course of the outbreak (Clarke and Ghani, 2004; Bishop et al., 2006) So far one MV patient has been diagnosed as a possible vCJD case. Two others—each exposed to a blood donor who went on to develop vCJD—died without showing any symptoms of prion disease but were found to be carrying abnormal prion protein at post-mortem examination.

## Human-to-human transmission

The possibility that many people might be incubating vCJD without showing symptoms raised concerns about the potential for transmission from person to person. As this would require transfer of prion protein, potential routes include use of blood, blood products, tissues or organs sourced from an infected donor, and transmission via surgery. The latter risk would arise if instruments used on an infective patient were re-used. Unfortunately, the abnormal prion protein is extremely difficult to remove and is heat-resistant: current decontamination methods would not fully eliminate the risk of transmitting infection (Taylor, 2000; Weissmann et al., 2002; Sutton et al., 2006). These concerns are not entirely confined to vCJD, although the risks of spreading sporadic CJD appear to be confined to a smaller group of procedures involving brain and eye tissue (Bernoulli et al., 1977). Meanwhile, vCJD has been transmitted through donated blood in at least four instances, three of which have led to the recipient dying from vCJD (Llewelyn et al., 2004; Peden et al., 2004). The scale of person-to-person transmission risks is very difficult to evaluate, given the uncertainty as to how many people are already carrying vCJD infection. All risk assessments have to incorporate very wide ranges of scenarios (Department of Health, 2000; 2005; NICE, 2006; Bennett et al., 2005; Bennett & Dobra, 2006). A further concern is that, in the worst case, person-to-person transmission could lead to vCJD becoming self-sustaining within the population, rather than gradually disappearing once the original foodborne source of infection is removed.

In dealing with such risks, key lessons of the Phillips inquiry remain valid:

- Although the likelihood of a risk to human life may appear remote, where there is uncertainty all reasonably practicable precautions should be taken and strictly enforced
- All pathways by which vCJD may be transmitted between humans must be identified and all reasonably practicable measures taken to block them
- The needs of victims of vCJD and their families have special features. Consideration should be given to how best the health and welfare services can meet them. (The Report noted that patients for whom a care plan had been carefully arranged received better managed care.)

## Risk communication and the CJD Incidents Panel

The CJD Incidents Panel ('the Panel') is an expert committee set up in 2000 by the Chief Medical Officer for England. Its remit is to advise hospitals, trusts, and public health teams throughout the UK on the management of incidents involving possible transmission of CJD (of any type) from person to person. The Panel is accountable to the Department of Health, and has a secretariat based at the Health Protection Agency (HPA). It has a key role both in dealing with the consequences of identifiable individuals having been put at risk of prion infection and in minimizing the risks of onward transmission.

Members of the Panel contribute on a personal basis, rather than as representatives of a trust, university, or other institution. They are drawn from a range of backgrounds. Today, there is strong representation from transfusion medicine, various branches of surgery, anaesthesia, infection control, instrument management and decontamination, public health, and dental and medical general practice. There are lay members, patient representatives, and members with expertise in medical ethics and health psychology.

Typically, 'incidents' occur because there is no reason to suspect that an individual is incubating a prion disease. For example, if a patient who has undergone invasive surgery is subsequently diagnosed with CJD, the instruments may already have been re-used many times, creating a risk to subsequent patients. For sporadic CJD, any appreciable risk would be confined to procedures involving the brain or back of the eye. But with vCJD, infectivity is more widely distributed, so concern attaches to a wider range of surgical procedures—and to the possibility of an infected person having donated blood, tissues or organs.

Incidents involving surgery require decisions with regard both to the instruments involved, and to subsequent patients on whom they have been used. Instruments are generally quarantined (pending diagnosis of the index patient) or disposed of. This may impose considerable costs on the NHS Trusts involved—an impact that the Panel must be cognisant of but not restricted by when giving advice. However, the more difficult decisions typically involve notification of the patients involved.

## 'At risk' status and the notification dilemma

If there is reason to think that someone may be at increased risk of being infected with CJD, it is clearly important to minimize the risk of the infection being passed on to others. Ways of doing so typically include preventing him or her from donating blood or tissues, and not re-using surgical instruments that might be capable of passing on the infection. However, such precautions require the person to be informed that they are considered to be 'at risk'. This is not a step that can be taken lightly, given that the individual is being told that they might have an incurable and fatal disease, for which there is as yet no reliable test. This could be devastating news, in both psychological and practical terms. Furthermore, the scientific uncertainties make it impossible to quantify the risk adequately: even if infected, they might never develop symptoms. The need to protect public health thus needs to be balanced against the risk of harming individuals.

The Panel has managed this dilemma by applying a threshold (CJD Incidents Panel, 2005). Those found to be at additional risk of carrying any form of CJD (as compared with the general public) are notified and treated as 'at risk' for public health purposes unless that additional risk falls below 1%, even if calculated using pessimistic assumptions. This helps to provide a consistent way of balancing public health and individual distress. The use of a threshold for notification is not new. Similar approaches have been used in relation to other public health problems; for example, HIV infection. However, this dilemma in the context of CJD—and especially vCJD—has rightly focused very serious consideration owing to the potential impact on the individual, and, if inappropriately used, potentially causing unnecessary public disquiet. Notification of individuals considered to be 'at-risk' of CJD by the Panel has primarily been motivated by concern for public health, as well as for fair and open communication with the individuals about their exposure and risk.

In general, the Panel has judged that a risk of 1% (above background population risk) warrants telling individuals of their risk and giving advice to take precautions that may protect others. The Panel recognizes the need to be cognisant of the impact of this information on 'at-risk' individuals, and to recognize the need for good clinical governance arrangements for those affected. Advice packages are constantly updated to meet the needs of persons 'at-risk'.

The Panel receives a stream of requests for advice on individual incidents. Where advice has already been given on similar incident(s), the Panel advises through the secretariat based on the precedent previously agreed. Where the circumstances are new, or new issues are raised, then the incident is brought to the Panel for discussion. The Panel also advises on more generic issues involving substantial groups of individuals.

Clearly, the Panel has an absolute need to provide effective communication. This has raised a number of challenges, not least in the need to communicate to different audiences, including:

◆ The public at large
◆ Known individuals and groups being notified as 'at risk for public health purposes'
◆ Health professionals providing care to these individuals, always including general practitioners (GPs)

- Other people who may see implications for themselves in whatever is announced
- Secretary of State and other Health Ministers (who have given an undertaking that any significant developments will be made public through statements made directly to the House of Commons)
- Chief Medical Officers (as health is a devolved responsibility, there are separate lines of responsibility for England, Wales, Scotland, and Northern Ireland)
- Media
- NHS Trusts
- Blood, tissue, and organ transplant services
- Royal Colleges and other professional bodies (whose practice may well be affected by Panel advice).

These challenges are particularly apparent in considering possible transmission via donated blood, owing to the large numbers of people who are donors or recipients, and the high public interest in blood safety. For example, one question is 'who should be informed first?' If news goes first to the individuals affected—who have the most obvious 'right to know'—they may immediately seek advice from health professionals who have not yet been briefed. Nobody would want to learn about their risk status via stories in the media, yet failure to inform the media can give the appearance of secrecy. The following section provides four examples of how these issues have been managed in practice, and some of the lessons learnt.

## Notification exercises: some examples

### Recipients of blood components from vCJD cases

In the early days of existence of the Incidents Panel, the UK Blood Services asked for advice on the management of recipients of blood components (e.g. red cells) from donors who later developed vCJD. The Panel's initial advice was these recipients should be notified, but recognized the need to develop mechanisms for the notification itself and for providing ongoing support. Work on these aspects was progressing when, in December 2003, surveillance identified a link between a donor and recipient, both of whom developed vCJD (Llewelyn et al., 2004). This was the first direct evidence of transmission of vCJD through blood transfusion, and in 2004 led to anyone who had received a *blood transfusion* since 1980 being excluded from donating blood within the UK.

The Secretary of State announced to the House of Commons in December 2003 that all living recipients of blood components from donors who subsequently developed vCJD would be notified, as already advised by the Panel. To give information to the affected individuals as soon as possible, and with the Christmas and New Year period fast approaching, they were to be notified without delay. The Secretary of State also undertook to keep the House of Commons informed of any future major developments in relation to vCJD and blood.

Records showed that there were 16 living recipients. Notification was carried out through local Health Protection Teams (HPTs). Local Consultants in Communicable Disease Control (CsCDC) worked with others to satisfy themselves that the correct recipient had been identified, usually by reviewing hospital medical records, before contacting each patient's general practitioner (GP). Generally, the GP called in the patient for a consultation and gave the information, backed up with written information provided by the Health Protection Agency (HPA). This latter information was extensive, and GPs often had little time to familiarize themselves with it before passing it on to their patient. Support from the local CCDC and others (for example, a local neurologist, or CJD Section, HPA) was offered and taken up by some GPs. Although the timing of this notification, so close to a major holiday, was less than ideal, most living recipients were notified within a short space of time.

A review of the exercise was conducted through questions to the GPs who were involved. Generally, the very short timeframe and the efforts to conduct the notification before the Christmas holiday season led to GPs feeling pressurized to comply. Many GPs believed that waiting 1 or 2 weeks until surgeries were fully staffed and able to provide the sometimes extensive support needed would have ultimately been in patients' best interests. As against this, any delay might have been seen as trying to conceal bad news or to keep relevant information from those affected.

## Recipients of fractionated plasma products

In contrast to the small numbers involved in the notification just described, a much larger exercise concerned recipients of fractionated plasma products, e.g. coagulation factors such as factor VIII, widely used to treat haemophilia.

The key point here is that these products are manufactured from pools of many thousand donations. This greatly increases the chance of exposure to an infected donor—though it also means that the amount of infected material received may be very small. As an early precaution against vCJD transmission had been to switch from UK- to US-derived plasma in manufacturing these products from late 1998, all notifications related to batches manufactured before then.

The earliest cases of vCJD in former blood donors had triggered notification exercises and product recalls in 1998 and 2000. Because some albumin products had been used outside the UK in other final products, these notifications had international repercussions. Many recipients, exposed to minute quantities of the affected product, were informed that they had been put at risk of vCJD. The current UK risk assessment, not available at the time of these earliest notifications, would not class such individuals as 'at risk'.

However, patients with bleeding disorders may have repeated, long-term exposure to plasma products. Many haemophiliacs had coagulation factor treatment from one or more of the pre-1998 affected batches. Others may have been exposed to batches not yet identified as a risk. Despite very great uncertainties as to the infectivity persisting in these products, a precautionary view suggested that a significant number of recipients could have been exposed to a cumulative risk warranting an 'at risk' classification. Meetings were held with relevant groups (the Haemophilia Centre Doctors Organisation, the Haemophilia Society, and the Immunodeficiency Association), involving medical professionals and patient representatives. Options for notification were explored, bearing in mind that more 'historical' blood donors might develop vCJD in the future. As a result of these consultations, the decision was made to consider all haemophiliacs who have received UK-derived plasma products as being 'at risk' as a group, an umbrella approach that takes care of future notifications. They are all treated accordingly when requiring surgery. This comprises by far the largest 'at risk' group identified to date, numbering about 5000 people. Of the patients with primary immunodeficiency, many fewer had received sufficient product to fall within the 'at risk' classification, and they were managed by individual notification. The two groups were thus treated differently, but they and their clinicians had input into these decisions.

Haemophiliacs were informed by haemophilia centre clinicians, by whom they were known. Staff in these centres had previously been involved in communicating information, when this became known, about risks of HIV and HCV transmission. This experience was invaluable, in addition to that gained with earlier vCJD notifications. Furthermore, these clinicians were well informed about both individual patients and the issues relating to the notification. Staff likely to be involved could be identified in advance (by association with defined patient groups), were invited to a training session to gain background information, and were given opportunities to provide input into the conduct of the exercise. Past exposure to other bloodborne infections heightened the risk of exacerbating patients' existing concerns for their health. So the process was constructed so that patients would be given full information about vCJD and its risk of transmission by plasma products and then allowed to choose whether or not they wished to know if they had received an implicated batch. This allowed them to determine the approach that would enable them to cope best with this further and new uncertainty. In addition, they were informed that precautions would be taken in any case if instruments were used to conduct certain investigations or surgery on themselves. Thus, public health measures would be invoked whether or not the patient chose to know, and the whole group is considered at risk of vCJD for public health purposes. This approach has the advantage of limiting secondary spread should further patients be identified in the future as recipients of an implicated batch.

By the time of this notification, the information resources had been reviewed and amended, partly in response to comments after the first (blood recipient) notification. Different information needs were identified for these plasma product recipient groups. Extensive consultation took place. Nevertheless, timing of the notification was problematical. Because of the previous undertaking given by the then Secretary of State for Health, the notification was to be publicly announced through a statement to the House of Commons. While there was no wish to delay unnecessarily, notification over the peak summer holiday months was not ideal, and would not lend itself to a statement in the House of Commons. Eventually, notification took place in September 2004.

## Donors whose blood was transfused to a patient who later developed vCJD[1]

The notifications outlined above concerned individuals who may be at increased risk of vCJD owing to possible receipt of blood/blood products from an infected donor. Because the incubation period for vCJD may be long, and variable between individuals, the reverse question also arises. A donor whose blood had been transfused to someone who later develops vCJD might be the possible source of their recipient's infection, if no other source has been identified. By implication, such donors are at some additional risk of carrying vCJD, even though they have not shown any symptoms of the disease. DH analysts produced a 'reverse risk assessment' to quantify this risk (Department of Health, 2004; Bennett et al., 2006). The Incidents Panel judged that in the three incidents of this type seen so far—one of which involved 103 donors to a single

---

[1]  This section on notification of blood donors has been adapted from a previous publication (Hewitt, Moore & Soldan, 2006)

vCJD case—the increased risk warranted considering such donors to be 'at-risk' for public health purposes.

In taking this decision, striking the balance between the potential for individual distress and the protection of public health was particularly challenging. It could be argued that those donors who were no longer donating blood presented very little risk to public health and that no further action was needed. On the other hand, they could become organ or tissue donors in the future, or need medical interventions through which other patients could be put at risk. Notification was therefore necessary. For active blood donors, the balance was clearer. The option to leave these donors to continue donating blood, and to discard their blood without their knowledge, was briefly considered. Most would agree that this is not only unethical, but is in complete contrast with a climate of openness and honesty in the blood services' dealing with donors. Such action would almost certainly amount to an illegal assault. Furthermore, although some donors would be distressed by the notification, it was considered that many would be concerned, or angry, had they not been informed.

As this exercise involved donors, the UK blood services felt strongly that they should take responsibility for the initial contact. The notification—though not the actual risk—was a direct result of donating blood, and the duty to give the 'bad news' relating to their blood donation was therefore seen as a responsibility best placed with the blood service. Indeed, donors might think it strange if the message came from anywhere else.

The blood services have a long history of communicating results of blood tests to donors, experience that was obviously relevant. The most usual method used is by letter with back-up in the form of a personal interview either by telephone or face to face according to the donor's needs/preferences. Where the concern is over a disease conventionally recognized as sexually transmitted, however, the donor is invited either to attend an appointment or to telephone without any prior knowledge of the test results. There are obvious disadvantages to this approach: the donor is usually ill-prepared for the news, and lacks any written information until the appointment itself. The opportunity to prepare questions and assess personal implications of the information is lacking, and this limits the value of the personal interview. For HIV and syphilis infections, however, the blood services can arrange rapid referral to local specialist services, which helps to ensure that appropriate clinical care and other support is accessible.

For the donor vCJD notification exercise, options included asking donors to see their GP, calling them in to be told face to face by blood service staff, or notification by letter. Consideration was given to the numbers involved, their location, when, and where they could be seen, the impact of delay, and the anxiety caused by not knowing what the call to an appointment was about. It was concluded that calling donors for an interview without providing any information was unacceptable. It would put the donor at a disadvantage, provoke anxious telephone calls asking for further information, and could lead to greater distress than a well planned written notification. It was decided to follow the procedure in which the blood services have most experience: notification by letter accompanied by written information, with support available from special helplines, GPs, HPA consultants, and CJD experts.

It was recognized that some donors would immediately turn to their GP. The exercise was managed so that GPs always had advance notice of the notification of their patients, were provided with supporting literature, and had information on the support available from health protection units (HPUs). For lapsed donors, the GP was always asked about the current health/circumstances of the ex-donor before any notification letter was sent, although it was made clear that, as this was a public health exercise, non-notification was not an option. As a precaution, GPs were reminded that they should not inform their patient until the blood service had confirmed that the letter had been sent to the donor. One of the two cases of reported distress in a recipient of the notification letter was a donor who was contacted by her GP before she had received the letter from the blood service.

The main message to the donor was contained in a letter identifiable as a communication from the blood service. Its content was identical throughout the UK, differing only in the contact telephone numbers. It was important to make the letter clear, concise, and relevant: including too much information might distract from the key message. It was supplemented by an information document containing facts about vCJD, explanation of the rationale for the notification, questions and answers, and other sources of advice. Although this document was adapted from those used in patient notification exercises, it was 'customized' for blood donors.

Donor helplines generally provided a direct telephone number for the clinical staff office during normal working hours, with a suitably experienced member of staff available to take calls. After hours, calls were transferred to an on-call consultant, suitably briefed and able to deal with enquiries. In the event, only one donor made a call outside normal office hours. Nevertheless, the arrangement remained in place until the last donor notification letters had been sent many weeks later. Because all other calls were received during normal office hours, the blood services were able to ensure that they were dealt with by a small core of clinical staff experienced in dealing over the telephone with anxious or distressed donors. In the event, most calls involved requests for information in an effort to assess personal risk, together with helpful suggestions. The response to the notification suggested that this was a workable and generally acceptable method of communicating difficult information to a fairly large group of people, when information had already been put in the public domain. The public announcement was in many ways helpful, as some donors heard it on the day they received the letter, so that the news was not exactly out of the blue. Contrary to predictions, there were more calls from active donors (who received their letter on the day of the public announcement), than from lapsed donors (who heard some weeks later). Perhaps active donors were more likely to turn first to the blood service for further information. As the main implication for these healthy individuals was that they could no longer act as blood donors, it is possible that the lapsed donors saw the notification as largely irrelevant. Unlike the active donors, they were unlikely to feel disappointed and 'rejected'. Not surprisingly, the blood services also received many calls from unaffected donors who heard the announcement and wanted to check whether they were 'on the list' to be notified.

Although the outcome in respect of donors' experiences was not evaluated at the time, every contact with a donor, GP, or HPU was logged. A formal evaluation is now under way. The information to date indicates that most donors, although anxious, understood the notification and its implications, and had received the information with equanimity. This could reflect the fact that blood donors generally volunteer because of a wish to help others and are conscientious about their responsibility to fellow citizens.

Nevertheless, the timing of the exercise was again problematic. The notification of donors and their GPs had been planned over the early summer of 2005, and was announced by a public statement in the House of Commons on 20 July 2005. An earlier provisional date had been agreed, but other political events brought about a postponement. Not only did this affect critical dates such as posting of letters to the affected individuals and release of press statements and staff briefings both within blood services and in hospitals, it also brought into jeopardy the timing of the exercise. No mass communication exercise such as this should be launched at the end of the week, since letters would be received at the weekend, possibly when immediate support would be less readily available. Yet the Commons announcement was twice delayed from the start of a week, leading to immense concern for those responsible for the exercise. Ultimately, the announcement was made and the exercise was launched, but the undertaking given to the House of Commons was increasingly seen to be an additional difficulty for those planning this type of complicated exercise.

## Other recipients of the donors whose blood was transfused to a patient who later developed vCJD

The identification and notification of a cohort of donors as 'at risk' because they had donated blood which could have been the source of vCJD infection in a recipient raised a further issue. If these donors could have been infected with vCJD, then other patients who had received blood from them could also be at risk. In practice, the risk assessment for these 'other recipients' led to the conclusion that where there had been a small number of donors to the infected recipient, then the other recipients also came within the 1% additional risk threshold. Where the infected recipient had been exposed to a large number of donors (as noted, in one case over 100 donors were identified), the risk for other recipients of these donors fell below the threshold requiring public health measures. Following on from the 2005 donor notification, therefore, was a much smaller exercise to notify the 'other recipients' of the donors involved in the small exposure cases. This exercise followed the model set earlier for transfusion recipients.

## Current and future challenges

As can be seen, much of the Incidents Panel's role has involved working retrospectively to deal with risks of infection following the confirmation of an incident. Nevertheless, some of the current agenda is more forward looking. For example, the DH has sought advice on the management of individuals who might be identified following the introduction of a test to screen blood donations for vCJD. Such tests are currently under development. While a test holds out the promise of reducing the risks of vCJD transmission, the number of false positive results could be high, and could have severe implications for the individuals concerned. This poses great challenges for effective risk communication (Department of Health, 2009).

The Panel has also grappled with the question of how best to deal with 'highly transfused' patients who have received many units of blood components, given by many different donors. Statistically, exposure to more donors puts patients at increasing risk of vCJD, even if there is no reason to suspect that any specific donor is carrying infection. Eventually, this risk will meet the 1% threshold used by the Panel, raising the question of whether such recipients should be regarded as 'at risk'. The difficulty here is that any such calculation depends entirely on the prevalence of vCJD infection. In other contexts, the Panel has dealt with 'incidents' in which a person has been or may have been exposed to infectivity (whether iatrogenically through surgery or through donated blood or tissues). Despite the scientific uncertainties, it is at least possible to establish and explain a tangible link between those potentially 'at risk' and someone with CJD or vCJD. For the 'highly transfused', the link is less tangible, but the risk may be no less real.

The key unknown here is the prevalence of infective donors. As already noted, the appendix tissue survey of Hilton *et al.* (2004) gives a best estimate of about one person in 4000 having signs of subclinical vCJD infection. If the same figure applies to blood donors, and if all those infected have infective blood and if such blood would infect the recipient for certain, analysis suggests that anyone who has received blood components from 40 or more donors will have reached the 1% risk threshold. The difficulty since this credible piece of work was reported is that no other prevalence study has been completed with strong enough results to either prove or disprove its conclusions. Although a large scale prospective survey of tonsillar tissue has shown no similar evidence of infection, advice from the Spongiform Encephalopathy Advisory Committee is that the Hilton *et al.* study provides the best evidence on prevalence available (SEAC, 2008). The analysis provided by the Department of Health has been in-depth and thorough, but the fact remains that the one in 4000 prevalence scenario is based on just one study, not supported by the incidence of cases year on year.

The Chief Medical Officer asked the Panel for its view, which was that a risk as outlined above must exist for the highly transfused. However, the Panel also concluded that, without stronger prevalence data, there should be an exception to the 1% risk threshold and a threshold of 2% would be more appropriate. This would imply taking action with regard to those who had received 80 or more donor exposures, estimated to comprise approximately 30 000 people.

During late 2007 and 2008, the Panel was tasked to work in partnership with the Transmissible Spongiform Encephalopathies Working Group of the Advisory Committee on Dangerous Pathogens to determine the best way to identify and manage this group. Under current proposals, most of the highly transfused will be identified only when their risk status becomes a matter of public health, e.g. when about to embark on surgery to the brain, central nervous system, or posterior eye. However, a more proactive approach is proposed for patients who have gone well beyond 80 exposures, and a proposal stands to notify them, starting with those who have had the most (over 800) exposures. However, this is not a static position, as regularly transfused patients will continue to break through the 80 and 800 exposure ceilings. Very careful consideration continues to be given to balancing the need to notify strata of people affected, given the potential negative effect on their wellbeing versus the need for a precautionary approach to public health.

There is thus the potential for much higher numbers of people being identified as 'at risk for public health purposes'. To advise on the appropriate clinical governance arrangements for individuals identified as 'at risk', including follow-up care and support, the DH convened the vCJD Clinical Governance Advisory Group chaired by Sir William Stewart (CGAG, 2007). It proposes the creation of patient-focused clinical governance arrangements to standardize the care that patients at risk of vCJD receive across the country. It recommends that GPs should take the lead in commissioning care for them, supported by consultant neurologists and the specialist national centres—the National CJD Surveillance Unit and the National Prion Clinic.

The Incidents Panel has commissioned research to learn more about the impact of notifications. Throughout, the concern for those 'at risk' is prompted not only by the chance of their having vCJD or CJD (given the precautionary nature of the 1% threshold, most of those notified will not be infected). It is also prompted by the need for communication to an individual previously unaware of the potential risk of a fatal brain disease. Depending on the individual's reaction, this communication may affect the way they look at and manage the rest of their life. The potential for a negative health impact on someone unlikely to develop the illness itself is obvious. Yet such communication is unavoidable if we are to prevent the risk of prion infection spreading though the population.

## References

Bennett, P. G. & Dobra, S. A. (2006). Risk assessments for vCJD and blood transfusion: a perspective from the United Kingdom. In: Turner M. L. (ed.). *Creutzfeldt-Jacob Disease: Managing the risk of transmission by blood, plasma and tissues.* Bethesda, MD, AABB Press.

Bennett, P. G., Dobra, S. A. & Gronlund, J. (2006). The implications for blood donors if a recipient develops vCJD. *OR Insight,* 19(4): 3–13.

Bennett, P. G., Hare, A., Townshend, J. (2005). Assessing the risk of vCJD transmission via surgery: models for uncertainty and complexity. *Journal of the Optical Research Society,* 56: 202–13.

Bernoulli, C., Siegfried, J., Baumgartner, G. *et al.* (1977). Danger of accidental person-to-person transmission of Creutzfeldt-Jakob disease by surgery. *Lancet,* i: 478–9.

Bishop, M. T., Hart, P., Aitchison, L. *et al.* (2006). Predicting susceptibility and incubation time of human-to-human transmission of vCJD. *Lancet Neurology,* 5: 393–8.

Bruce, M. E., Will, R. G., Ironside, J. W. *et al.* (1997). Transmissions to mice indicate that 'new variant' CJD is caused by the BSE agent. *Nature,* 389: 498–501.

CGAG. (2007). *vCJD Clinical Governance Advisory Group: Independent Review for the Department of Health.* London, Department of Health, March 2007.

CJD Incidents Panel. (2005). *Management of possible exposure to CJD through medical procedures, Framework Document.* August 2005. London, Health Protection Agency.

Clarke, P. & Ghani, A. C. (2004). Projections of the future course of the primary vCJD epidemic in the UK: inclusion of subclinical infection and the possibility of wider genetic susceptibility. *Journal of the Royal Society* (J R Soc Interface doi:10.1098/rsif.2004.0017).

Department of Health. (2000). Risk assessment for transmission of vCJD via surgical instruments: a modelling approach and numerical scenarios. http://www.dh.gov.uk/en/Publicationsandstatistics/Publications/PublicationsPolicyAndGuidance/DH_4075387

Department of Health. (2004) Assessing the implications for blood donors if recipients are infected with vCJD. http://www.dh.gov.uk/en/Publicationsandstatistics/Publications/PublicationsPolicyAndGuidance/DH_4115311

Department of Health. (2005). Assessing the risk of vCJD transmission via surgery: an interim review. http://www.dh.gov.uk/en/Publicationsandstatistics/Publications/PublicationsPolicyAndGuidance/DH_4113541

Department of Health. (2009). Mapping out the consequences of screening donated blood for PrPSc. http://www.dh.gov.uk/en/Publicationsandstatistics/Publications/PublicationsPolicyAndGuidance/DH_094804

Department of Health and Ministry of Agriculture, Fisheries and Food. (1989). *Report of the working party on Bovine Spongiform Encephalopathy (the Southwood Report).* London, DH/MAFF.

Food Standards Agency. (2008). *Meat Hygiene Service Annual Report 2007/8.* London, Food Standards Agency.

Hewitt, P. E., Moore, C. & Soldan, K. (2006). vCJD donor notification exercise: 2005. *Journal of Clinical Ethics,* 1: 172–8.

Hilton, D. A., Ghani, A. C., Conyers, L. *et al.* (2004). Prevalence of lymphoreticular prion protein accumulation in UK tissue samples. *Journal of Pathology,* 203: 733–9.

Llewelyn, C. A., Hewett, P. E., Knight, R. S. *et al.* (2004). Possible transmission of variant CJD by blood transfusion. *Lancet,* 363: 417–21.

Maxwell, R. J. (1997). *An Unplayable Hand? BSE, CJD and the British Government.* London, King's Fund.

NICE. (2006). Patient safety and the risk of transmission of Creutzfeldt–Jakob disease (CJD) via interventional procedures. Available at http://www.nice.org.uk/guidance/IPG196/guidance/pdf/English

Peden, A. H., Head, M. W., Ritchie, D. L. *et al.* (2004). Preclinical vCJD after blood transfusion in a PRNP codon 129 heterozygous patient. *Lancet,* 363: 527–9.

Phillips, L., Bridgeman J. & Ferguson-Smith, M. (2000). *The BSE Inquiry,* Vol. I–XVI. London, Stationery Office.

SEAC. (2008). Prevalence of subclinical variant Creutzfeldt-Jakob disease infections. Position statement, Spongiform Encephalopathy Advisory Committee, http://www.seac.gov.uk/statements/statements.htm

Sutton, J. M., Dickinson, J., Walker, J. T. & Raven, N. D. H. (2006). Methods to minimise the risk of CJD transmission by surgical procedures: where to set the standard? *Clinical Infectious Diseases,* 43: 757–64.

Taylor, D. M. (2000). Inactivation of transmissible degenerative encephalopathy agents: A review. *Veterinary Journal,* 159: 10–17.

Weissmann, C., Enari, M., Klohn, P. C. *et al.* (2002). Transmission of prions. *Journal of Infectious Disease,* 186 (Suppl. 2): S157–S165.

Will, R. G., Ironside, J. W., Zeidler, M. *et al.* (1996). A new variant of CJD in the UK. *Lancet,* 347: 921–5.

Chapter 12

# Contesting the science: public health knowledge and action in controversial land-use developments

Eva Elliott, Emily Harrop, & Gareth H. Williams (Cardiff University)

## Introduction

In the USA and UK, public health assessments of environmental developments and incidents have been based typically on a network of professional experts working through local and national statutory agencies. However, in recent years, in the context of a loss of trust in scientific expertise and political fidelity, traditional approaches to the assessment of health hazards have struggled to connect with the concerns of local communities, resulting in conflict and dissonance in the interpretation of risk. This contestation may concern different aspects of risk: whether or not a particular disease actually exists (such as in Gulf War syndrome); the causal pathway of a particular disease (such as breast cancer or asthma); and the standards of proof and scientific methodology used to investigate a hazard (Brown, 2007).

Protests by local citizens against what they perceive to be exposure to environmentally induced diseases and hazards have recently been of interest to social scientists working in the health field (Brown, 2007). These protests have included mobilizations around the impact of landfill waste sites, opencast mines, chemical weapons, and contaminated water on illnesses or diseases such as asthma, breast cancer, leukaemia, and congenital birth defects (Brown, 2007; Couch & Kroll-Smith, 2000; Futrell, 2003; Moffatt & Pless-Mulloli, 2003; Williams & Popay, 2006). Brown (2007) highlights the way in which public protest has had an important historic role in identifying emerging disease clusters and in challenging the role, methods, and values of science itself. He argues for the development of a 'critical epidemiology', which takes a socio-structural and health inequalities approach and connects this to arguments about social justice. While this 'lay knowledge' is often used to refer to 'common misconceptions' (Moffatt *et al.*, 1995), it is more useful, for some of the reasons Brown has highlighted, to view such knowledge as data rather than as a barrier to knowledge about environmental hazards.

From the perspective of scientists and public agencies, it is increasingly argued that professionals need to communicate risk more effectively, and develop methods of engaging citizens at all stages of their work. Collins & Evans (2002), for example, argue for a special 'third wave' rationale for science and technology, which recognizes the value of expertise while also recognizing the contribution which can be made by 'experience-based expertise' alongside specialist 'accredited experts'. However, such arguments fail to acknowledge the role of citizen protest in challenging claims to scientific neutrality and objectivity (Brown, 1992). Others have argued that we need to pay more attention to the alternative forms of reasoning (Alaszewski & Horlick-Jones, 2002) that citizens bring in disputes over technical questions, such as safe thresholds where the issue for local residents may not just be about avoiding the risk of increased cancer levels but assaults on their ability to live well in their home environments (Moffatt & Pless-Mulloli, 2003; Pless-Mulloli *et al.*, 2001; Northridge & Shepard, 1995; cf Wakefield *et al.*, 2005). What is also of interest in recent disputes, though, is that citizens are now also arming themselves with the conceptual and evidential resources of toxicology, risk assessment, and biomedicine to gain credibility in the eyes of traditional scientists (Couch & Kroll-Smith, 2000; Epstein, 1995).

## Forms of contention and epistemic legitimacy

This relatively new phenomenon, whereby ordinary people contest and challenge the work and judgement of experts, has been explained in terms of epistemological differences between scientific and lay approaches to understanding illness, which cause somewhat inevitable tensions (Brown, 1992; Moffat & Pless-Mulloli, 2003; Potts, 2004); perceptions of flawed science, and the power and hegemonic status of scientific practices, which pose a threat to social identities and ways of knowing (Wynne, 1996a, b). Case study research of these kinds of environmental dispute have illustrated how experiences of flawed or discredited science act as an important source of contention in conflicts over environmental health issues. This body of literature suggests that official accounts which attempt to deny local claims made by virtue of scientific 'fact' will be contested and fought over in often localized contexts. Where 'bad science' is perceived as grounded in the practices of experts and then placed alongside the sophisticated accounts being developed by local groups, official claims pertaining to objectivity and superiority are questioned. This leads to the corrosion of public trust in the credibility of scientific accounts

(Brown, 1992; Couch & Kroll-Smith, 2000; Potts, 2004; Williams & Popay, 2006; Wynne, 1996a, b), although the need to acknowledge the influence of experiences of dependency on trust relationships, alongside this kind of critical, reflexive 'awakening' has also been stressed (Wynne, 1996b). This phenomenon has been termed 'popular epidemiology' (Brown, 1992), and can be seen as part of a process by which people become 'citizen scientists' (Irwin & Wynne, 1996).

This chapter builds on this literature through exploring two different forms of public protest against land developments which were considered by local people to threaten public health. However, they diverged in terms of their means of struggle and, no doubt connected to this, the different opportunity structures open to them. In the first example, a protest group, known as 'Rhondda Against Nanty-y-Gwyddon Tip' or RANT, came to pursue an oppositional course in their struggle to close and make safe a local landfill site. In the second, local residents used the process of a health impact assessment (HIA), through a university-based HIA support unit and the national public health service for Wales, to present evidence on possible risks to public health in an appeal against an application to extend an opencast mine.

Although there are a number of definitions of HIA, the one which is most often cited is known as the Gothenburg Consensus which describes it as:

> . . . a combination of procedures, methods and tools by which a policy, programme or project may be judged as to its potential effects on the health of a population, and the distribution of those effects within the population

(European Centre for Health Policy, 1999, p. 4).

Although, on this definition, HIA sounds like a technocratic tool, the use of HIA sets up a process of dialogue that brings to the table policy-makers, scientific experts, and, increasingly, members of relevant publics to engage in analysis and discussion of evidence and theory (Kemm & Parry, 2004). Whilst a tension between the aims of improving scientific prediction and addressing the democratic deficit has been acknowledged (Parry & Wright, 2003), HIA has the potential to create deliberative spaces through which contestation of evidence can take place. Our preferred definition of HIA would be something like:

> Health impact assessment is a process through which evidence (of different kinds), interests, values and meanings are brought into dialogue between relevant stakeholders (politicians, professionals, and citizens) in order imaginatively to understand and anticipate the effects of change on health and health inequalities in a given population.[1]

---

[1] Presented by Gareth Williams, South East Asian and Oceania Regional Health Impact Assessment Conference, Sydney, Australia, November 2007.

The two case studies are not part of a single research study and make use of different forms of data. The first case study draws on documentary evidence, drawing on data underpinning scientific and public investigations, letters to public officials and the media, council minutes, and press releases to investigate the history of the protest from the perspective of the residents who turned into local activists[2]. The second acknowledges data from the HIA report itself but draws mainly from interviews conducted with residents just over a year after the assessment was completed. The two studies offer complementary insights into the processes available to citizens to voice alternative modes of reasoning about risk and the implications this has at a local level for efforts to manage and communicate contested views of evidence between local citizens and public authorities.

## Public protest and toxic waste

The Nant-y-Gwyddon waste disposal site is on a mountain (Mynydd-y-Gelli) above the adjacent communities of Clydach Vale, Gelli, Ystrad, and Llwynpia in the Rhondda Valley of south Wales. It is located in a region with a long history of coal mining and a population struggling with the social and economic legacy of the industry's demise. Waste disposal operations at the site began in 1988 and in the mid 1990s their licence was amended to the disposal of industrial in addition to domestic waste. The site was shut down in March 2002 on the recommendations of an Independent Investigation carried out on behalf of the Welsh Assembly, following 5 years of concerted and highly publicized protest action by RANT and others.

The earliest community efforts at investigating the suspected health problems associated with the site can be traced to the first survey sent out by local activists in December 1996, which found an increasing frequency of a range of symptoms, including headache, sore throat, fatigue, and general malaise. Residents linked these to 'the obnoxious fumes and poor air quality we are experiencing since the . . . company took over management of the Nant-y-Gwyddon refuse site'[3]. In the public meetings that followed, more serious illnesses such as gastroschisis and sarcoidosis also started to be detected and suspected of being linked to the tip[4]. As observations of these symptoms and

---

[2] The research project only focused on the period up to the closure of the tip in March 2002, although RANT remained, and are still active today.

[3] Letter to Council, Environmental Services, 13/12/1996.

[4] Letter to MP, 10/2/1997.

their possible connections accumulated, a medical committee within RANT was set up to research and campaign on these problems[5].

## Official studies: friend or foe?

In the period 1997 to 2001, various official investigations were commissioned and undertaken. RANT was actively engaged with several of these studies at different stages of the research process, but most actively in the two epidemiological studies which took place in the summer of 1997 (Fielder *et al.*, 2000) and Autumn 1998 (Welsh Combined Centres for Public Health, 2000), and the 'health clinics', led and coordinated by the then health authority in the summer of 1998 (Bro Taff Health Authority, 1999). However, although RANT campaigned for and actively cooperated and participated in these official efforts, from the start they also experienced frustration and disappointment in terms of both implementation and outcome. This frustration was expressed in a letter written to the appointed epidemiologist following the publication of the inconclusive findings of the first epidemiological survey, which was recognized to have put them 'in a "Catch 22" situation from which we are having problems extricating ourselves'[6]. That RANT continued to engage with official efforts, in spite of these frustrations, seems not only due to their perceived dependency on these bodies and their 'accredited' studies, but also to a perceived (albeit slim) opportunity to influence the methodology and, by implication, outcomes of the research. This in turn seems to have been inspired firstly by a growing confidence that RANT seemed to develop in their own knowledge in the face of contradictory 'official' claims, and second, by some detection of sympathy and possible allegiance amongst the scientists themselves.

A third important factor shaping RANT's continued engagement with official studies was, somewhat ironically, their experiences of poor and apparently fallible scientific practices. For example, in their meetings with the team of epidemiologists, RANT was made acutely aware of the poor quality of routine data used by the first epidemiological study, and the severe limitations this would place upon any conclusions to be drawn from the study[7]. In their evidence to the investigation, numerous examples were also given by residents of what a resident described as 'Environment Agency cock ups' with regard to sampling practices; e.g. how water testing was carried out when it was pouring with rain, and hence diluted, or a sample was taken and then forgotten about for

---

[5] Resident, oral evidence to investigation, 2001.

[6] Letter to epidemiologist, Wales College of Medicine, 18/11/97.

[7] Letter to Council (Environmental Services), 18/11/1997.

a week.[8] The failure of the respective authorities to coordinate simultaneously the air quality testing and health clinics was similarly seen at best to be an example of incompetence but also, at worst, an intentional move to undermine any chances of conclusive findings.[9]

Residents also recalled experiences which they felt demonstrated more directly how 'science' might be applied selectively to support political objectives. On discussing how a report into gas and leachate management was presented to councillors, one activist explained; 'I mean they come out with the conclusions at the end and they use that lovely word "unlikely". I really do think it's quite an enormous word for them . . . the summary hasn't mentioned problems with burn-off, or the design fault with valve chamber and discharge of leachate into river . . . the members weren't told of this'. Another RANT member similarly explained how, at a meeting with the Environment Agency, it was noted that water sample readings of Nant-y-Gwyddon stream on average were satisfactory, but when asked about individual readings, two readings were found to be exceptionally high, the problem thus being that the 'average is low but peaks are high—pollution is pollution even if it only happens once. The Environment Agency should have said so and not used average figures to draw attention away from high readings'.[10]

## A critical cooperation

Through their continuing engagements with official experts, RANT was not only compelled to press for further investigations, but also to steer and keep a check on them. One of the ways in which they saw a role for themselves here was in their endeavours to impress as much of their local knowledge upon the respective bodies, who were seen to be overly reliant on 'official' information sources, which in turn were seen to be at odds with their own experiences. For example, whilst the local health authority, drawing on a local health profile, initially reported no unusual illness clusters in the area[11], RANT countered these claims in a letter to the local Director of Public Health by providing details of the number and names of confirmed cases of sarcoidosis, gastroschisis and 'bad abscesses', and called for a more 'in-depth' investigation.[12] Similarly, in a letter to the council the following year, RANT expressed 'delight'

---

[8] Resident, oral evidence presented to the investigation, 2001.

[9] Resident, oral evidence presented to the investigation, 2001.

[10] Resident, oral evidence presented to the investigation, 2001.

[11] Bro Taff Health Authority, Local Health Profile, April 1997.

[12] Letter to Director Public Health, Bro Taff Health Authority, 13/8/1997.

that the council were going to carry out their own dust sampling, enclosed a map highlighting distances from the tip which might be of assistance, and suggested that villages further afield should be sampled. By way of compromise, RANT proposed that they observe the sampling and suggested the streets 'that appear to have suffered the most severe problems from the gases but that the council chooses the houses'.[13]

A further dimension to this engagement activity was through a more overt critique of official methods and conduct. With respect to the first epidemiological survey, RANT were quick to point out a fundamental methodological limitation with the study; namely, that it did not incorporate a door-to-door survey, and hence 'The number of reported cases to us of the exacerbation of children's asthma, sticky eyes and ear infections is not going to be picked up by this study and this will be a very sad day for the people of the Rhondda'.[14] In a similar vein, in a letter to the epidemiologist, RANT expressed their unhappiness with the methodology of the 'time to pregnancy study' on the grounds that, by interviewing women who were 20–40 weeks' pregnant, the study would fail to identify the large numbers of women who had undergone spontaneous or medically induced abortions (owing to congenital abnormality) prior to this date. To back this criticism, they used a combination of local knowledge on women in the area who fell into such a category, combined with the findings of a paper in the *Lancet* reporting the 'Eurohazcon' (Dolk *et al.*, 1998)[15]. When the findings of such studies failed to go their way, RANT were then well placed to draw attention to these methodological criticisms, as part of a damage limitation strategy intended to undermine official claims[16]. Spurred on by their experience-based convictions (regarding the tip) and doubts (regarding official claims), RANT also embarked on their own alternative research programme, independent of official efforts, examples of which included surveys, extensive literature searching, analysis of available datasets, and dust and water sampling programmes.

This case study shows the way in which conflict can give rise to research activity, and quite sophisticated contestation and collaboration over the forms of evidence employed, the robustness of the methodology on which it is based, and the political context in which research is used. In the next case we take another example of public concern, but one which was channelled and facilitated through an expert-led process of health impact assessment.

---

[13] Letter to Council, Environmental Services, 9/3/98.

[14] Letter to Director Public Health, Bro Taff Health Authority, 13/8/1997.

[15] Letter to epidemiologist, Wales College of Medicine, 9/9/98.

[16] Letter to Council (Environmental Services) 18/11/1997.

## Health impact assessment and opencast mining

The origin of this particular HIA was a request by a resident to examine the impact of a proposed extension to an existing opencast mine (Welsh Health Impact Assessment Support Unit). A group of residents living in villages bordering existing opencast operations and the proposed extension believed that opencast mining in the area had already had a negative impact on their health, and that future operations would result in more years of living with the cumulative effects of exposure to hazards such as particulate matter, dust, and noise. Promised land treatment and rehabilitation would take at least a further 5 years, but, after what was felt to be a series of broken promises from the company, the residents expressed doubts that the company would restore land in the foreseeable future.

Various attempts at improving communication between the company and local residents by the local planning authorities were felt to have failed. For instance, two consultation meetings were organized, but representatives from the company did not attend (Golby & Elliott, 2007). A local action group was set up to appeal against the application and approaches were made to an HIA support unit based at a university. Following discussions between the researcher based at the unit and the residents' group, a steering group was formed which included the researcher from the Welsh Health Impact Assessment Support Unit (WHIASU), representatives, including a researcher from the National Public Health Service (NPHS), and community members representing relevant interest groups. Two officials with specialist knowledge, one from the local public health team and the other from environmental health, declined to be part of the steering group but attended as observers at meetings and provided technical advice on particular issues regarding public health, pollution control, and environmental monitoring. These officers provided this support with the full agreement of their respective Chief Executives. Although the researchers met with representatives from the mining company, these representatives refused to take part in the process.

Initial steering group meetings identified key health concerns which most commonly included respiratory problems, including asthma, cardiovascular problems, and stress-related illness but also included diabetes, brain tumours, skin diseases, eye irritation, and congenital abnormalities. These were largely perceived to be related to particulate matter, dust, and noise produced by the site.

In terms of the process, the HIA itself consisted of a review of published research literature and relevant local and national reports and documents, a 'guided' visit to the site, and six focus groups with groups of residents identified as being 'at risk' from opencast operations. These included residents living near the present opencast, older people, residents involved in outdoor pursuits, local business representatives, and parents of young children. There was also one mixed group of local residents. Draft versions were checked for both technical inaccuracies and local salience and finally agreed by the steering group. Material from the HIA was considered by the relevant planning authorities and, though it is unclear what part the HIA played, the planning application was refused in its existing form.

## Credibility and control

This simple sounding process was beset by conflict and disagreement about definitions of legitimate evidence, fair processes, and power and control. Whilst for the researchers and the statutory representatives the concern was to consider the evidence using accepted methodological standards of robustness and impartiality, residents wanted to present data which they felt demonstrated unequivocally the health problems that they experienced and their perceived links to the opencast operations. The request by residents for a survey of self-reported health complaints in the area was rejected by the researchers on the basis that the results would not meet the statistical standards required for valid sample surveys. In any case, the decision- making timescale was such that there would not be time for it to be considered as material evidence. Other pieces of research evidence that residents had found over the internet were also rejected for various reasons concerning the soundness of the results and their lack of application to the local context:

> And of course they [the residents] were swamping them with material, they were looking on the net and all sorts of places. The other thing as well is that the net isn't a very good primary reference source—you can find evidence of all sorts on there and what you don't get is the context. So you get one paper that says one thing and if it suits your argument you will latch onto it, but forgetting that there are 95 papers that say completely the contrary. So there was a lot of that we had to filter out.
>
> Local authority officer

Similarly, there were concerns about the methods of data collection that the researchers themselves employed. On the one hand there was a concern about the reliability of the data that would be generated from focus groups as only small numbers, and possibly unrepresentative groups, of residents were involved. On the other hand, they were concerned that focus group participants, who may not have been active in opposing the application, would express views that would not confirm that their own fears had any validity. Whilst the advertising for volunteers to participate in focus groups was carried out by local activists, the identification of participants and the process of conducting the groups were controlled by the researcher. This meant that, whilst HIA provided a recognized mechanism through which their concerns about impact could be considered, it was a process over which they felt they had little control.

> We didn't have a clue who was going to turn up to these focus groups, so we tended to take a back seat totally and just listen, and hope that people said the things we wanted them to—which they did, it was all very positive towards our fight. It was nerve racking, because we didn't know the people. We might have known one or two but a lot of people we had never met or anything. And you get this young chap coming in speaking against it. The focus groups were very, very positive.
>
> Resident activist

Sometimes these debates resulted in open hostility to the researcher who reflected that much of the HIA process involved managing and responding to deeply felt emotions (Golby & Elliott, 2007). Interviews with residents and officials who participated in the HIA about a year after the report was submitted indicate that the HIA provided a fragile attempt to sustain a process that attempts to be both democratic and scientifically credible. For residents this meant that there was a constant need to consider the pay-off between having control of the process and the end product being seen as credible in the eyes of the decision-makers.

> But if we got up and did our own HIA, that would have absolutely no standing, no worth and wouldn't even be useful for the time it would take up . . . We just took part like zombies—because we didn't have a clue what it involved or what was going to come out of it . . . I think we were lucky to have had one that was organized and led by somebody else who wasn't one of us.
>
> Resident activist

The HIA required often uncomfortable deliberations between residents, officials, and the researchers as to what should be considered legitimate and what was not in terms of evidence. For the researcher, good qualitative evidence had its own power to communicate the meaning of risk, though residents were wary of this, believing that a survey documenting perceptions of ill-health would be more convincing than data obtained through in-depth discussions with small groups of people.

To a certain extent they were right. Resident activists were aware of the way in which HIA attempts to embrace conflicting views of what is considered credible evidence. In a memorandum submitted by another opencast company on the role of coal production in future energy supply in Wales, they criticized HIAs which they saw as drawing on qualitative evidence and the views of the vocal few:

> Whilst community engagement in health impact assessments can have significant benefits, efforts need to be made to engage with the silent majority of the community

as well as the vocal members of that community. Additionally, it needs to be recognized that the more vocal members of communities often have ideas which are poorly founded in fact and there may be a role for those conducting the HIA in educating them and reducing the prejudices that they have gained from ill-informed media reports and other sources.

Supplementary memorandum submitted by company[17]

One resident, in response to some of the responses to the HIA, reflected on the way in which lay knowledge is framed as anecdote to reduce its claims to 'truth'.

> What I feel with the HIA as well is when it does get discredited for not being scientific and it gets discredited for being anecdotal. Well if you are going to have a public consultation process as part of the community's involvement and community-based decisions, everything is going to be anecdotal, so you either don't take any notice and don't have consultation, or you do; and if you do you don't negatively describe it as anecdotal. They say it's anecdotal if its positive, but what we have found is that it is recorded as being anecdotal in a negative way—'just anecdotal'.

Resident activist

This places residents with concerns about impact in a 'double bind' where, because residents are anxious and stressed about possible threats of local hazards, they are seen as sensitized and therefore all data which draws on these concerns and actions, such as qualitative data on individual experiences and quantitative data such as GP consultations, are dismissed as bias. As other researchers have noted, this results in concerns about health effects among people who experience the effects to be systematically overlooked (Moffat et al., 1995).

## Meaning and perspective

Although concern about the opencast mine was framed in terms of its potential impact on identifiable disease or illness, many of the focus group discussions about the impact of living with opencast revolved around the assault of coal dust on the senses—its taste, its feel—and its impact on the everyday life—dirty washing on the line and 'dust sandwiches'. However, one lever for local residents in the HIA was the broad social definition of health that the process operationalized. This was seen as legitimizing their experiences of the impact of opencast on their everyday lives within a public health frame.

---

[17] http://www.parliament.the-stationery-office.co.uk/pa/cm200607/cmselect/cmwelaf/ucenergy/m13.htm. Accessed 19 September 2008.

> It says . . . the WHO [*World Health Organization*] . . . its not just impact on physical health, its total health and that comes out in it, and I learned from that because I didn't know that at the time. And I thought this is a good way of looking at it, because they say that there is no scientific proof that dust from the site will harm you and that's it for them as far as health is concerned, and anyway they say 'we're not breaching guidelines' and they have these set thresholds. Its affecting us—people can see it, feel it, touch the dust, but because it's within them it's as if you are complaining about nothing and that makes you feel terrible.
>
> Resident activist

This reframing of the 'health impact' meant that different forms of knowledge and evidence could be brought together into a meaningful understanding of people's personal and community concerns. In an uncomfortable, often conflictual deliberative process, HIA provided the beginnings of a collective *verstehende* theorizing creating 'new knowledge spaces' for the development of a more civic epistemology (Elliott & Williams, 2008). For at least one of the specialist experts involved in the HIA, the process developed his own appreciation that it was 'what matters' that was meaningful, and not just evidence:

> There have been occasions in the past where a good number of the houses have been peppered by black dust, there have been occasions where there have been noise problems, there have been occasions where there has been over pressure from the blasting going on—still within tolerable limits, but enough to disturb people. So I think if someone was to turn round and just dismiss what the residents have got to say then that is completely the wrong thing to do.
>
> Local authority officer

## Conclusions

Both case studies could be seen as presenting possible ways for citizens both to contest and produce new forms of possible reasoning about the effects of controversial land developments on the health of local populations. Although the extent of public influence is difficult to discern, both groups could claim to have had some success: for RANT in the closure of the tip and for the opencast activists a rejection of the application put forward by the company. However, both these consultations provided challenges for public health officials charged with managing risk communication in contentious environments.

The first case study illustrates how communities caught up in more oppositional kinds of protests might engage with science as a means to advance their cause. Somewhat ironically, the increasingly oppositional and instrumental nature of this campaign meant that the activists were compelled to accept the terms of a scientific epistemology which they felt was problematical. It meant that they were essentially required to focus on whether toxic waste was responsible for causing particular identifiable diseases and had to collude with an underlying acceptance that their concerns were legitimate only if they could identify a connection between levels of hazardous waste and serious illness. The very acceptance that the argument was about whether minimum thresholds for the protection of human subjects against identifiable disease had been breached meant that other concerns about health impact were largely outside the sphere of discourse in the struggle to secure a public inquiry. Such concerns were clearly important, however, and were widely articulated during the investigation itself. They included more everyday and mundane health complaints such as headaches and nausea as well as upset caused by foul smells, flies, and other issues such as stress and loss of enjoyment of their homes and surrounding area.

The HIA, on the other hand, perhaps because it incorporated a broader notion of wellbeing, embraced what might be seen as a more hermeneutic model of risk assessment. That is, the meanings of risk in terms of residents' own lived experience were accepted as having validity in their own right albeit reported alongside what was known about the extent of risk to specific diseases. What was important about the process is that it provided a sometimes emotionally charged deliberative space through which to contest and debate the validity and salience of the impacts within a particular local context. For public health and other statutory officials, HIA provides an opportunity to identify, debate, respond, and therefore better manage concerns raised by local people about controversial land developments.

However, the activists in the HIA, like RANT, also 'submitted' to processes that they felt failed to illuminate the risks as they saw them. This selective 'silence' by activists in favour of a sustained but critical engagement with the dominant scientific epistemology supports Wynne's emphasis on the role of dependency in shaping lay–expert relationships (Wynne, 1996b). In this respect, RANT found themselves trapped within the prevailing orthodoxy, even though they, like protestors in other studies, were frustrated by failures to establish clear links, let alone causal connections, between a 'hazardous' site and a particular illness or disease (Moffatt et al., 1995; Moffatt & Pless-Mulloli, 2003). The advantage for activists involved in the HIA is that the process at least provided an opportunity for questions about the nature of scientific method to be debated within the process itself, though one could argue that the dominant *social* science epistemology is what ultimately shaped lay and professional relationships in this case.

This is not to downplay the importance of local activists' efforts. It has been pointed out that communities are usually the first to identify a connection between toxic hazards and health, hence the importance of maintaining this kind of focus (Brown, 2007; Moffatt *et al.*, 1995). Furthermore, although there would be a danger in a perspective which panders to or flatters publics through an uncritical privileging of lay perspectives, we would argue that the development of social and physical scientific methods and theories themselves are tested and developed through an engagement with civil society (Elliott & Williams, 2008). Far from being 'duped', RANT, in particular, exposed fundamental flaws in scientific epistemology and practice, and, in their espousal of the precautionary principle, both groups of activists challenged the status of dominant risk management approaches in public life. Not least, the favourable outcomes secured for both groups also lends credence to this aspect of their struggle.

Both case studies emphasize the importance of seeing knowledge about public health issues in the round, and recognizing that 'science' is often flawed and inadequate, that it does not ask the questions that are of importance to those most severely affected, and it is very often used to exclude the legitimate and well informed perspectives of local people.

## Acknowledgements

The studies here were reviewed by Cardiff School of Social Sciences Ethics Committee. The Nant-y-Gwyddon study is part of a case studentship funded by the ESRC and supported though a partnership between the Wales Centre for Health and Cardiff University School of Social Sciences. WHIASU is commissioned by, and works in partnership with, the Wales Centre for Health. Interviews with HIA participants were part of a study by WHIASU to explore public engagement in HIA. Many individuals have given their support to this study. We would like to thank in particular Chloe Chadderton, Alison Golby and Carolyn Lester.

## References

Alaszewski, A. & Horlick-Jones, T. (2002). Risk and health: review of current research and identification of areas for further research. http://www.kent.ac.uk/chss/docs/riskandhealth.PDF. Accessed 19 September 2008.

Bro Taf Health Authority. (1999). Report on complaints of ill health perceived due to exposure to Nantygwyddon landfill site: A descriptive survey. *Archives of Welsh Assembly Independent Investigation into Nantygwyddon Landfill Site.* Welsh Assembly Government.

Brown, P. (1992). Popular epidemiology and toxic waste contamination: lay and professional ways of knowing. *Journal of Health and Social Behaviour,* 33: 267–81.

Brown, P. (2007). *Toxic Exposure: Contested Illnesses and the Environmental Health Movement.* New York, Columbia University Press.

Collins, H. M. & Evans, R. J. (2002). The third wave of science studies: studies of expertise and experience. *Social Studies of Science,* 32: 235–96.

Couch, S. & Kroll-Smith, S. (2000). Environmental movements and expert knowledge: Evidence for a new populism. In: S. Kroll-Smith, P. Brown, & V. J. Gunter (ed.). *Illness and the Environment: A reader in contested medicine*. New York, New York University Press, pp. 384–404.

Dolk, H., Vrijheid, M. & Armstrong, B. *et al.* (1998). Risk of congenital anomalies near hazardous-waste landfill sites in Europe: the EUROHAZCON study. *Lancet*, 352: 423–7.

Elliott, E. & Williams, G. H. (2008). Developing public sociology through health impact assessment. *Sociology of Health and Illness*, 30: 1101–16.

Epstein, S. (1995). The construction of lay expertise: AIDS activism and the forging of credibility in the reform of clinical trials. *Science, Technology & Human Values*, 20: 408–37.

European Centre for Health Policy. (1999). *Health Impact Assessment: Main concepts and suggested approach (Gothenburg Consensus)*. Brussels, European Centre for Health Policy.

Fielder, H. M. P., Poon-King, C. M., Palmer, S. R., Moss, N. & Coleman, G. (2000). Assessment of impact on health of residents living near the Nant-y-Gwyddon landfill site: retrospective analysis. *British Medical Journal*, 320: 19.

Futrell, R. (2003). Framing processes, cognitive liberation, and NIMBY protest in the U.S. chemical-weapons disposal conflict. *Sociological Inquiry*, 73: 359–86.

Golby, A. & Elliott, E. (2007). Community participation in a controversial planning application: a challenge for research practice. *Qualitative Researcher*, 6: 7–9.

Irwin, A. & Wynne, B. (1996). Introduction In: Irwin, A. & Wynne, B. (eds). *Misunderstanding Science? The Public Construction of Science and Technology*. Cambridge, Cambridge University Press, pp. 1–18.

Kemm, J. & Parry, J. M. (2004). The development of HIA. In: J. Kemm, J. Parry, & S. Palmer (eds). *Health Impact Assessment*. Oxford, Oxford University Press, pp. 15–23.

Moffatt, S. & Pless-Mulloli, T. (2003). 'It wasn't the plague we expected.' Parents' perceptions of the health and environmental impact of opencast coal mining.' *Social Science & Medicine*, 57: 437–51.

Moffatt, S., Phillamore, P., Bhopal, R. & Foy, C. (1995). 'If this is what it's doing to our washing, what is it doing to our lungs?' Industrial pollution and public understanding in north-east England. *Social Science and Medicine*, 41: 883–91.

Northridge, M. E. & Shepard, P. M. (1995). Environmental racism and public health. *American Journal of Public Health*, 87:730–731.

Parry, J. & Wright, J. (2003). Community participation in health impact assessments: Intuitively appealing but practically difficult. *Bulletin of the World Health Organization*, 81: 388.

Pless-Mulloli, T., Howel, D. & Prince, H. (2001). Prevalence of asthma and other respiratory symptoms in children living near and away from opencast coal mining sites. *International Journal of Epidemiology*, 30: 556–63.

Potts, L. (2004). An epidemiology of women's lives: the environmental risk of breast cancer. *Critical Public Health*, 14: 133–47.

Wakefield, S., Elliott, S., Eyles, J. & Cole, D. (2005). Taking environmental action: the role of local composition, context, and collective. *Environmental Management*, 37: 40–53.

Welsh Combined Centres for Public Health. (2000). Report on the study of time to pregnancy. *Archives of Welsh Assembly Independent Investigation into Nantygwyddon Landfill Site*. Welsh Assembly Government.

Welsh Health Impact Assessment Support Unit. Health Impact Assessment of the Proposed Extension to Margam Opencast Mine. Available at http://www.wales.nhs.uk/sites3/ Documents/522/Kenfig%20Hill%20Final%20%2D%20Dec%2005.pdf. Accessed 19 September 2008.

Williams, G. H. & Popay, J. (2006). Lay knowledge and the privilege of experience, 2nd edn. In: D. Kelleher, J. Gabe & G. Williams (eds). *Challenging Medicine*. London, Routledge, pp. 122–45.

Wynne, B. (1996a). 'May the sheep safely graze? A reflexive view of the expert-lay knowledge divide'. In: S. Lash, B. Szerszynski, B. Wynne *et al.* (eds). *Risk, Environment and Modernity: Towards a New Ecology*. London, Sage, pp. 27–43.

Wynne, B. (1996b). Misunderstood misunderstandings: social identities and the public uptake of science. In: A. Irwin & B. Wynne (eds). *Misunderstanding Science? The Public Construction of science and Technology*. Cambridge, Cambridge University Press, pp. 19–46.

Chapter 13

# A precautionary tale—the role of the precautionary principle in policy-making for public health

Denis Fischbacher-Smith & Kenneth Calman
(University of Glasgow)

## Introduction

> Our age is not more dangerous—not more risky—than those of earlier generations, but the balance of risks and dangers has shifted. We live in a world where hazards created by ourselves are as, or more, threatening than those that come from outside (Giddens, 1999, p. 34).

Much of the debate within the social sciences in recent years has centred on the relationship between risk and modernity and the emergence of the so-called 'risk society' (Adam, 1998; Beck, 1992; Bulkeley, 2001; Giddens, 1990; 1999). One thesis is that modern society, whilst it has overcome many of the difficulties that faced its predecessors, has begun to create problems as a function of its own activities—especially around sociotechnological issues and the role of 'science' in society (Angell, 1996; Erikson, 1994; Irwin, 1995; 2006; Lupton, 1999; Perrow, 1984; Tenner, 1996). This in turn has generated considerable issues for public health policy (Edwards & Elwyn, 2001; Petersen & Bunton, 2002; Rhodes, 1998; Tulloch & Lupton, 1997). The manner in which we deal with uncertainty (Taleb, 2007; Wynne, 1992) has transcended many aspects of modern life, and some have argued that the resultant fear that society often displays does not reflect the 'true' nature of those risks (Bauman, 2006; Robin, 2004; Shiloh et al., 2007; Siegrist et al., 2007; Trumbo et al., 2007).

In describing the 'liquid fear' of modern society, Bauman (2006) argues that:

> Fear is at its most fearsome when it is diffuse, scattered, unclear, unattached, unanchored, free floating, with no clear address or cause; when it haunts us with no visible rhyme or reason, when the menace we should be afraid of can be glimpsed everywhere but is nowhere to be seen. (p. 2).

Bauman sees our current concerns as the 'greenhouse of fears' and argues that modernity was believed to move us away from that fear. Post-modernity, however, seems to have returned us to a more fearful condition in which we are acutely aware of our susceptibility to danger (Bauman, 2006; Beck, 1992; Giddens, 1990) and where the perceptions that we hold of risk are perhaps more important in our construction of reality than are the attempts of 'science' to determine those risks. Take the recent example of the outbreak of H1N1 influenza (swine flu) in Mexico (McVeigh & Tuckman, 2009). The spread of the virus and the communication of that hazard are both influenced by the speed of our 'communication' processes. Those who are exposed to the hazard are able to travel by aircraft all over the world, thereby exposing new victims to the virus at a speed that would have been impossible for influenza outbreaks in the early 20th century. At the same time, the speed of modern communications means that we are quickly made aware of this 'risk'[1] and that compounds the sense of dread associated with the event.

Uncertainty and our abilities to 'manage' it have ultimately become the focus of our fears. When accidents occur then there is a sense that those charged with the management of that risk have failed in their duty—even though it is impossible to manage out the risk in every human endeavour. All too often, failures in one set of activities have the effect of 'perceptively irradiating' other areas by undermining the confidence that people have in the management of the system. This can even occur where there is no apparent crossover between the activities or where the accident took place in a different location (see Chapter 16). Where outcomes have a significant potential to cause harm and where there is uncertainty around the calculation of the probabilities associated with those outcomes, then there is a need to recognize the impact that this 'double uncertainty' of both cause and effect will have on perceptions and the generation of fear. Within this set of discussions, the precautionary principle has emerged as a potentially important policy tool for environmental protection and, more recently, public health management.

Our aim in this chapter is to examine some of the issues that arise from the relationship between fear and perceptions of risk and the implications that the precautionary principle might have in shaping the conflict that ensues in risk debates. We also explore the nature of the precautionary approach in practical terms and the nature of uncertainty as a core element in the process of public health risk management.

---

[1] See also the coverage of the problem by the BBC at http://news.bbc.co.uk/1/hi/world/americas/8019566.stm (Accessed 27th April 2009)

## Uncertainty—unpicking a construct

> The message is that there are no 'knowns'. There are thing we know that we know. There are known unknowns. That is to say there are things that we now know we don't know. But there are also unknown unknowns. There are things we don't know we don't know. So when we do the best we can and we pull all this information together, and we then say well that's basically what we see as the situation, that is really only the known knowns and the known unknowns. And each year, we discover a few more of those unknown unknowns— Donald Rumsfeld (2002), Press Conference at NATO Headquarters, Brussels, Belgium[2].

Uncertainty, as exemplified by Donald Rumsfeld's now infamous quote, is seen to have multiple dimensions (Knight, 1964), and the dynamics of the construct have, in turn, considerable implications for risk communication and public health. Before exploring the precautionary principle in more detail we need to consider its relationship with the nature of uncertainty, as it is our contention here that the two are symbiotic.

In popular usage we tend to consider risk and uncertainty as related. Perhaps a more useful categorization would be to consider those elements that have a degree of predictive validity (Rumsfeld's known unknowns) as separate from those that are unpredictable or unknown. Clearly these issues generate considerable problems, in both policy and risk communication terms, as Rumsfeld's attempts to distinguish between the various elements of uncertainty testify. If we try to disentangle the construct of uncertainty, then several strands emerge that relate to the manner in which humans try to deal with the 'unknowns' they face[3].

The most obvious element of uncertainty relates to the manner in which particular hazards become realized. Key elements here are the processes by which relatively minor issues can escalate into major catastrophic events. Perrow, for example, argues that the complex interactions that take place between elements of the system can allow failures to migrate from the original triggering event and to do so in ways that create problems for those charged with managing the system. At the same time, he argues that the speed of this

---

[2] There are several accounts of this speech. This is taken from the US Department of Defence official transcript of the speech and is available on line at: http://www.defenselink.mil/transcripts/transcript.aspx?transcriptid=3490

[3] This draws on the elements identified by Knight (1964) along with some additional elements that are seen to be relevant to our current discussions here. Knight argues that uncertainty needs to be separated from risk as the latter has a measurable dimension to it. Uncertainty can be indeterminate by its very nature. As such, a true 'risk' is not uncertain as it can be quantified and may even have a degree of predictive validity. Knight distinguishes between measurable and unmeasurable forms of uncertainty.

interaction will be such that it also creates problems for control owing to the manner in which the event escalates. This 'tight coupling' and 'interactive complexity' (Perrow, 1984) represent a significant source of uncertainty within organizations. The weaknesses this generates are frequently masked by the assumptions made by those responsible for managing the system (Pauchant & Mitroff, 1992; Turner, 1976). We can term this as 'causal uncertainty'—we do not necessarily understand the mechanisms by which these failures occur and we certainly cannot predict them.

In addition to this *causal uncertainty*, there are also problems that arise out of the *emergence* that occurs within sociotechnical systems. Here the interaction between various elements of the system produces non-linear effects—that is, it will create a situation where cause does not equal effect. This emergence can arise from the design or operational characteristics of the system and the conditions it generates will present managers and operators with problems that may exceed their experience base or management protocols. The impact of their decision-making process within the uncertainty generated by these conditions will add a further layer of emergence to the point that the system may well spiral beyond its contingency limits (Smith, 2005; 2006). This 'escalation uncertainty' interacts with issues around the uncertainty present in causal underpinnings to create conditions that are confounding and difficult to control.

A third element of uncertainty concerns the *uncertainty of outcome* (Knight, 1964). This is important when we consider those activities which are moved from the controlled environment of the laboratory into the 'real world'. Again, processes of emergence play a significant role here. The uncertainty of outcome can be seen to lie at the heart of a number of public health scares in the UK (notably BSE, genetically modified crops, and mobile telephone masts), where the relationships between 'exposure' and response were generally scientifically unknown (in real world settings). These types of problems have been termed 'trans-scientific' (Weinberg, 1972) in that they go beyond the abilities of science to prove. It is important to note that in some cases this may be a relatively temporary problem and that science may, with further advances in knowledge, be able to provide a burden of proof. Other problems may, however, be intractable (Johnson, 1972). The fear associated with the uncertainty around causality, escalation, and outcome interact together to create a complex mosaic of fear that is difficult for policy-makers and those charged with risk communication to penetrate.

A fourth element is seen in terms of the *perceptual uncertainty* (Knight, 1964) that may arise. Whilst there is recognition that public perceptions of risk are potentially problematic in policy terms, it should also be noted that experts may be subject to 'perceptual blindness', particularly in terms of any challenges to their dominant paradigmatic views of the world. Similarly, a consensus within the scientific community is no guarantee that this is based upon the result of universally accepted research. Rather, other political factors may play a role in shaping that consensus (Collingridge, 1992; Collingridge & Reeve, 1986; Smith, 1990). Thus, and in the context of risks that are trans-scientific (Weinberg, 1972), perceptions can play an important role in shaping and escalating fears about certain forms of risk and the evidential base that is associated with claims of 'safety'.

The fifth element identified by Knight concerns the uncertainty inherent in the *implementation* of policy and managerial decisions. The potential for uncertainty here is considerable as we can embed 'error cost' (Collingridge, 1992) into the decisions and policies such that the true costs of the error will only be recognized and realized (in financial or physical terms) at a later date. It is also possible that we can inhibit innovation in such a way that the costs of introducing the innovative product or process later on will be more expensive. It is also conceivable that how we implement policy can also be problematic and might increase uncertainty (especially the perceptual uncertainty) surrounding a particular hazard. An example can be used from the BSE crisis to illustrate this process. Here, a policy decision was taken to remove all specified offal from the human food chain as this was seen as the main source of the transmission risk from cattle to humans. It appears that some abattoirs interpreted this policy as meaning the removal of the majority of the material (most notably in the removal of the spinal cord where it was difficult to ensure that all of the material was removed from the carcass)[4]. Thus, whilst the policy was precautionary in its scope, its implementation may have generated problems around the maintenance of a source of potential hazard that policy-makers had assumed had been removed.

In an attempt to deal with various forms of uncertainty, policy-makers have turned to a precautionary approach to try to minimize the potential for conflict and risk generation. The 'principle' can be seen as a means of framing the actions of managers and policy-makers in and around risk-based activities where there is no clear 'evidence of safety'. This notion of 'evidence of safety' as opposed to 'evidence of harm' is a fundamental shift in the approach taken to dealing with such issues and is likely to become more prominent in

---

[4] This point was made in a BBC programme detailing the BSE crisis. See also http://www. mad-cow.org/~tom/BBC.html (Broadcast in 1996, transcript accessed 27th April 2009). Reference is also made to this practice in the BSE inquiry. See http://www.bseinquiry.gov. uk/report/volume13/chapterf.htm#245024 (Accessed on line, 27th April 2009)

policy-making[5] over the next decade across a range of public health debates around risk. Whilst medicine has long adopted a precautionary approach, it can be argued that this has been somewhat limited in its scope, and this paper seeks to open up a debate concerning the role of the principle, as configured in other disciplines, within healthcare in general and public health in particular.

## The precautionary principle—elements of the abstract

The origins of the precautionary principle are commonly seen to lie in German environmental legislation of the 1980s (Boehmer-Christiansen, 1994; Stebbing, 1992), although its use has widened to include other areas within the broad set of societal concerns around risk. Within German environmental debates, the concept of *Vörsorgeprinzip* (precautionary principle) emerged to describe the process of state intervention in areas where the potential for harm existed (Boehmer-Christiansen, 1994). Precautionary approaches, in their broadest sense, are not new. Public health legislation, for example, has long taken a precautionary and preventative approach around areas where there is a (relatively) clear relationship between activities and harm. It is this notion of providing a burden of proof on the part of the risk generators, and the need for them to communicate that risk to those who might be affected by the activity or product, that marks the precautionary principle as an important departure in policy terms. However, the use of the principle in practice has not been without its critics, and the USA in particular has been seen as one of the main objectors to its use (Boehmer-Christiansen, 1994; Jordan & O'Riordan, 1999; O'Riordan & Cameron, 1994; Tickner & Raffensperger, 2001).

The core elements of the precautionary principle require that action is needed around problems where there is a lack of clear evidence that can be used to inform policy, and where action needs to be taken to deal with the potential consequences of an activity rather than proven outcomes (Deville & Harding, 1997). In essence, the precautionary approach is about making certain that any decisions taken are reversible and that the potential impacts associated with the activity do not cause catastrophic damage (Deville & Harding, 1997). In that respect, the principle advocates an approach that many would simply see as good management practice or appropriate ethical behaviour (Tombs & Smith, 1995). So what differentiates the precautionary principle from good management practice?

---

[5] The recent banking crisis has done little to salve public concerns about the decisions of 'experts' and may yet create even greater calls for the use of a precautionary (or at least a more cautious) approach to management decision making and policy making.

Boehmer-Christiansen (Boehmer-Christiansen, 1994) outlines a number of central elements within the principle. The first element is the notion of precaution itself in which those charged with managing the problem are required to show that the hazards associated with the activity are not considered to be unacceptable when set against the benefits that arise from the activity. This first element raises three key issues. The first relates to the question of who is deemed sufficiently expert to make the diagnosis of safety? This puts the power of expertise at the centre of debates concerning the use of the precautionary principle (Calman & Smith, 2001). Secondly, the cost–benefit dynamic of this process is potentially open to abuse by those in positions of power who can manipulate any evidence to suit their own agendas (Collingridge & Reeve, 1986; Irwin, 1995; 2006). Thirdly, the manner in which risk is communicated and the extent of trust that public groups have in the messenger, become centrally important in shaping the context in which risk debates take place. The inherent uncertainty underpinning those calculations and the 'boundaries of consideration' (Jackson, 1996; 1999) that are used to frame risk invariably become important areas of contention.

The second element outlined by Boehmer-Christiansen relates to the notion of proportionality within the judgement of cost–benefit relationships. Boehmer-Christiansen highlights the issue of irreversibility—that is, when the potential for harm cannot be remediated. In such cases, the initial policy approach within Germany was to ensure that 'there should be no action before there is full understanding' (Boehmer-Christiansen, 1994). A central issue here is the notion of 'error cost'—the manner in which we embedded the costs of mistakes within policies that only become obvious many years later (Collingridge, 1992). The difficulties here concern the manner in which we can identify the costs and the benefits at the point at which the 'policy' decision is taken. On the one hand, taking no action may generate significant costs later on as the impact of the decision becomes apparent, whilst on the other, excessive cost may be borne at the outset by creating controls that are based on a potential for hazards that is inaccurate. In policy terms both are problematic and have led to accusations of the 'nanny state' interfering excessively (Calman, 2009; Fitzpatrick, 2001).

In addition to the elements outlined above, Jordan and O'Riordan (1999) suggest additional themes that are commonly considered important within the precautionary principle. The first of these relates to the *burden of proof* within risk debates. The manner in which the 'state' assumes a proactive (and preventative) approach as regulator is a key dynamic in the effectiveness of the precautionary principle. The second theme concerns the related issue of the *proportionality of response* that has to be taken around the hazards that are identified. Thirdly, Jordan and O'Riordan highlight the importance of ecological space and the importance of non-human entities in the process. This is a potentially problematic area as many previous approaches to environmental problems have taken a largely anthropocentric view of issues. A shift here would require a fundamental re-casting of societal values and assumptions about the relative importance of non-humans and the societal desires around the consumption of goods and services. Fourthly, they argue that there should be a shift in the burden of proof towards the risk generator and a greater consideration of the margins that exist for errors within any determination of harm. Finally, they raise the issue of the intergenerational effects of certain types of risk and the need to recognize existing ecological debts in the overall process. The latter also includes an important element of international cooperation around the creation of global hazards or where the implementation of environmental or health policies requires effective international collaboration (Jordan & O'Riordan, 1999). Obvious examples here would include issues relating to climate change, pandemic influenza, and cross-border environmental pollution.

Table 13.1 seeks to relate the various elements of the precautionary principle to the elements of uncertainty identified earlier and highlights some of the resultant issues. These issues are raised speculatively as we lack the space here to deal with them in detail. They also serve as signposts for further areas of research and investigation around the implications that the precautionary principle has for public health policy.

**Table 13.1** Potential problems associated with the precautionary principle

| Core Elements of the Precautionary Principle | Elements of Uncertainty | Issues arising out of these elements |
| --- | --- | --- |
| 1/Proactive precaution | Emergent Uncertainty | ◆ *Centrality of expertise in raising the issues to a level of policy awareness*<br>◆ *Power of interested parties to manipulate the agenda*<br>◆ *Role of trust and communication in the expression of risk*<br>◆ *Direct vs Indirect precaution and difficulties in determining the success of intervention strategies*<br>◆ *Requires intervention at the outset on the part of the regulatory mechanisms - pro-action is a key component of the process* |

**Table 13.1** (continued) Potential problems associated with the precautionary principle

| Core Elements of the Precautionary Principle | Elements of Uncertainty | Issues arising out of these elements |
|---|---|---|
| 2/Proportionality of Cause and Effect | Uncertainty of Outcome | • *Difficulties associated with emergence in non-linear systems*<br>• *Difficulties around the use of techniques in cost-benefit analysis*<br>• *Inter-generational and spatial issues around cause and effect*<br>• *Burden of proof issues around the effectiveness of intervention*<br>• *Requires a widening of our boundaries of consideration around*<br>• *Problems associated with determining cost and benefit - especially in terms of intergenerational impacts* |
| 3/Causation, burden of proof, and margins of error | Causal Uncertainty | • *Problems associated with non-linear systems create difficulties for proving cause and effect relationships*<br>• *Limitations of science and knowledge and the potential for new knowledge to be made available*<br>• *A required shift in the burden of proof to those who generate the potential risk and their need for proof of safety* |
| 4/Consensus | Perceptual Uncertainty | • *Problems around the relative weightings that may be given to expert opinion and the legitimacy of various forms of knowledge*<br>• *Abilities of groups with less access to power to mount compaigns and garner support around highly technical issues*<br>• *Role of the media in shaping the nature of the debate* |
| 5/Common Burden | *Implementation Uncertainty* | • *Notion that the burden of damage is collectively carried - raises questions about subsidies and inducements*<br>• *Equity issues between risk generators and potential victims - especially in terms of their relative abilities to shape policy agendas*<br>• *Question of who bears the cost of in-action in those cases where all policy outcomes have costs associated with them*<br>• *Difficulties associated with inter-generational effects*<br>• *Possibility that risk may be 'exported' and result in the exploitation of other communities*<br>• *Global risks require globally based precautionary actions (eg climate change)* |

**Table 13.1** (continued) Potential problems associated with the precautionary principle

| Core Elements of the Precautionary Principle | Elements of Uncertainty | Issues arising out of these elements |
|---|---|---|
| 6/Role of non-human entities and the safeguarding of ecological space | Emergent and Perceptual Uncertainty | ◆ Non-humans may play a significant role in causation (eg pandemic flu) or may be the victims of human actions<br>◆ Requires a shift away from anthropocentric approaches to risk towards a more inclusive approach<br>◆ Difficulties associated with the relative weightings of 'victims' in terms of cost-benefit calculations |
| 7/Recognition of environmental debt | Perceptual Uncertainty | ◆ Difficulties around liability for long-standing environmental problems<br>◆ Issues around burden of proof for certain forms of impact would require a careful approach to proportionality of liability |

Adapted from information in Boehmer-Christiansen, 1994; Jordan & O'Riordan, 1999; Knight, 1964; O'Riordan & Cameron, 1994.

## Risk communication and precaution

> The precautionary approach focuses on the need for more effective preventive action and the introduction of control measures not requiring proof of causality between contaminants and their effects . . . At the same time they require a shift in the burden of proof, expecting dischargers to prove that their effluents would cause no harm (Stebbing, 1992, p. 287).

The quote from Stebbing illustrates one of the key components of the precautionary principle—namely the changes around the burden of proof and the introduction of controls. This is a difficult issue in terms of the communication of risk. A recent example of the use of the precautionary principle within the UK illustrates the problem. The issue concerns the advice given to government on the use of mobile phones. The publication of the report by the Stewart Committee (Stewart, 2000) makes a number of references to the need for a precautionary approach. The committee observes that:

> . . . it is not possible at present to say that the exposure to RF radiation, even at levels below national guidelines, is totally without potential adverse health effects, and that the gaps in knowledge are sufficient to justify a precautionary approach. . . . we recommend that a precautionary approach to the use of mobile phone technologies be adopted until much more detailed and scientifically robust information on any health effects becomes available (Stewart, 2000, p. 3).

In advocating such an approach, the committee recognized that it brings with it a number of costs, in terms of financial implications for the industry, the loss of benefits to individual users, and the considerable benefits that arise to society as a whole. There is recognition of considerable controversy around the relationships between mobile phone use and health effects, and that only the risks from driving whilst using the phone were proven (Maier *et al.*, 2000). Cause and effect relationships are far from clear in dealing with such issues and it is precisely the non-linear nature of the problem that takes it beyond the normal sphere of influence provided by scientific knowledge. The problem is essentially trans-scientific in that it goes beyond the ability of science to prove cause and effect relationships. The response by the Department of Health (DH, 2000) welcomed the precautionary approach advocated within the Stewart Report and has confirmed the government's intention to continue to support further research into the health risks from mobile phone use.

Several issues around risk communication emerge here. In the first instance, there is a need to impress upon the 'population at risk' that the hazards they face from mobile phone use are varied and that there are also interaction risks (for example, when related to driving or walking across the road). A key problem in changing behaviour is that the changed behaviours have to provide a material benefit to the user. This can be in terms of clear positive benefits in health terms or by making the costs of the behaviour prohibitively high. There are some residual questions as to whether the ban on the use of mobile phones whilst driving (without the appropriate hands-free systems) has changed behaviour. Given the relatively low risk of detection by the police, it is not uncommon to see drivers using telephones in their hand-held mode whilst driving.

A second issue concerns how information is communicated. The issues around mobile phones are not just related to the physical damage that may be caused by the exposure to RF radiation but whether the use of the phone itself may cause problems relating to the individual's cognitive abilities to process information whilst driving or crossing the road. This distraction element of the activity may well prove to be the most significant health effect through the generation of accidents. However, if RF radiation is subsequently shown to have deleterious health effects, then there would be clear implications for the mobile telecommunications industry as a whole. The communication of these hazards raises several elements of uncertainty, most notably around causal, emergent, perceptual, and implementation uncertainty. Each element should be incorporated into any communications strategy to make it effective.

Thirdly, the processes around the encoding of the message, the selection of channels used to communicate the message, and processes around feedback verification, also need to be considered to ensure that the communication is effective. The problem here centres on the issue of feedback verification. How does the sender of the message know that the information has been received and decoded in the manner that was intended? A further difficulty here concerns how the communicator can incorporate the uncertainty that s/he has into the message itself. This has proved to be a problem in several public health scares, as indicated by other contributions to this collection, including the MMR vaccine, BSE, foot and mouth, and pandemic influenza. Admitting that there are margins of error in the scientific understanding of a problem is one thing but capturing that in a communication strategy that seeks to change behaviour in a precautionary manner is considerably more problematic. A major problem here centres on the amplification of risk (usually by the media) and the implications that this generates for risk communications strategies.

At its core, the precautionary approach tries to ensure that uncertainty is dealt with in a more effective, open, and honest way. As we have argued here, uncertainty is itself a multifaceted construct, and the various elements of uncertainty need to be incorporated into the use of any precautionary approach as well as the manner in which we communicate that uncertainty. The complex mosaic of issues will remain a challenge for public health practitioners, managers, and policy-makers. They will also require society to make some fundamental changes to its core values and assumptions if we are to move beyond the current state of fearfulness that is generated by the uncertainty that we face.

## Conclusions

In many respects, the emergence of the precautionary principle within a public health context can be seen as part of wider concerns and discourses surrounding risk and, in particular, around the process of stewardship (Calman, 2009; Hart, 1999). There is little doubt that honesty and openness in risk communication is a goal to which organizations should aspire. As such, it sits within the wider framework of governance and ethical behaviour that have been part of the policy agenda for several years. However, some significant problems remain for the implementation of the precautionary principle in practice, and many of these centre on the processes by which we communicate hazard and uncertainty. The philosophical change that is required by some organizations to recognize the limitations of their own knowledge is considerable. When combined with the requirement to communicate that uncertainty to others, a quantum shift is required in the core assumptions and values of the organization and its senior managers.

These issues are not just related to the issues of health and environment. Had the financial industry been more willing to recognize the limits of its own knowledge and understanding of the nature of markets, or had it been willing to communicate those uncertainties to its customers, then the current global economic crisis might well have been averted.

A precautionary approach has widespread implications for the ways in which our organizations deal with risk. By being more precautionary in the ways that we 'manage', we may go some way towards preventing future crises.

The precautionary principle, whilst obviously an important move forward in terms of how risk is managed and communicated, generates problems concerning how organizations seek to engage with their stakeholders. The principle requires the development of a degree of honesty around issues of uncertainty and hazard that has not always been forthcoming from business or from government. In the age of 'political spin', one might conclude that the precautionary approach may well prove to be a principle too far for some organizations.

## References

Adam, B. (1998). *Timescapes of modernity. The environment and invisible hazards.* London, Routledge.

Angell, M. (1996). *Science on trial. The clash of medical evidence and the law in the breast implant case.* New York, NJ, W.W. Norton and Company.

Bauman, Z. (2006). *Liquid fear.* Cambridge, Polity.

Beck, U. (1992). *Risk society. Towards a new modernity* (M. Ritter, Trans.). London, Sage.

Boehmer-Christiansen, S. (1994). The precautionary principle in Germany—enabling government. In: T. O'Riordan & J. Cameron (eds). *Interpreting the Precautionary Principle.* London, Earthscan, pp. 31–60.

Bulkeley, H. (2001). Governing climate change: the politics of risk society? *Transactions of the Institute of British Geographers,* 26(4): 430–47.

Calman, K. (2009). Beyond the 'nanny state': Stewardship and public health. *Public Health,* 123(1): e6–e10.

Calman, K. & Smith, D. (2001). Works in theory but not in practice? Some notes on the precautionary principle. *Public Administration,* 79(1): 185–204.

Collingridge, D. (1992). *The management of scale: Big organizations, big decisions, big mistakes.* London, Routledge.

Collingridge, D. & Reeve, C. (1986). *Science speaks to power: the role of experts in policy-making.* London, Francis Pinter.

Deville, A. & Harding, R. (1997). *Applying the precautionary principle.* Sydney, The Federation Press.

DH. (2000). Mobile phones and health: Stewart Report—the government's response. London, Department of Health. Accessed at http://www.doh.gov.uk/mobile.htm on the 14 May 2000.

Edwards, A. & Elwyn, G. (2001). Understanding risk and lessons for clinical risk communication about treatment preferences. *Quality in Health Care*, 10 (Suppl. I), i9–i13.

Erikson, K. (1994). *A new species of trouble. Explorations in disaster, trauma, and community*. New York, W. W. Norton and Company.

Fitzpatrick, M. (2001). *The tyranny of health—doctors and the regulation of lifestyle*. London, Routledge.

Giddens, A. (1990). *The consequences of modernity*. Cambridge, Polity Press.

Giddens, A. (1999). *Runaway World. How globalisation is reshaping our lives*. London, Profile Books.

Hart, G. (1999). Risk and health: challenges and opportunity. *Health, Risk and Society*, 1(1), 7–10.

Irwin, A. (1995). *Citizen Science: A study of people, expertise and sustainable development*. London, Routledge.

Irwin, A. (2006). The politics of talk: coming to terms with the 'new' scientific governance. *Social Studies of Science*, 36(2), 299–320.

Jackson, W. (1996). Natural systems agriculture (on 'nature as standard'). *The Land Report* (55/56), 60–1.

Jackson, W. (1999). Foreword. In: C. Raffensperger & J. Tickner (eds). *Protecting public health and the environment. Implementing the precautionary principle*. Washington DC, Island Press, pp. xv–xix.

Johnson, H. G. (1972). Science and trans-science. *Minerva*, 10(3), 484–6.

Jordan, A. & O'Riordan, T. (1999). The precautionary principle in contemporary environmental policy and politics. In: C. Raffensperger & J. Tickner (eds). *Protecting public health and the environment. Implementing the precautionary principle*. Washington DC, Island Press, pp. 15–35.

Knight, F. H. (1964). *Risk, uncertainty and profit*. New York, A. M. Kelly.

Lupton, D. (ed.) (1999). *Risk and sociocultural theory. New directions and perspectives*. Cambridge, Cambridge University Press.

Maier, M., Blakemore, C. & Koivisto, M. (2000). The health hazards of mobile phones. The only established risk is of using one while driving. *British Medical Journal*, 320, 1288–9.

McVeigh, T. & Tuckman, J. (2009). Global flu fears as 68 die and virus spreads. *The Observer*, 26th April 2009: pp. 1 & 5.

O'Riordan, T. & Cameron, J. (1994). The history and contemporary significance of the precautionary principle. In: T. O'Riordan & J. Cameron (eds). *Interpreting the precautionary principle*. London, Earthscan, pp. 12–30.

Pauchant, T. C. & Mitroff, I. I. (1992). *Transforming the crisis-prone organization. Preventing individual organizational and environmental tragedies*. San Francisco, Jossey-Bass Publishers.

Perrow, C. (1984). *Normal accidents*. New York, Basic Books.

Petersen, A. & Bunton, R. (2002). *The new genetics and the public's health*. London, Routledge.

Rhodes, R. (1998). Deadly feasts. *The 'prion' controversy and the public's health*. New York, NY, Touchstone.

Robin, C. (2004). *Fear. The history of a political idea*. Oxford, Oxford University Press.

Shiloh, S., Guvenc, G. & Onkal, D. (2007). Cognitive and emotional representations of terror attacks: a cross-cultural exploration. *Risk Analysis*, 27(2), 397–409.

Siegrist, M., Keller, C., Kastenholz, H., Frey, S. & Wiek, A. (2007). Laypeople's and experts' perception of nanotechnology hazards. *Risk Analysis*, 27(1), 59–69.

Smith, D. (1990). Corporate power and the politics of uncertainty: Risk management at the Canvey Island complex. *Industrial Crisis Quarterly*, 4(1), 1–26.

Smith, D. (2005). Dancing around the mysterious forces of chaos: exploring issues of complexity, knowledge and the management of uncertainty. *Clinician in Management*, 13(3–4), 115–23.

Smith, D. (2006). The crisis of management—managing ahead of the curve. In: D. Smith & D. Elliott (eds). *Key readings in crisis management: Organisational systems and structures for prevention and recovery: forthcoming.* London, Routledge.

Stebbing, A. R. D. (1992). Environmental capacity and the precautionary principle. *Marine Pollution Bulletin*, 24(6), 287–95.

Stewart, W. (2000). Mobile phones and health. *Report of the Independent Expert Group on Mobile Phones (Stewart Committee).* Didcot, National Radiological Protection Board.

Taleb, N. N. (2007). *The Black Swan. The impact of the highly improbable.* London, Penguin.

Tenner, E. (1996). *Why things bite back. Technology and the revenge effect.* London, Fourth Estate.

Tickner, J. & Raffensperger, C. (2001). The politics of precaution in the United States and the European Union. *Global Environmental Change*, 11(2), 175–80.

Tombs, S. & Smith, D. (1995). Corporate responsibility and crisis management: some insights from political and social theory. *Journal of Contingencies and Crisis Management*, 3(3), 135–48.

Trumbo, C. W., McComas, K. A. & Kannaovakun, P. (2007). Cancer anxiety and the perception of risk in alarmed communities. *Risk Analysis*, 27(2), 337–50.

Tulloch, J. & Lupton, D. (1997). *Television, AIDS and risk: A cultural studies approach to health communication.* London, Allen & Unwin.

Turner, B. A. (1976). The organizational and interorganizational development of disasters. *Administrative Science Quarterly*, 21, 378–97.

Weinberg, A. M. (1972). Science and trans-science. *Minerva*, 10(2), 209–22.

Wynne, B. (1992). Uncertainty and environmental learning: Reconceiving science and policy in the preventive paradigm. *Global Environmental Change*, 2(2), 111–27.

# From the inside, looking out at those looking in—organizational issues around preparation and response for public health risks

Chapter 14

# Changes to food risk management and communication

Sue Davies (Chief Policy Adviser, *Which?*)

## Introduction

The past decade has been a period of dramatic change to the way food issues are managed and communicated. Now easily taken for granted, new institutions have been formed and new approaches adopted with the aim of ensuring greater public protection and confidence.

In the aftermath of bovine spongiform encephalopathy (BSE) and a series of food poisoning outbreaks, a new UK Food Standards Agency (FSA) was created with a clear remit to put consumers first and to operate openly and transparently (Food Standards Act, 1999). Wide-ranging reform at European level has also seen the separation of risk assessment and communication from the political aspects of risk management through to the creation of a European Food Safety Authority (EFSA) (Regulation EC 178/2002). New principles for analysing and handling food risks have also been adopted to guide decisions at global level, through the United Nation's body, the Codex Alimentarius Commission (Codex Alimentarius Commission, 2007).

Central to these across-the-board changes has been a much greater focus on risk communication. Although there have been differences in approach and level of ambition, at the heart of the new approaches has been far greater emphasis on transparent and inclusive decision-making.

Ten years down the line, it is timely to review whether the changes have lived up to expectations and whether decisions about managing food risks are more robust, providing lessons for other areas. It is also important to consider whether the reforms have created greater public confidence in the risk assessment and management process as a result of greater involvement and clearer, more relevant, information to UK consumers.

What may have been relevant several years ago also needs to be looked at in the context of the ever more complex and multifaceted risks that face consumers today—not merely food safety scares, but also the increased focus on choosing healthier diets and making more sustainable food choices.

## The way we were

In the first edition of this book, *Which?* (then known as the Consumers' Association) set out the arguments for why we needed a fundamental change to the way that food issues were handled. We had campaigned for an independent food agency to put public health first and ensure decision-making was more open, transparent, inclusive, and, therefore, precautionary. Risk communication needed to become a two-way process, ensuring that consumers were involved throughout the decision-making process. The goal was to ensure more socially acceptable decisions and relevant information for consumers.

Although BSE was the main impetus for change, it was not the only driver. A series of food scares, such as the rise of *E. coli* O157 and salmonella in eggs, as well as concern that nutrition policy was overly politicized, led to a breakdown in trust (Consumers' Association, 1997). This was fuelled by a lack of openness over the real motivations for the government's decisions. There was concern that crucial decisions were often taken in a substructure of apparently unaccountable bodies. As a result, there was a lack of confidence in the objectivity of science coupled with concern that there was over-reliance on science. Political motivations all too often seemed to be wrapped up in scientific justification but without a clear explanation of where science ended and other factors, economic or social, came into play.

These issues received greater prominence as a result of the Phillips Inquiry into BSE (Phillips, 2000), which highlighted the need for much greater openness:

> When responding to public or media demand for advice, the government must resist the temptation of attempting to have all of the answers in a situation of uncertainty ...
> If doubts are openly expressed and publicly explored, the public are capable of responding rationally and are more likely to accept reassurance and advice if and when it comes.

A lack of openness about any conflicts of interest behind the scientific advice that government received, and the over-reliance on a narrow range of disciplines, also helped to create mistrust. We also highlighted the apparently changing nature of risk as a result of an ever more globalized, complex, and technological food supply chain, requiring a careful consideration of how to reach socially acceptable decisions and a greater dependency on institutions outside the UK.

## A period of change

These problems led to a broad consensus around the need for a new approach. The food industry, as well as consumer and public health groups, recognized that change was needed if consumers were to have confidence in its products. In the UK, the FSA was established with responsibility for all three stages of risk analysis: assessment, management, and communication. Its clear responsibility is 'to protect public health from risks which may arise in connection with the consumption of food and otherwise to protect the interests of consumers in relation to food' (Food Standards Act, 1999). Its remit covers food safety and standards, but also nutrition, and it works according to three core values: putting the consumer first; openness and independence; and being science- and evidence-based.

At arms' length from government, the FSA has unique powers to publish the advice that it gives to ministers. It is also governed by an independent board appointed through open competition to reinforce this independence. From the outset, the FSA Board has been distinguished by the way it holds its meetings in open session so that the basis for its policy decisions are clear. These meetings are also web-streamed, enabling stakeholders to understand how it works and also to put questions directly to the Board members.

Of particular significance, the FSA has also opened up the scientific advice that underpins its decisions to scrutiny. The network of independent scientific committees now hold their main meetings in public, enabling stakeholders to understand and directly question their advice. The FSA guidance on how its scientific committees operate (Food Standards Agency, 2002) also specifies the importance of multidisciplinary expertise, including two public interest or consumer representatives.

These changes have led to a far more open and inclusive approach to risk communication than we saw previously. Scientific advice has become more open and the approach to determining risk management decisions is generally more inclusive, with greater involvement of different stakeholders through working groups and consultations, and a greater focus on consumer research and engagement.

## International aspects

Mirroring the UK situation, a breakdown in confidence in the EU's ability to handle food risks as BSE spread through member states also led to a review of its role. Greater responsibility for food legislation was transferred to the Directorate-General for Health and Consumer Protection. However, diverging from the UK, the EU focus was on administratively separating responsibility for risk assessment from responsibility for risk management. The EFSA was set up, with responsibility for providing scientific advice. But to confuse matters, responsibility for risk communication is shared with the European Commission, and, ultimately, with the Member States. As with the UK FSA,

EFSA is governed by a Management Board made up of 'a broad range of relevant expertise', including four members with a 'background in organizations representing consumers and other interests in the food chain' (Regulation EC 178/2002).

Since its creation, successive food legislation has transferred everything from food packaging materials to health claims away from Member States to the EFSA. The intention is to ensure a consistency of approach, but in practice there can still be conflicts between Member States and the EFSA, for example, around the assessment of GM foods. The dual responsibility for risk communication can also cause some confusion, with consumers potentially hearing different messages from their national governments, EFSA, and the European Commission on the same issue, as seen with the issue of cloning, for example (see below).

EFSA has taken steps to ensure it works transparently, although these are not as far-reaching as those adopted by the FSA. EFSA Management Board meetings are also open to the public and are web-streamed. There has been emphasis on ensuring openness about the potential interests of Panel and Board Members through rules on declaration of interests and in communicating the opinions of EFSA's experts, including minority opinions. However, transparency does not yet extend to holding open meetings of the scientific panels or overarching scientific committee or to the appointment of lay or consumer representatives as members or even as observers.

The international standards body, the Codex Alimentarius Commission, which works through a series of committees made up of member governments, has also become much more significant in terms of the way that food risks are handled. Codex standards are used as reference texts in dispute settlements of the World Trade Organization, and so these standards can be the ultimate arbiter of the level of protection UK consumers may expect (World Trade Organization, 1994). This was reinforced in the EU–US beef hormones dispute, for example, where, based on a Codex standard, the EU ban was considered an illegal barrier to trade and resulted in reparations to the US. However, being far removed from most people's daily lives, Codex has often been criticized for its lack of transparency and consumer representation compared to participation by commercial sector interests. It depends on FAO/WHO expert committees and consultations, such as the Joint Expert Committee on Food Additives (JECFA), for scientific input. These have taken some steps to improve transparency, such as declaration of interests, but generally these operate at a level removed from most people's consciousness.

However, after many years of debate, Codex recently adopted a standard on *Working Principles for Risk Analysis for Food Safety for Application by*

*Governments* (Codex Alimentarius Commission, 2007). The use of the precautionary principle was the main stumbling block. However, the principles do recognize precaution and emphasize the importance of transparency and inclusivity. They advise, for example, that:

> Risk communication should be more than the dissemination of information. Its major function should be to ensure that all information and opinion required for effective risk management is incorporated into the decision-making process.

The Codex Working Principles also recognize the importance of asking the right questions, emphasizing the importance of 'risk assessment policy' to ensure that the risk assessment is 'systematic, complete, unbiased and transparent.' This is an issue still rarely dealt with explicitly and consistently within UK and EU processes.

## Communicating uncertainty

There has therefore been a significant change in approach at all levels. There has, for example, been a noticeably different approach to the way that information is communicated to UK consumers. Whereas the public were given reassurances about the safety of beef in the past, the remaining uncertainties around BSE are now made much more explicit. FSA advice on the difficult issue of whether BSE may have passed to sheep, for example, spells out what is and isn't known:

> BSE has never been found in the UK sheep flock. However, some sheep were fed the same feed that is thought to have given cattle BSE and laboratory research has shown that sheep can be artificially infected with BSE (Food Standards Agency, 2008a).

A similar approach was adopted in relation to atypical scrapie:

> Atypical scrapie is not BSE, and there is an absence of scientific evidence that it can be transmitted to humans or that it is of any risk to humans. However, a risk can't be ruled out (Food Standards Agency, 2008b).

The FSA's approach to handling the discovery of acrylamide in baby food was also notably different to some member states, with the FSA making clear that:

> Acrylamide is known to cause cancer in animals and its presence in some foods may harm people's health (Food Standards Agency, 2008c).

The policy of openness can come into conflict with other interests. The FSA was, for example, criticized by the food industry for its handling of contamination of foods with illegal dyes, including Sudan I, leading to a large food product withdrawal. It was accused of over-reacting, using emotive language, and creating unnecessary public concern given the scale of the risk. The FSA argued that it was the appropriate action to take given that the contaminant was illegal and a known carcinogen. The Panel set up to review the handling of the incient recommended that the FSA should consider the potential for devising a range of simple messages to the public, giving in non-scientific language different examples of risk relating to everyday life (Food Standards Agency, 2007).

Food incidents have not disappeared as a result of this new approach to risk communication. Even some of the food hazards that have been with us for many years, such as food poisoning bacteria, including *Campylobacter* and *Listeria*, remain poorly understood. An Inquiry set up by the Welsh Assembly to try and understand the circumstances of the largest ever *E. coli* O157 outbreak in Wales, affecting over 150 people and killing a 5-year-old boy, highlights just how serious the consequences can be (National Assembly for Wales, 2008; Pennington, Chapter 6, this volume). However, on the whole there is no longer the constant cycle of food scares that dominated the late 1980s and early 1990s.

The FSA certainly feels that there is greater confidence. Its most recent survey of consumer attitudes to food reported that there had been a drop in the level of concern about food safety since 2006, while there was growing awareness of issues around nutrition and health.

## Risk communication as risk management

When faced with a great deal of uncertainty, as seen in the case of BSE, the government often has to fall back on risk communication as a key risk management measure. It may not be possible to eliminate the risk as it may not even be fully understood whether there is a risk at all—and therefore consumers are provided with information to, at least in theory, enable them to make more informed choices. The risk of BSE in sheep is an example of this. Current measures would reduce the risk, but not eliminate it. The FSA has therefore been open about the potential risk and has also provided more targeted information to particular groups. Despite these efforts, it is questionable whether most people are aware of its advice—and the effective dissemination of information is often very reliant on accurate media coverage as the main route to the public.

The move towards publication of hygiene scores on food premises or local authority websites is a more direct way by which the public is able to take action according to the particular risk presented and, as evidence from other countries suggests, drives up standards in the process. In some situations, however, the FSA has been criticized for intervening too slowly and relying too much on providing consumers with information instead—as initially seen in relation to food colours associated with hyperactivity in children.

The establishment of EFSA adds a new dimension and a new challenge for effective risk communication, with the potential for EFSA opinions to differ from those of national authorities. Given that opinions are often based on expert judgements, EFSA Panels may reach different conclusions to national scientific committees involving other experts. This has been seen in relation to advice on BSE issues, for example.

## Broader than science

Part of the FSA's remit is to 'protect other consumer interests in relation to food'. EU legislation (Regulation EC 178/2002) also recognizes the importance of other factors besides science. These issues particularly come into play when dealing with new technologies, such as GM foods or animal cloning. Although some of the public's reluctance to accept GM foods is because of concern about the long-term health consequences, it also stems from failure on the part of consumers to see any benefits for themselves and outrage at the way that the first crops were introduced into food products without any effective consumer choice. There was a failure to take account of the public's views sufficiently early in the process and to talk about the risks in a way that recognized the source of people's concerns. Despite efforts to communicate uncertainty in relation to other risks, the FSA was heavily criticized for failing to understand that the public's concerns went beyond issues that could be resolved by reiteration of the conclusions of the risk assessment.

Debates about other new technologies are now becoming more prominent. The European Commission is currently deliberating over animal cloning in food production, which shows how different values, such as animal welfare and ethics, sit alongside the science. A *Which?* survey in February 2008 showed strong consumer opposition to the use of cloning for food production (*Which?*, 2008). A European Commission Eurobarometer survey shows that this applies across the EU, with many citizens stating that cloning could never be justified for food production (European Commission, 2008). An EFSA opinion, published in July 2008 (European Food Safety Authority, 2008a), concluded that the food safety risks were unlikely to differ from those of conventionally bred animals, although the data available are limited, but highlighted the potential for animal health and welfare problems. A concurrent report produced by the European Group on Ethics, however, advised that there was currently no ethical justification for the use of cloning in food production (European Group on Ethics, 2008).

A broad range of factors will therefore influence the way that the public views risk. The FSA seems to have learnt from the GM experience and has attempted to gain an understanding of consumer attitudes to cloning early in the decision-making process. Deliberative workshops held in 2007 highlighted how people's attitudes to the use of cloning in food also related to their concerns about it being a step away from cloning of humans (Food Standards Agency, 2008d).

The same approach has yet to be seen in relation to the use of nanotechnologies in food production. This new technology appears to have more obvious and wider ranging benefits for food products, but may also raise a range of social and ethical questions which will affect consumers' perception of the risk and its acceptability. Policy-makers face the challenge of determining an appropriate form of regulation and effective communication when faced with fundamental uncertainties about how materials produced and manipulated at the nanoscale behave. EFSA's draft opinion on nanotechnologies (European Food Safety Authority, 2008b) pointed out that:

> Current uncertainties for risk assessment of nanotechnologies and their possible applications in the food and feed area arise due to presently limited information in several areas.

Despite many positive statements about the need for public engagement, the government still appears to be struggling with how to do this in a meaningful way in practice. A lack of food industry transparency about the research already underway in this area makes communication difficult and exposure to any possible risks impossible to assess. A *Which?* Citizens Panel, held at the end of 2007 (*Which?*, 2007), found that consumers appear open to the benefits on offer, but expect to be fully informed about where the technology is used and want effective safeguards in place before products come to market. Failure to respond openly and proactively, involving consumers at this early stage, risks undermining this.

## Effectively involving consumers

Despite concerns about the approach to nanotechnologies, there has generally been a much greater emphasis on involving consumers in decision-making in the UK, and innovation in terms of the way that this is done. This has been seen at the risk management stage, as well as in relation to representation on the UK scientific committees, as already described.

While there are differences of approach in different policy areas, the past few years have seen the use of a wide range of working groups and other stakeholder fora to involve and understand consumer views as well as the perspectives of other stakeholders. Greater emphasis has been placed on consumer research, including the use of deliberative techniques, such as citizens' panels, juries, and workshops, to address more complex issues.

While there is a risk of complacency, given that several years have elapsed since the FSA was set up with a clear steer to adopt a new approach, the setting up of a new Social Science Research Committee and an FSA Committee on Public Engagement is a positive sign.

At European level, many cultural aspects come into play. However, formal mechanisms for hearing the views of consumer organizations and other stakeholders on a range of food issues and risk have also been established in recent years. The European Commission chairs an Advisory Group on the Food Chain and Animal Health. EFSA has established a Stakeholder Consultative Platform, chaired by the European Consumer Organization.

## New challenges

There have therefore been a lot of positive changes over the past few years which have helped to ensure that risk assessors and managers, as well as consumers, are now far more aware of the complexities of food risks than in the past. There is no doubt that efforts to involve consumers have been enhanced and consumer views have increasingly informed food policy decisions.

However, since the reforms of 10 years ago and the greater emphasis on risk communication have come into effect, the relative priority of food risks and the public health challenges that we face have also changed, demanding a continuing assessment of whether the changes that have been made go far enough.

Ten years ago, foodborne diseases were the main issues of concern, whether these were new, poorly understood diseases such as BSE, or continuing unacceptable levels of food poisoning bacteria. Widespread contamination of foods with carcinogenic chemicals, including PCBs, acrylamide or, more recently, melamine, have become prominent in recent years, reflecting the difficulty of controlling food hazards along an ever-lengthening food supply chain. New technologies regularly come to the fore and may raise new challenges for how we assess, regulate, and inform consumers about any potential risks—as well as how to balance these against potential benefits.

Perhaps most striking has been the much greater focus now placed on the nutritional quality of our diets, e.g. the longer term risks of consuming too much fat, sugar, and salt, and too few fruits and vegetables, as well as the short-term health effects of contaminated food. While the effects of food poisoning can be devastating, diet-related diseases are now recognized as the major killers across the UK and the rest of Europe, including cancers, heart disease, stroke, and type 2 diabetes. Obesity rates are rising dramatically, with around a quarter of the UK population now obese and estimates that 70% of boys and 55% of girls will be obese or overweight by 2050, based on current trends (Government Office for Science, 2007).

This demands a different type of approach. Although harmful if consumed to excess, the risks cannot be regulated in the same way. The 2008 obesity strategy for England (Department of Health, 2008) describes the government as having a significant role:

> not in hectoring or lecturing but in expanding the opportunities people have to make the right choices for themselves and their families; in making sure that people have clear and effective information about food, exercise and their wellbeing; and in ensuring that its policies across the piece support people in their efforts to maintain a healthy weight.

The traditional approach was to educate people, but this has not worked. The past few years have seen much greater emphasis on the government as having an enabling role through a range of complementary actions aimed at improving diets, alongside physical activity. In practical terms this has involved steps to provide much more direct risk communication to try to bring about behavioural change, such as the development of a simplified 'multiple traffic light' food labelling scheme showing whether levels of key nutrients are high, medium or low. The government's focus on the 'five a day' message is also an example of other efforts to provide clear, simple information to consumers. FSA consumer research suggests that 78% of people are at least aware of the message (Food Standards Agency, 2008e). The FSA has also invested heavily in a campaign to highlight the need to reduce salt intakes. The initial message emphasized that salt was bad for your heart and that adults should aim to eat no more than 6 g a day. An integrated approach of setting salt targets for industry and encouraging traffic light labelling on the front of packaging to influence consumer demand has seen a reduction of salt levels in foods as well as in individual diets. The campaign has already seen a reduction in average population salt intakes in adults from over 9 g to 8.6 g (Food Standards Agency, 2008f).

The government is also in the process of developing a broader campaign to encourage behavioural change in England. Branded 'Change4Life', the social marketing campaign with a £75 million government investment will cut across many areas and will involve the government working with a range of stakeholders, aiming to establish a movement for change.

Obesity and diet-related disease has also become a much greater priority at European and international level, through the creation of stakeholder bodies such as the EU's Platform for Action on Diet, Physical Activity and Health, which encourages voluntary commitments from stakeholders. A White Paper on Nutrition, Overweight and Obesity has set a deadline of 2010 to review progress in key areas. EFSA is also focusing more on nutrition-related issues, providing EU-wide nutrition guidelines and assessing health claims to ensure that they can be substantiated—and therefore do not mislead consumers.

## Joining up the messages

While issues around diet and health—and some of the positive messages about eating certain beneficial foods—have come to the forefront and are receiving much greater attention, they illustrate a tendency to compartmentalize risks which is inconsistent with the way consumers make decisions about what to eat. Issues around food safety, food standards, healthy eating—and now increasingly food sustainability—are often dealt with in isolation, rather than in the broader context of how consumers make their choices and shop for food, particularly in the current climate, with an increasing concern about the cost of food and many consumers on a more limited budget.

This issue of 'joined up' communication was one of the core themes of a recent report from the Cabinet Office, 'Food Matters' (Cabinet Office, 2008), which highlighted the need for more consistent and coordinated advice for consumers and saw the government playing a vital role as a 'choice editor'. A plethora of different ethical schemes and conflicting messages, as seen for example with the issues of food miles and fair trade, leave consumers unable to take action even if they are committed to making more sustainable food choices. A specific example included in the report was advice around fish. While consumers are being encouraged to consume fish for nutritional reasons, concerns about depleting fish stocks indicates a need to limit our intake. A similar conundrum has previously arisen in relation to balancing the benefits of consuming more oily fish because it contains long chain omega 3 fatty acids that have a role in maintaining heart health, with concern about levels of dioxins and PCBs in fish linked to increased cancer risk.

There has been an increased focus on the need to tackle contradictory messages that can undermine government advice. Some measures, although limited, have been introduced to limit less healthy food marketing to children on TV. Action over the wide range of non-broadcast techniques, from food packaging to internet promotions, used to target foods high in fat, sugar and salt to children, is starting to happen, but is also too limited in scope.

## Putting consumers first

As well as new risks, such as obesity and climate change, that impact on the way that food risks are communicated, political challenges could also impact on the lessons that have been learned from previous crises. There is now an increasing focus on better regulation and reducing administrative burdens on industry. While this should benefit consumers as well as businesses, there is also a danger that, if taken too far, some of the positive changes that have been made could be undermined. The FSA has agreed to a target to reduce the burden of its regulations on businesses by 25%.

A recent report by the Better Regulation Executive (Better Regulation Executive, 2008) reviewing FSA's progress in this area highlights just how full circle things could come if too short term an approach is adopted. While recognizing the FSA's statutory duty to protect consumers, it concluded that the FSA has taken this further and in some circumstances presents itself more as championing the consumer interest as distinct from protecting. It advised that: 'This pro-consumer stance, we believe, can complicate the Agency's engagement with and understanding of business.'

## Where next?

'Food Matters' (Cabinet Office, 2008) clearly presented the challenge of making sure that communication from government is joined up so that ultimately consumers are in a position to make safe, healthy, and more sustainable food choices. While the examples described highlight that we have come a long way in terms of risk communication, there is still a need to try to put food risks in context and explain how different food safety incidents relate to each other. While the risk of different hazards can rarely be quantified, food safety advice must recognize the nature of people's concerns and needs to be more coherent, linked up with broader advice about what we should be eating. The introduction of new technologies and emerging risks as a result of a more complex supply chain will raise new challenges. Individual issues flare up and then appear forgotten—at least by the media, and do not remain in the public eye. While efforts are still being made to involve consumers and consumer representatives more in food policy decision-making, it is important that the lessons of the past are not forgotten and that this continues to be a priority and an area of further development and innovation.

The FSA's independence and consumer-focused remit remains essential for its credibility. It is therefore important that this is not undermined by the focus on cutting red tape, leading back to a more short-term approach, where economic interests become the driver for policy to the detriment of consumer protection and public health. We learnt at huge public cost, through the BSE crisis, what can be the result. Overall, we have come a huge way as a result of that terrible breakdown in food policy. It is essential that the key principles that guided the changes a decade ago remain the conrnerstones of food policy: putting public health first, openness and transparency, and ensuring that risk communication is a two-way process which leads to more robust and socially acceptable risk decisions.

## References

Better Regulation Executive. (2008). *Effective inspection and enforcement: implementing the Hampton vision in the Food Standards Agency*. Better Regulation Executive, Department for Business, Enterprise and Regulatory Reform. London, National Audit Office.

Cabinet Office. (2008). *Food Matters, Towards a strategy for the 21st Century*. The Strategy Unit, Admiralty Arch, The Mall, London.

Codex Alimentarius Commission. (2007). *Working Principles for risk analysis for food safety for application by Governments*, CAC/GL 62-2007.

Consumers' Association. (1997). *A National Food Agency*.

Department of Health. (2008). *Healthy Weight, Healthy Lives: A cross-government strategy for England*. London, HM Government.

European Commission. (2008). European attitudes towards animal cloning. Analytical Report. *Eurobarometer*, October 2008.

European Food Safety Authority. (2008a). Food safety, animal health and welfare and environmental impact of animals derived from cloning by somatic cell nucleus transfer (scnt) and their offspring and products obtained from those animals (Question No EFSA-Q-2007-092). Adopted on 15 July 2008. *The EFSA Journal*, 767: 4–49.

European Food Safety Authority. (2008b). Draft opinion of the scientific committee on the potential risks arising from nanoscience and nanotechnologies on food and feed safety (Question No EFSA-Q-2007-124). European Food Safety Authority, Endorsed for public consultation 14 October 2008.

European Group on Ethics in Science and New Technologies to the European Commission. (2008). *Ethical aspects of animal cloning for food supply*, Opinion No 23.

Food Standards Act 1999. London, House of Commons.

Food Standards Agency. (2002). *Report of the Review of Scientific Committees*. Available at: http://www.foodstandards.gov.uk.

Food Standards Agency. (2007). *Report of the Sudan I Review Panel*. Available at: http://www.food.gov.uk.

Food Standards Agency. (2008a). *BSE and sheep*. Available at: http://www.food.gov.uk.

Food Standards Agency. (2008b). *Atypical scrapie*. Available at: http://www.food.gov.uk.

Food Standards Agency. (2008c). *Acrylamide*. Available at: http://www.food.gov.uk.

Food Standards Agency. (2008d). *Animal cloning and implications for the food chain*. Available at: http://www.food.gov.uk.

Food Standards Agency. (2008e). *Consumers Attitudes Survey 2007: UK Report*. Available at: http://www.food.gov.uk.

Food Standards Agency. (2008f). *Proposals to revise the voluntary salt reduction targets*. Available at: http://www.food.gov.uk.

Government Office for Science. (2007). Foresight, Tackling obesities: Future Choices— Project Report.

National Assembly for Wales. (2008). E. coli *Public Inquiry*. Available at: http://new.wales.gov.uk/ecoliinquiry

Phillips, L. (2000). Report, evidence and supporting papers of the Inquiry into the emergence and identification of bovine spongiform encephalopathy (BSE) and variant Creutzfeldt–Jakob Disease (vCJD) and the action taken in response to it up to 20 March 1996. Lord Phillips of Worth Matravers.

Regulation EC 178/2002 of 28th January 2002 laying down the general principles and requirements of food law, establishing the European Food Safety Authority and laying down procedures in matters of food safety.

Which? (2007). The Nano Citizens' Panel. Opinion Leader Research conducted a Citizens' Panel on behalf of Which? with 14 members of the public. Panellists were selected broadly to reflect the general public and sat for three days from 29th November to 1st December 2007.

Which? (2008). 1968 members of the public representative of the general population of the UK were interviewed by telephone about attitudes to cloning for food production in February 2008.

World Trade Organization. (1994). Agreement on the application of sanitary and phytosanitary measures.

## Chapter 15

# Communicating risk across publics and between organizations: the case of childhood accidents

Moira Fischbacher-Smith (Centre for Health, Environment and Risk Research, University of Glasgow)

## Introduction

Communicating risk around issues relating to health and wellbeing or health promotion, like so many aspects of the organization and delivery of health and social care, has become the provenance of interagency activity. The health promotion agenda and the public(s) it must address create a level of complexity in terms of messages and target audiences that is further complicated by the multi-organizational context through which such communications are channelled. Communications must relate to adults and children across the demographic and cultural spectrum, and are often concentrated on the behaviours of populations within economically deprived areas where the population has multiple health and social needs, and where there is often a disinclination towards positive health messages and/or behavioural change. Moreover, the social circumstances in many areas mean that, where behavioural change is achieved, it may be short-lived. Risk communication around public health must therefore address psychological, physiological, social, and economic behaviours, and seek to induce behavioural change amongst individuals and groups over the longer term such that health inequalities might be reduced and risk mitigated. As such, health promotion messages, and more specifically those messages targeted at particular types of risk, need to be carefully targeted at specific groups within the population. This chapter begins by considering the nature of the public(s) at whom health promotion is targeted, and illustrates the issues in relation to one particular area of risk—unintentional injuries. The chapter then discusses the nature of this particular risk, the problem of communication with the target group(s), and highlights the particular challenges faced by healthcare, social care, and voluntary organizations in creating interagency (or joined up) communication strategies.

## The population at risk

Unintentional childhood injuries (UCIs) are the leading cause of death amongst children in Europe and the US (Garzon, 2005; Garzon et al., 2007; Morrison et al., 1999; Towner & Towner, 2001). UCIs also account for many disabilities amongst children, and the physical and social impacts of injury, rehabilitation, and disability are often given too little consideration by governments and society more generally (Peden et al., 2008). There are many sources of injury, ranging from drowning, road traffic accidents, poisoning and burns, to injury involving pets (such as dog bites). Similarly, there are many locations in which such accidents can occur, including public places, playgrounds, the home, and shopping areas. Many countries have seen a reduction in injuries following effective lobbying, policies concerning equipment safety, fire prevention, labelling of medications, and childproof packaging (Klassen et al., 2000). Sweden in particular has witnessed significantly reduced numbers of UCIs following years of sustained coordinated and fully resourced strategies and interventions aimed at various age groups of children (Jansson et al., 2006). Sweden's success has involved environmental policies, product modifications, legislative change, interagency strategies, changes to urban planning, and government action in relation to funding and priority setting. Despite the success in Sweden and elsewhere, however, UCIs remain significant in terms of mortality and morbidity, and constitute one element of the fourth objective of the Millennium Development Goals—'to reduce by two-thirds the mortality of children under 5 years of age by 2015' (Peden et al., 2008, p. 145).

The term 'unintentional' suggests that these injuries are not simply 'a result of carelessness, stupidity or indifference' (Garzon et al., 2007). Rather, they 'result from a predictable interaction among host (person factors), environment (external factors), and injury agents (physical forces that result in bodily harm)' (Garzon et al., 2007). A similar view is taken by Deal et al. (2000b) and Reason (1990; 1997), who consider how various latent factors combine with 'active' errors, creating the conditions in which accidents occur. Potential (or latent) factors can erode the multiple layers of defences that are in place to prevent or mitigate damage and allow errors or violations to go undetected. In other words, whilst adult supervision, fire prevention, childproof packaging, and safety equipment (amongst others) all exist as layers of defence against accidents, none is flawless and, even in combination, these layers of defence may have gaps or shortcomings. Equipment can be faulty (even at the point of purchase), a supervisory adult may not know how to use the equipment, and smoke alarms are regularly left without a battery. Thus in a home where the smoke alarm battery has not been replaced, and the fire safety equipment is either broken or unfamiliar to the adult, a fire may escalate out of control before the emergency services have any chance of reaching the site of the incident. All of this may arise from a child discovering a box of matches or from a teenager leaving their hair straighteners plugged in and lying on the carpet. Reason refers to layers of defences as layers of 'Swiss cheese'. Where the holes can become aligned (as illustrated above), this allows a set of factors to combine to create an accident. Accidents are, therefore, not random, unexplained or unpreventable occurrences but instead can be anticipated and prevented. A key public health challenge is to ensure that people at risk, or those responsible for the population at risk, have an appreciation of the nature of unintentional injury risk (Garzon, 2005; Naidoo & Wills, 2000).

The interactions between these risk factors can also create latent pathways of risk that erode the existing defences. For example, safety equipment may be faulty and in reach of the inquisitive child, thereby creating a potential hazard pathway that erodes defences. Variability in the situational contexts adds further complexity to the problem of UCIs. As they grow, children's motor skills improve, as does their ability to link consequences with their own behaviour. However, when they are particularly young, their natural inquisitiveness, combined with a lack of awareness of what constitutes a hazard (e.g. failing to realize that a pile of books is not a safe platform from which to access something at a higher level), as well as their ability to respond physically either in terms of strength or speed in the event of an incident, all vary. Similarly, their environment varies, and hosts a range of potential hazards that may vary over time. Agent factors—defined as the 'means through which injuries occur' (Garzon, 2005)—again are myriad in nature, and range from the sharpness or size of a toy, to the speed of a heavy item falling from a shelf. Table 15.1 highlights findings from several studies (Garzon et al., 2007; Peterson et al., 1995; Ramsay et al., 2003; Russell, 1998; Towner et al., 2001b) that are indicative of the range of risks and hazards.

Adult (most commonly parental) supervision is of particular importance in mitigating the risk of accident given many 'normal' household items are a source of risk. As very young children are largely ill-equipped to recognize hazards, they rely on mediating factors—their parent/carer/older sibling's ability to recognize, avoid, and/or mediate the risk. This in turn is heavily influenced by the supervisor's perception of risk, supervisory diligence, and physical capabilities. Much attention has been paid to this aspect of childhood

**Table 15.1** Factors associated with unintended childhood injury

**Child factors**

*Behavioural and developmental*: natural curiosity, desire to manipulate things, impulsive natures, no awareness of risk or consequence, an innate desire to copy adults or older siblings, limited ability to learn from mistakes

*Physical*: changing motor skills, inability to 'combat inertia' (Garzon, 2005) (prevent a fall), tendency to be top-heavy and prone to falling, limited physical strength, small and pliable airways, rapid metabolic rates (problematic when ingesting a poisonous substance), less physical resilience to injury, limited ability to distinguish between visual and auditory signals/warnings

**Supervisory factors**

*Cognitive*: levels and sustainability of those levels of concentration, awareness of hazards and risk, familiarity with the environment (e.g. a baby-sitter may not know the home environment well)

*Physical*: physical strength and speed to keep up with a child's whereabouts (indoors or outdoors), speed of response (e.g. limited speed of movement due to pregnancy or injury), impaired hearing or vision such that audio or visual warnings go unnoticed

**Environmental factors/hazards**

Unguarded stairs, accessible window ledges/balconies, poorly lit or crowded spaces, busy roads, damaged/narrow paved areas, ungated gardens near busy roads, multiple occupant buildings with cluttered stair wells or no fire prevention equipment, poorly designed living space, small spaces/gaps

**Agent factors**

*In the home*: plugs, plug-in air fresheners, cables, household plants, candles, cosmetics, perfumes and hair sprays, cleaning products, medication, toys for older children, scissors, hobby/craft items (e.g. knitting needles, tools), and curtain and blind drawstrings/cords. *Outside*: uneven pavements, discarded bottles, needles, obstacles from fly tipping, unsafe play equipment such as trampolines and junior skateboards

**Social factors**

In addition to the factors noted earlier, there are further 'social' risk factors: *gender* (boys experience twice as many accidents as girls); *deprivation* and *socioeconomic status*; and in terms of *supervision*, the age and marital/cohabiting status of the parent(s), young parents and their substance abuse behaviours, and their level of educational qualifications and maternal health

injury within the literature (Morrongiello *et al.*, 2006; 2007). For the purposes of this discussion, it is sufficient to identify supervisory considerations as both sources and mitigators of hazard and to recognize that different supervisory groups (older siblings, grandparents, and baby-sitters for example) may also need to be targeted in different ways in terms of risk communication.

At this point in the discussion, it is therefore clear that there are a number of risk pathways that exist, many of which have a common mode potential for failure around the role played by the supervisor as both the originator of the hazard and as the key point of mitigation. There are several points of intervention in any accident (Reason, 1997), and adults and siblings can play an important role in risk mitigation (Child Safety Action Plan, 2007; Morrongiello *et al.*, 2006; 2007).

Preventing accidents is, however, just one layer of defence. Where there are gaps in other layers of defence, a key issue is how, and under what conditions, they may align. An understanding of how situations can escalate is also important. For example, a harassed mother who is carrying a baby may become distracted if the baby wriggles, letting an ill-positioned kettle slip from her hand and injuring a toddler at her side. The injury may derive from the kettle and/or from the boiling water. In an effort to assist, the mother may remove clothing in the case of a burn, causing further pain and skin damage, thereby escalating the event further. Dealing with the injury, also an element of risk communication, is a further point of risk mitigation. However, this requires a knowledge base around the nature of burns and how they should be handled. For example, an awareness of how to deal with such accidents in the home may have meant the mother responding differently and reducing the effects of the burn rather than exacerbating them by removing the child's clothing.

Such errors (holes in Swiss Cheese) may take different forms. They may include a lack of knowledge around the particular forms of hazard (as suggested above), poor supervisory practice, ill-prepared supervision (e.g. from older siblings), or the intervening effects of alcohol and drugs that, if taken by the supervisor, adversely affects his or her decision-making capabilities and impairs the supervisor's cognitive and physical responses. Some of these errors are preventable through a mix of education, advice, and behavioural change, albeit those related to problems of drug and alcohol addiction are more complex to resolve and may be embedded within concomitant personal and familial problems that raise further issues of risk and safety. In the following section, by combining Reason's work (Reason, 1990; 1997) with Naidoo and Wills' (2000) approaches to health promotion, the discussion goes on to identify points of intervention and mitigation that are available to public health practitioners, and discusses the particular characteristics of risk communication that arise.

## Public health interventions and risk communication

Where there is an identifiable risk (in this case UCI) and risk factors, two public health challenges arise: (1) designing an effective health improvement programme or, in this case, accident prevention programme with specific interventions; and (2) designing effective communications associated with the intervention. There are a number of approaches to health promotion (Naidoo & Wills, 2000) that can and have been used in efforts to improve child safety. These are shown in Table 15.2.

**Table 15.2** Approaches to health promotion: reducing UCIs

| Approach | Aims | Methods |
|---|---|---|
| Medical | To identify those at risk of injury or death from injury | Use of paediatric nursing staff in assessing the nature of injuries and the potential for ongoing risk |
| Behaviour change | Encouraging parents to take greater responsibility for child safety in the home and outside | Risk analysis and subsequent physical adaptation, e.g. child gates, smoke alarms as well as encouraging greater supervision |
| Educational | Raising awareness among parents, carers, and siblings of risks to children under 5 years old | Efforts to raise awareness of risk and prevention, e.g. fire safety programmes, school education |
| Empowerment | Working with communities to improve community safety | Road campaigns enabling communities to identify and create safer zones in residential areas and improve education concerning safety (among parents and children). The Scottish 'Twenty's Plenty' initiative is a good example |
| Social change | To address particular issues of injury associated with deprivation | Implementation of medicine labelling and childproof packaging. Parenting skills classes for new parents that include issues of supervision and injury prevention |

Developed from Naidoo & Wills, 2000, p. 102.

In the case of injury amongst the under-5 age group, a particular difficulty is that of addressing this target group directly in terms of the approaches set out in Table 15.2. As such, any intervention needs to be achieved through surrogates, of whom there are many—parents, guardians (some of whom may be foreign au pairs), siblings, nursery staff, extended family members, etc. These surrogates have very different characteristics in relation to potential 'holes' in this layer of defence. Nursery staff, for example, may be more knowledgeable about sources of hazard and, unlike a parent, can dedicate all of their time to supervision. A grandparent may have considerable knowledge of potential hazard and what to do in the event of an accident. But he or she may not have the physical energy to keep up with a small child that runs freely and nimbly around furniture, possibly falling against a table corner whilst ostensibly playing a game of chase. These surrogates thus vary considerably in terms of their knowledge of potential hazards, the quality of their supervision, their diligence as supervisors, their perception of and experience of risk, and their use of alcohol and drugs. They therefore require different messages about accident risks, supervisory responsibilities, and ways of mitigating and dealing with accidents.

Evidence on public health programmes and their specific individual and group level interventions suggests that, whilst each of the approaches in Table 15.2 can be effective in isolation, the results are greater when approaches are used in combination (Garzon, 2005; Towner et al., 2001). Community-based interventions, for example, whilst not a panacea (Naidoo & Wills, 2000), are more effective where multiple strategies are combined with an understanding and incorporation of behavioural change models (Klassen et al., 2000) as well as with visits to homes and physical/engineering interventions (e.g. installation of free smoke alarms). Where such actions are/can be combined with legislative changes such as laws on seatbelt use in cars, the effects are greater. Thus, a multistrand intervention with multifaceted communications is required (see also (Peden et al., 2008)). A key element of any such multistrand intervention is the need to create amongst the target population (or its surrogate) an awareness of the risk and the concomitant need for attitudinal and behavioural change.

It is notable, however, that not all community programmes are equally effective. Thus, in addition to effective risk communication, there needs to be effective emphasis on 'improved skills, changes in social norms, a supportive environment, and reinforcement that encourages behaviour change' (Klassen et al., 2000). It is particularly important to alter parental behaviour through both education and behaviour modification, especially in the case of the under-5 age group, although some studies have focused on education and behavioural change amongst 3–5–year-olds (Towner et al., 2001). Older siblings have also been the focus of education and behavioural change. Children may, for example, 'be trained to serve as monitors' (Klassen et al., 2000), e.g. in terms of 'buckling up' in the car. This message, where reinforced in school or nursery, can be transposed to the home environment and educate both parents and younger siblings. However, the scope for educating such relatively young children is limited. Younger children, for example, do not have suitably developed spatial awareness to deal with traffic and so cannot perform a monitoring role in broader road safety situations (Klassen et al., 2000).

Within public safety programmes and risk communication, it is also important to balance the rights of a child to a healthy, active, inquisitive lifestyle with the need to ensure they are safeguarded against unnecessary risks (Child Safety Action Plan, 2007). This balance therefore must become a central theme of a communications strategy. Whilst public health messages need to convey issues of road safety (e.g. when using bicycles, scooters, roller blades, and skateboards), parents, guardians, and children must be made aware of the need for and benefits of outdoor activity and exercise. At the same time, they can be encouraged to recognize that there are choices and risks associated with play within public and home environments. These choices centre on decisions about where it is safe to play, and at what point children (particularly within groups) might need to be supervised so that they do not take unnecessary risks when overexcited.

Where a programme is proposed, the risk needs to be spatially defined, and the communications targeted to the particular target group and through the relevant programme agencies. In areas of high deprivation, for example, where there are often a number of projects targeting a range of behaviours and problems, an intervention around UCIs will be most effective if incorporated with wider initiatives around child health and wellbeing and if it combines education, behavioural change, social change, and empowerment. Indeed, the WHO report (Peden *et al.*, 2008) considers it essential to have integrated children's strategies as no one measure is effective in isolation. Injury prevention should therefore be a part of a wider strategy around child health, wellbeing, and education, with health agencies taking a lead. One might also argue that within this approach, the UCI element should also address childhood injuries in a holistic way, recognizing common mode issues across several hazard pathways. In other words, addressing education and advice, design-related issues (e.g. play areas, car speeding policies), and wider social considerations (including social norms)—the common mode issues—needs to be done alongside several hazard pathways, such as traffic accidents, accidents in the home and playground, and secondary hazards such as alcohol and drugs. The intervention should also draw on, or signpost, resources already available through a range of organizations that provide advice, community resources, inspection, and/or promote particular initiatives such as Child Safety Week (RoSPA, 2008; Child Accident Prevention Trust, 2008; Safe Kids, 2008; The Scottish Good Egg Guide, 2008). At the same time, interventions need to be embedded within, and sensitive to, the particular population concerned.

## Integrated risk communication: the multi-agency challenge

Interventions are more effective when they are integrated into the community and when approaches are tailored to address unique community characteristics such as ethnicity or socioeconomic status . . . [and] involve community stakeholders in the programme development (Klassen *et al.*, 2000, p. 85).

As noted earlier, delivering health and social care services, and, more recently, promoting health and wellbeing, has increasingly become the provenance of multi-agency activity. Related developments around the area of social marketing (see below for further discussion) further illustrate the collective approach that is being taken towards understanding and influencing health-related behaviours where the approach is initiated through partnerships (such as the Department of Health and the National Consumer Council), and where changes are designed and delivered through public, private, and voluntary sector organizations. Indeed, interagency collaborations (referred to as partnerships or networks) have particular salience in public health where, in order to address complex multifaceted problems, an interagency perspective is necessary (Craig & Fischbacher, 2007).

Partnership working between agencies has consistently been regarded as readily accepted amongst agencies in principle, relatively easy to agree in broad terms, but problematic to implement and particularly problematic to evaluate in terms of both short- and long-term effectiveness (Craig & Fischbacher, 2007; Mandell & Keast, 2008). In relation to risk communication, particular challenges arise around communicating with the population/public at risk, the wider population or public(s), and between the agencies involved in designing and implementing specific public health interventions. These issues exist at a number of levels. In the first instance, a key challenge concerns the ability of professionals from different agencies to communicate effectively—overcoming professional conventions, cultures, and languages—to assess priorities and agree on key interventions. Whilst on the surface ensuring a collective approach to identifying and solving problems around public health might be readily achieved, research suggests that interprofessional barriers frequently jeopardize joint working (Glendinning, 2003; Huxham & Vangen, 2005; Mandell & Keast, 2008). With the exception of child protection where, as a result of legal requirements, professional considerations are overlooked in the interest of information sharing and ensuring that vulnerable children are not placed at further risk, many interagency partnerships are characterized by debate over alternative, discipline/profession-specific approaches to problem-solving and resistance to changing professional behaviours. This problem is compounded by the fact that additional resources to support interagency working are frequently short-term and do not convince staff that longer term activity will be sustainable. This is in contrast to the approach in Sweden where architects, urban planners, government agencies, transport agencies, and others have been collectively addressing the design of safer urban spaces for some time.

There is also the matter of the way in which expertise is recognized and heeded amongst the 'target groups'. There are issues associated with the level of trust that publics place in scientific evidence (see, for example, Bleich et al., 2007) and there can be confusion about what messages to heed, and how to weigh up the complex, sometimes conflicting, evidence that is portrayed through various forms of media, as the MMR debates recently showed (Petts & Niemeyer, 2004). Much of the evidence in relation to risk and health is reliant on the role of experts to interpret and communicate the underlying science. Such communications will need to be tailored for the many constituent groups that comprise general categories of broad interest groups. Policymakers, for example, may in fact be made up of elected members, consultants, politicians, think tanks, and so forth (Garvin, 2001). Similarly, the public is heterogeneous in terms of aspects such as education, scientific knowledge, and demographics: each of these influences the form and content of communication that is likely to have meaning to them. As we have already considered within this chapter, simply communicating to those responsible for supervising children would require differing methods and messages for siblings as for nursery nurses, grandparents, parents, au pairs, and so forth. Many studies also show that because of the difficulties of assessing evidence and seeking clarity and coherence amongst many conflicting 'expert' views, members of the public are in reality often more influenced by information that comes from their own social networks (Bleich *et al.*, 2007; Garvin, 2001; Petts & Niemeyer, 2004). This particular form of communication is both an opportunity and a problem for public health agencies. Personal stories can be convincing in either a positive or negative way: there are always 20-a-day smokers, drink drivers, drug takers, and other risk takers who defy the odds and whose personal accounts can be unhelpful reference points and behavioural influences. On the other hand, community-based interventions can benefit hugely from the involvement of a few, well integrated, members of the community whose capacity to spread evidence-based messages and to be heeded by that community can be crucial to effective communication strategies. Social networks are, however, not necessarily coterminous with the geographical areas in which many public health interventions occur and so there will need to be coordinated communications between the various bodies that interact nationally with different target groups. For example, teenagers (older siblings) have social networks through school, clubs, and internet sites, whereas grandparents may have very different social networks. Such messages need to acknowledge, or at least survive amidst the otherwise competing narratives often portrayed within the media. As Table 15.3 shows, the analytical paradigms of different interest groups potentially serve to undermine coherent risk communication. The more socially oriented needs of many members of the public may be at odds with the scientific and/or political paradigms of those seeking to promote particular lifestyles or communicate around issues of risk.

**Table 15.3** Conflicting analytical paradigms

|  | Scientists | Policy-makers | Public |
| --- | --- | --- | --- |
| Origin of evidence | Scientific studies | Availability | Popular sources |
| Legitimization of supporting evidence | Adherence to scientific method | Political, social, and economic implications | Received wisdom |
| Dismissal of conflicting evidence | Adherence to scientific method | Expediency | Common sense |
| Conceptualization of certainty and uncertainty | Probabilistic | Context-specific | Polarized (either certain or uncertain) |
| Understanding of complex issues | Compartmental | 'Need to know' | Limited by sources |
| Resultant knowledge | Specific and limited | Political, contextual, instrumental | Tacit, experiential, individual |
| What is done with the knowledge | Added to cumulative body of knowledge | Applied to current situation and context only | Added to body of personal experience |
| Analytical paradigm | Scientific | Political | Social |

Source: Garvin, 2001.

With regard to specific risks—such as those of UCI—agencies need to agree on the relative priorities in terms of hazard pathways and the means by which these might be addressed. The language and method of communication is likely to vary from one organization to another and so much discussion needs to take place around what risks must be addressed and how they might be presented both to colleagues in other agencies and to the public(s). The heterogeneity of the target groups for particular forms of communication becomes key and in the case of risks to child health, the need to reach the target group through surrogates further complicates the interagency element of risk communication and public health.

## Creativity and conflict

In bringing together staff from a range of organizations, there is potential for both creativity and conflict. There is also considerable scope for service (re)design and emergence in terms of strategies and ideas. It is a long-held rationale that complex problems need complex solutions (Alter, 1990; Alter & Hage, 1993). Whilst collaboration amongst a range of public health and related providers may draw attention to differing professional philosophies and a range of strategies from preventive to curative, there is also huge scope for generating variety in decision-making that can allow new ideas and approaches to emerge (Smith & Fischbacher, 2005). A key issue in getting to this stage is the effectiveness with which agencies involved in public health communicate with one another. If the message they put to the public(s) is to be unified and consistent, then there needs to be a common understanding between these agencies of the issues that they can tackle collectively and the ways in which they may do so. There then also needs to be a clear strategy for targeting communications. In this respect, the approach of social marketing may assist organizations in targeting their communications, drawing on well founded marketing approaches (Stead et al., 2007). Recently considered by the UK government as being a key means of improving public awareness as well as leading to changes in behaviour (Department of Health, 2004), social marketing draws on marketing approaches normally seen in commercial settings and uses them within the context of changes in relation to health and wellbeing. The approach has been shown to have benefits within several settings to date, such as in relation to smoking cessation, drug taking, and healthy eating. There may be considerable mileage, particularly in relation to addressing children, to consider ways in which the social marketing approach might be adopted in relation to issues of safety, accidents, and injury.

Irrespective of the adoption of any particular approach (such as social marketing), governments and health agencies faced with the responsibility of reducing UCIs in all children need to contend with several key interagency challenges around communicating and mitigating risk. These include:

- *Defining the public(s)* that is of concern. In this case, there are the risk group, the siblings who are key conduits of behavioural messages, parents or carers who are usually responsible for monitoring behaviour and creating the environment in which hazards may exist. Then there are those whose behaviour is a key determinant of the increased or decreased risk of injury, such as drivers and cyclists, dog owners, those responsible for public places, urban planners, law enforcement agencies, transport agencies, schools, and so forth

- *Creating an interagency framework* in which multiple organizations can come together, signal a coherent and united message that is then consistently communicated to the public(s) within school, home, and a range of community settings

- *Blending a national and local approach* that allows key players within communities (in particular those who are socially integrated) to provide reliable and consistent messages to the population at risk and within the settings that are important. This in itself requires collective action on the part of health and social care agencies, education, local libraries and other providers of information, and local businesses

◆ *Explicitly tackling the often competing priorities and philosophies of professionals.* The various analytical paradigms (Table 15.3), languages, and approaches of professional groups associated with the many organizations that could contribute to reducing UCIs present particular challenges. As with child protection for those children deemed at risk, injury prevention should be an area in which conventional barriers are removed, and professional interests given reduced priority. This is far easier said than done, but remains a priority. There is, for example, a great deal that could be learned from careful assessment of the success in places like Sweden and the ways in which agencies can cooperate effectively.

The matter of interagency partnership generally, and interagency cooperation and communication around UCIs is vexing. The exponential growth in the volume of publications on the matter of partnership working is sufficient to indicate the particular difficulties that organizations face. However, in matters of UCIs, there is a need to overcome interagency difficulties both to enable change within communities and indeed to raise awareness of the scale and impact upon children and families of the consequences of injuries. As Deal *et al.* recently noted:

> The twentieth century saw huge successes in healthcare in the United States. Immunizations, antibiotics, and public health initiatives have combined to lower the infant mortality rate and lengthen lifespan. Unlocking the secrets of the human genome promises more advances. Despite these advances, we remain stymied by the steady drumbeat of death and disfigurement attributable to childhood injuries. Injuries, both violent and unintentional, are one of the most significant public health issues facing children today, but public outrage is absent. As a result, proven solutions go unused, and thousands of children die each year (Deal *et al.*, 2000a, p. 4).

From this quote, and from other work cited in this chapter, the risk communication challenge begins with assembling and disseminating the data in relation to UCIs amongst those responsible for their reduction. Thereafter, the issues raised in this chapter come to the fore and represent a significant challenge for health and social care organizations nationally and internationally.

## References

Alter, C. (1990). An exploratory study of conflict and coordination in interorganizational service delivery systems. *Academy of Management Journal*, 33(3): 478–502.

Alter, C. & Hage, J. (1993). *Organizations Working Together*. London, Sage.

Bleich, S., Blendon, R. & Adams, A. (2007). Trust in scientific experts on obesity: implications for awareness and behaviour change. *Obesity*, 15(8): 2145–56.

Child Accident Prevention Trust (2008). http://www.capt.org.uk. Accessed 20 May 2008.

Child Safety Action Plan. (2007). Child safety strategy: preventing unintentional injuries to children and young people in Scotland. http://www.capt.org.uk/pdfs/css_dec07.pdf.

Craig, P. & Fischbacher, M. (2007). Collaborating for health. In: S. Cowley (ed.). *Community Public Health in Policy and Practice*, 2nd edn. London, Elsevier.

Deal, L. W., Gomby, D. S., Zippiroli, L. & Behrman, R. E. (2000). Unintentional injuries in childhood: analysis and recommendations. *The Future of Children*, 10(1): 4–22.

Department of Health. (2004). *Choosing Health: Making Healthier Choices Easier*. London, Stationery Office.

Garvin, T. (2001). Analytical paradigms: the epistemological distances between scientists, policy makers and the public. *Risk Analysis*, 21(3): 443–55.

Garzon, D. L. (2005). Contributing factors to preschool unintentional injury. *Journal of Pediatric Nursing*, 20(6): 441–7.

Garzon, D. L., Lee, R. K. & Homan, S. M. (2007). There's no place like home: a preliminary study of toddler unintentional injury. *Journal of Pediatric Nursing*, 22(5): 368–75.

Glendinning, C. (2003). Breaking down barriers: integrating health and care services for older people in England. *Health Policy*, 65: 139–51.

Huxham, C. & Vangen, S. (2005). *Managing to Collaborate. The theory and practice of collaborative advantage*. London, Routledge.

Jansson, B., Leon, A. P., Ahmed, N. & Jansson, V. (2006). Why does Sweden have the lowest childhood injury mortality in the world? The roles of architecture and public pre-school services. *Journal of Public Health Policy*, 27(2): 146–65.

Klassen, T. P., MacKay, J. M., Moher, D., Walker, A. & Jones, A. L. (2000). Community-based injury prevention interventions. *The Future of Children*, 10(1): 83–110.

Mandell, M. P. & Keast, R. (2008). Evaluating the effectiveness of interorganizational relations through networks. *Public Management Review*, 10(6): 715–31.

Morrison, A., Stone, D. H. & Group, E. W. (1999). Unintentional childhood injury mortality in Europe 1984–93: a report from the EURORISC Working Group. *Injury Prevention*, 5: 171–6.

Morrongiello, B. A., Corbett, M., Lasenby, J., Johnston, N. & McCourt, M. (2006). Factors influencing young children's risk of unintentional injury: Parenting style and strategies for teaching about home safety. *Journal of Applied Developmental Psychology*, 27: 560–70.

Morrongiello, B. A., MacIsaac, T. J. & Klemencic, N. (2007). Older siblings as supervisors: Does this influence young children's risk of unintentional injury? *Social Science and Medicine*, 64: 807–17.

Naidoo, J. & Wills, J. (2000). *Health Promotion: Foundations for Practice*. London, Bailliere Tindall.

Peden, M., Oyegbite, K., Ozanne-Smith, J. *et al.* (2008). *World Report on Child Injury Prevention*. Geneva, World Health Organization.

Peterson, L., Bartelstone, J., Kern, T. & Gillies, R. (1995). Parents' socialization of children's injury prevention: description and some initial parameters. *Child Development*, 66(1): 224–35.

Petts, J. & Niemeyer, S. (2004). Health risk communication and amplification: learning from the MMR vaccination controversy. *Health, Risk and Society*, 6(1): 7–23.

Ramsay, L. J., Moreton, G., Gorman, D. R. *et al.* (2003). Unintentional home injury in preschool-aged children: looking for the key—an exploration of the inter-relationship and relative importance of potential risk factors. *Public Health*, 117: 404–11.

Reason, J. T. (1990). The contribution of latent human failures to the breakdown of complex systems. *Philosophical Transactions of the Royal Society of London*, B 37: 475–84.

Reason, J. T. (1997). *Managing the risks of organisational accidents*. Aldershot, Ashgate.

RoSPA. (2008) R. S. f. t. P. o. A. http://www.rospa.com. Accessed 20 May 2008.

Russell, K. M. (1998). Preschool children at risk for repeat injuries. *Journal of Community Health Nursing*, 15(3): 179–190.

Safe Kids. (2008). http://www.safekids.co.uk. Accessed 20 May 2008.

Smith, A. & Fischbacher, M. (2005). Stakeholders in the service design process. *European Journal of Marketing*, 39(9/10/Special issue).

Stead, M., Gordon, R., Angus, K. & McDermott, L. (2007). A systematic review of social marketing effectiveness. *Health Education*, 107(2): 126–91.

The Scottish Good Egg Guide. (2008). http://www.protectchild.co.uk. Accessed 20 May 2008.

Towner, E. & Towner, J. (2001). The prevention of childhood unintentional injury. *Current Paediatrics*, 11: 403–8.

Towner, E., Dowswell, T. & Jarvis, S. (2001). Updating the evidence. A systematic review of what works in preventing childhood unintentional injuries: Part 2. *Injury Prevention*, 7: 249–53.

## Chapter 16

# Exporting Pandora's Box—exploitation, risk communication, and public health problems associated with the export of hazard

Denis Fischbacher-Smith (University of Glasgow) & Ray Hudson (Wolfson Research Institute, Durham University)

## Introduction

Globalization is by no means new, although processes of globalization have changed in form and emphasis with the passage of time. The processes of neoliberal globalization have attracted considerable attention in the academic literature, not all of which has been positive (Coe *et al.*, 2004; Dicken, 2004; Featherstone, 2003; Jones, 2008; Routledge, 2003). One particular aspect that critics have highlighted is the manner in which 'capital' has sought to exploit weakness in regulatory frameworks and labour costs. This has allowed organizations both to 'export' some noxious activities away from highly regulated western countries and to reduce operating costs by locating points of production in countries where environmental regulation is lax, labour unions are weak, and the costs of labour are low (Hudson, 2009; Smith & Blowers, 1992). In many cases, this 'export' of production has led to criticisms of western companies for their lack of social responsibility and their exploitation of 'developing' countries (Smith, 1993; Smith & Tombs, 1995; Tombs & Smith, 1995). This exploitation has led, in certain cases, to the creation of 'contaminated communities' (Edelstein, 1987) where high levels of pollution have generated concerns over public health, or where working conditions have led to worries about occupational safety and health. Processes of exploitation have also generated situations in which the power of the polluter has been used to exploit the relative weaknesses within the host communities to resist such developments. What has attracted less attention has been the impacts of these processes on public health and the problems that they create around expert judgement in decision-making and the processes of risk communication.

Whatever the underlying motivational forces may be, the process of hazard export can be seen as akin to the export of 'Pandora's Box'—by moving problems arising from hazardous activities out of highly regulated areas into zones where exploitation can occur. These exports take place without providing the appropriate set of knowledge(s) that would allow local communities to deal with the health and environmental problems that are generated. In some cases, these communities have little, if any, idea about the risks associated with these polluting or hazardous entities. As such, 'capital' (and its agents) can be seen to be exploiting imbalances in the knowledge, expertise, and power landscapes in which environmental 'decisions' are taken and the manner in which opposition to such activities can be bypassed. This raises some important issues for risk management and communication around public health issues.

Our aim here is to explore some of the processes that serve to generate the export of hazardous activities and to consider the manner in which the processes of production might impact upon the ways in which risk is 'consumed' by those groups that have little resilience to the hazards that they face. The implications for public health are considerable—those societies at risk will often neither have the resources to deal with a major pollution incident or accident, nor can they afford the costs of the chronic health impacts associated with polluting processes. In addition, these communities may lack the technical expertise to understand the nature of the risks they face or be incapable of 'resisting' environmental exploitation. The imbalance between corporate interests and potential victim groups is problematic enough in economically advanced countries (Irwin, 1995; Phillips, 2000; Rampton & Stauber, 2001; Smith, 1990), but the power gradient between these competing interests is even steeper in the global 'south' to which hazardous activities are exported. If the population 'at risk' lacks the technical literacy required to make sense of formal risk assessments, then they will be unable to mount an effective challenge to their findings or deal with the impacts of 'polluting' activities (Irwin, 1995; Irwin et al., 1996). To examine these issues in more detail, we need to contextualize the export of risk within the wider processes of globalization and to consider the nature of resilience within communities as a means of dealing with such problems. We also need to consider the role of science in both decision-making and risk communication. Before considering those issues in more detail, we first need to examine the drivers to risk exports.

# Capital flows, risk migration, and the erosion of public health

> ... one of the best predictors of the location of toxic waste dumps in the United States is a geographical concentration of people of low income and color (Harvey, 1996, p. 368).

Harvey's observation of the flow of risk into areas lacking power (both economic and political) remains an important issue for both the regulation of hazard and the management of public health. The areas to which Harvey refers can be likened to 'sinks' where the poor and the powerless, who already experience significant public health problems, are then exposed to increased levels of hazard without the necessary coping mechanisms. These coping mechanisms would include access to high quality healthcare (especially in the absence of state provision), political influence, access to expertise and knowledge about the nature of risk and the associated health effects, and the ability to move away from the source of the hazard. Such an underclass—to use Marx's term—deprived of economic and political power would inevitably lack access to good public health resources.

The combined consequences of a heightened level of risk and the lack of absorptive capacity[1] within their communities means that the 'export' of risk mirrors the hypermobility of capital. One can envisage a situation in which multiple flows of risk into these sink spaces will occur as capital exploits the evil twins of low cost and a weak regulatory regime. An initial flow of capital into these areas of relatively weak resource may be welcomed by the local population as jobs are created or wealth is generated. However, as capital has a strong tendency to pollute unless checked[2], then these initial benefits of (relative) wealth generation will be supplanted by environmental, health, or social costs associated with the production process. Capital investment in an area of relative poverty may also serve to attract itinerant groups to establish

---

[1] Absorptive capacity can be seen as the ability of a community to deal with the consequences of a hazard – both in terms of prevention and opposition but also with regard to dealing with the consequence of such risks.

[2] Pollution is often seen as an externality on the production process, which is 'ignored' by organizations unless they are forced to deal with the costs of prevention and clean-up. What has changed since the industrial revolution is the increased distances over which those hazards have been exported; the economic disparities between those who export the hazards and those who bear the costs associated with them; and the levels of complexity, expertise and knowledge that surround debates associated with the exploitation of those are exposed to these risks.

shanty developments close to such point sources of relative wealth. Witness the development of the shanty town next to the Union Carbide plant at Bhopal or the ribbon developments that have occurred close to oil pipelines in Nigeria and it is possible to see how these 'spaces of production' may generate unintended and hazardous consequences by attracting people to them, thereby increasing the population at risk. Irrespective of the failings of plant operators to manage the safety systems (which were considerable), the unregulated growth in the shanty town at Bhopal ensured that any failure would have serious off-site consequences. Attempts by shanty dwellers to 'break' into oil pipelines in Nigeria between 1998 and 2009 have had serious consequences, with the result that some 1500 people died[3] (Connors, 2008). We should perhaps not be surprised that those who are severely economically disadvantaged might be motivated by desperation to gain some sort of economic benefit by locating close to obvious 'corporate assets'. After all, extreme poverty and hunger are prime motivators within the human condition, especially when the discrepancies between rich and poor are extreme.

At a more abstract level, hypermobile flows of capital can result in increased environmental impacts that could, in extremis, have global consequences. Climate change and the generation of greenhouse gases have been policy issues for some 20 years, but without any effective resolution. Part of the problem has been the manner in which science has been used (and has failed) to reconcile opposing factions. In part, this has resulted from a set of problems around the scientific burden of proof and the manner in which large powerful interests can mobilize their power in the form of scientific 'evidence'. Similarly, the genetic modification of crops has been seen by some as an attempt by multinationals to control the world's food production—an allegation that has, of course, been refuted by companies, arguing that they are trying to address the issues of hunger and crop disease. For those poorer communities, which lack the educational and political means of engaging in discourse with powerful corporate elites, this creates an important element in the export of risk.

## Not in my backyard—the export of hazard

The processes by which risk is transmitted and the manner in which it can escalate to generate a crisis are important issues. The problems become more

---

[3] It has been suggested that in some cases this was for financial gain. The majority of Nigerians have to live on the equivalent of US$2 a day thus generating a powerful motivational factor in seeking to access the contents of pipelines despite the obvious hazards that they face. See Connors (2008) http://www.nytimes.com/2008/05/16/world/africa/16nigeria.html

acute in the highly globalized networks that organizations currently operate within, and this has led some to argue that we must now contend with a different set of environmental and societal settings within which risk has to be contextualized (Beck, 1992; Giddens, 1990; 1999; Gigerenzer, 2002). For some, this has led to the emergence of a whole new series of concerns within modern societies around the generation and transmission of risks (Erikson, 1994; Etkin, 1999; Fox, 1999; Lupton, 1999; Perrow, 1984; Tenner, 1996). 'Risk' can be seen as a social construction in which supposedly objective and scientifically determined risks are balanced by public perceptions of that risk (Beck, 1992; Collingridge & Reeve, 1986; Douglas & Wildavsky, 1983; Irwin, 1995). There is also an argument that sees effective risk management and regulation as a *partnership* process between the risk generators, the first responder organizations (whose job it is to mitigate those risks once they occur), and those who might be at risk from the activity (Barnes, 2001). Whilst this is achievable within wealthy western democracies, it is likely to prove problematic in much poorer countries where such partnership processes will not be possible owing to such issues as differentials in economic power, the nature of democratic processes, technical and scientific literacy rates, and the like. These imbalances simply add to the problems faced by those communities arising from the polluting activities themselves. Not only are they exposed to a range of additional risks (the benefits of which are felt elsewhere), but their communities also lack the resilience, expertise, and resources to mitigate the damage caused by those 'imported' hazards.

The problem is further compounded where the communication of those risks by the risk creators is absent or where it is couched in a language that is not readily understood by the receptors of the message. The technical literacy needed to oppose those who export these risks is inevitably high. Similarly, the level of economic and political capital needed to resist the import of these hazards is also considerable. We need to examine some of the underlying processes by which economic factors contribute to the drivers for such exports in order to provide a basis for considering the role of expert knowledge in shaping patterns of exploitation. In theory, processes of globalization could play a major role in improving public health and yet they are invariably seen as negative processes that generate, rather than ameliorate, problems. Perhaps one of the reasons why globalization has such a bad reputation in this regard can be traced back to the Bhopal tragedy.

The accident in the Indian subsidiary of Union Carbide at Bhopal in 1984, which killed in excess of 3500 people, had far-reaching implications for other chemical companies (Hazarika, 1987; Lapierre & Moro, 2002; Shrivastava, 1987; Smith, 1993). Bhopal was a watershed in the export of hazardous production from developed to developing countries as it highlighted the double standards that western multinationals seemed to be adopting in the distribution of those hazardous activities within their portfolio and the manner in which they managed those risks (Hazarika, 1987; Lapierre Moro, 2002; Shrivastava, 1987). The accident also exposed the limitations of the Indian healthcare system to cope with an accident on this scale along with the problems associated with the provision of both acute and long-term care for the victims. Bhopal highlighted the problems that local communities faced in terms of recognizing the nature of the hazards and mounting opposition to those activities. It also illustrated the difficulty that powerless groups can face when trying to obtain justice in the aftermath of an accident, even on such a large scale.

Union Carbide's initial response to the disaster was to claim that the Bhopal plant was designed to a high standard. In essence, it claimed that the 'resilience' within the system was engineered into the systems design. Union Carbide could not be seen to be exporting an inferior design or technology that failed to meet US standards for such a hazardous process. Carbide subsequently argued that there were 'differences' between the two plants, and that the Indian plant was designed and built by Indian engineers. The problem thus became one that was generated by the Indian subsidiary rather than the parent company (Browning, 1993: see also the statement at http://www.bhopal.com/ucs.htm). It also raised the prospect of sabotage as the initiating mechanism for the accident and, whilst never proven, this remains an element of Carbide's defence. The erosion of safety systems did, however, point to potentially lax and damaging managerial practices. The US parent claimed that it was unaware of these problems. One of the many narratives that emerged after the accident was that Union Carbide India managers had advised senior managers in the Union Carbide Corporation that the Bhopal plant needed investment in safety systems. However, this investment was not forthcoming and the plant continued operating with safety systems that were suboptimal. Union Carbide managers in the USA denied that they had received any warnings of suboptimal performance around the plant's safety systems. (See http://www.bhopal.com/faq.htm#faq5, which outlines a series of rebuttals to common criticisms made of Union Carbide.) This disagreement continues today as Union Carbide maintain their view that the plant was sabotaged.

Bhopal illustrates the importance of variability and unpredictability in shaping the manner in which organizations can fail. The manner in which shanty development was allowed to occur around the site points to the lack of effective regulation around these 'spaces of production'. The underlying reasons for these problems can be found in the manner that capital flows help to shape the landscapes of production (Hudson, 2001; 2002). It is our contention here that, by failing to generate greater resilience within the host communities where these activities are located, the export of hazard will erode the public and occupational health of those populations.

Bhopal served as a catalyst for a set of wider concerns about the export of risk (Smith, 1993; Smith & Blowers, 1991; 1992). Many of those concerns are still present today although the processes of risk exploitation have become more sophisticated. This includes the exploitation of workers and their exposures to high levels of occupational hazard, increased environmental degradation within local communities, and the use and exploitation of cheap labour and weak environmental legislation to ensure greater profit margins (Hudson, 2009). By widening the perspective that organizations take on crisis management to include more effective provision in the public health infrastructure in areas where they locate their production, organizations would be acting in a socially responsible way as well as seeking to contain the potential for crisis. However, the reality often is that this does not take place, or does so on a superficial level. Governments in the host countries are seen as having responsibility for providing healthcare capabilities and infrastructure—despite the fact that they invariably lack the resource to do so on the scale required to cope with a catastrophic accident. Put another way, these countries do not have the resilience that is needed to cope with the task demands of such accidents.

## Resilient communities—a challenge for multinationals?

The ability of communities to deal with the demands of hazardous events has proved to be an important issue for policy-makers. Both the Indian Ocean tsunami and Hurricane Katrina illustrated the problems that communities can face when dealing with major crisis events, and both illustrated the difficulties that the poorer and more vulnerable communities face in these circumstances. Similar problems will also be faced by communities around the long-term health impacts of pollution or occupational exposure—especially if there is a large population at risk.

Policy-makers in western nations have now begun to frame 'risk management' in terms of the notion of resilient communities. Resilience has emerged within the policy environment in the UK as a means of framing the ways in which organizations and elements of the state can deal with extreme events. However, whilst the term may be more politically acceptable than 'crisis management', it does raise questions about what the term 'resilience' means both in theory as well as in practice.

Resilience as a concept has a variety of origins across work in engineering, psychology, ecology, and the biological sciences. Each of these literatures tends to deal with the specifics of the term in different ways and this can be seen to shape the operationalization of the term in practice.

Holling and Gunderson (2002), for example, argue that the engineering approaches to resilience are typified by a search for:

> ... efficiency, control, constancy, and predictability—all attributes at the core of desires for fail-safe design and optimal performance. Those desires are appropriate for systems where uncertainty is low. (Holling and Gunderson, 2002, p. 27).

However, in those situations where levels of uncertainty are high—typical of organizational activities around sociotechnical systems—then the engineering approaches to framing resilience may prove limited. In contrast, Holling and Gunderson feel that 'biological' interpretations of resilience may provide a more appropriate perspective on the development of the concept. Here resilience is seen in terms of the:

> ... persistence, adaptiveness, variability, and unpredictability (p. 27),

that is associated with the impacts upon the community. Put another way, the ability of the population at risk to deal with such 'shocks' is seen as a key component of resilience. We argue here that the engineering approach to resilience is generally inappropriate when dealing with vulnerable communities—especially where the levels of technical literacy are low—and our approach is grounded within a systems view of resilience and resilient communities. It is our contention here that multinationals will generate the potential for catastrophic failure if they don't consider the public health infrastructure that is in place or fail to take account of the 'absorptive capacity' of the host population to deal with hazardous technologies and processes in a safe manner.

## Not in my backyard—your backyard is another proposition entirely!

> Risk determinations are an unrecognised, still undeveloped symbiosis of the natural and human sciences, of everyday and expert rationality, of interest and fact. They are simultaneously neither simply the one nor only the other. They can no longer be isolated from one another through specialisation, and developed and set down according to their own standards of rationality. They require a cooperation across the trenches of disciplines, citizens' groups, factories administration and politics, or—which is more likely—they disintegrate between these into antagonistic definitions and definitional struggles (Healy, 2001, p. 39).

Debates around the export of hazardous waste in the 1990s attracted a considerable amount of media and political attention in western countries, and also served to change elements of the regulatory environment in which 'toxic capitalism' operated. In some cases, the 'protests' at these polluting activities generated what have become known as patterns of resistance within local communities (Routledge, 1997). These patterns of resistance represent a challenge to the activities of what are seen as the dominant power elites within society:

> Resistances are assembled out of the materials and practices of everyday life and imply some form of contestation (Routledge, 1997, p. 361).

This contestation can take many forms, although in the case of risk-related issues, tends to involve the use of expertise to counter the claims of 'safety' made by corporate elites (Smith, 1990). In part, it was the emergence of patterns of resistance in the west that prompted the export of hazardous activities to countries with less developed mechanisms for opposition and where the revenues generated by such exports were extremely attractive. The low levels of technical and scientific literacy in these communities also served to compound the processes of exploitation. Resistance therefore becomes entwined in a series of discourses around knowledge and its interpretation.

Almost by definition, debates around hazardous activities create issues relating to the exploitation of those who are exposed to the risk. As such,

> ... practices of resistance cannot be separated from practices of domination: they are always entangled in some configuration. The practices and discourses of resistance require some form of coordination and communication, usually involving some form of collective action (Routledge, 1997, p. 361).

Concerns have been expressed about the role of expertise in this process and, in particular, about the role of experts in perpetuating the conditions that underpin the risk society (Cohen, 1997; Collingridge & Reeve, 1986). The utilization of science and its associated corpus of expertise is seemingly interwoven in the exploitation process (Smith, 1990) and Cohen observes:

> ... if society is unable to wrest control of its technology away from an increasingly discredited scientific-political establishment, the future takes on a much gloomier colour. Under these circumstances, the conditions that give rise to the risk society are likely to be prolonged indefinitely as science perpetuates its reductionist habits, dividing itself into still narrower specialisations and becoming further estranged from lay sentiment. The opportunity for democratic governance slips away as the scientific community, and the political institutions that depend on its input, struggles to preserve its legitimacy before an alienated public whose sense of alarm receives new justification with each periodic catastrophe. (Cohen, 1997, p. 108).

The 'normal' approach to deal with these problems is through the process of risk assessment. This invariably requires the issues to be mediated by technical experts and it is a process that can create difficulties around the burden of proof, error cost, and the exercise of powerful interests (Collingridge, 1992; Collingridge & Reeve, 1986; Smith, 1991; Smith & Elliott, 1992). Whilst there are well established tools and techniques for calculating risk and determining the consequences associated with a hazard, the evidential basis for such determinations and the extent to which the findings have predictive validity have proved to be contentious and a source of conflict. In many cases, experts' best estimates have been used as a means of bridging the information gap in determining the 'levels' of risk (in both probabilistic and consequential terms) (Smith, 1990). The problem in these cases is that the final determination of probabilities, on which policy-makers will make decisions, does not always highlight the degree of uncertainty and ambiguity in the data used. For poorer countries, this process can be heightened still further, as local communities are invariably unable to mount any serious and meaningful challenges to these risk determinations. The result is that expert knowledge and economic power combine to exploit local populations and also to undermine processes around risk communication.

Against this background, Collingridge and Reeve (1986) sought to develop a framework through which we could explain why some scientific debates generate controversy whilst others do not. They argue that there are two 'mechanisms' in which scientific arguments are fed into the policy-making process. The first of these, shown in Figure 16.1, they term the under-critical model. Here, organizations do not criticize any scientific information that supports the main policy objective. Any 'evidence' or argument that runs counter to the dominant view is criticized and marginalized. The result is an apparent scientific consensus that reinforces the policy consensus. The argument has been articulated that this state is possible when organizations have sufficient power to shape debates and to 'impose' their world view of

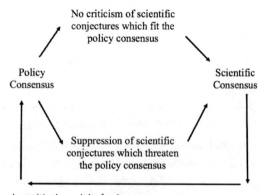

**Fig. 16.1** The under-critical model of science.
Reproduced from Collingridge & Reeve (1986), p. 33.

acceptable science on the scientific arguments (Collingridge & Reeve, 1986; Smith, 1990). Examples of such debates would include the early stages of the tobacco wars and debates around AIDS, climate change, and environmental impact (Davis, 2002; Epstein, 1996). In these cases, powerful corporate interests were able to provide their own scientific evidence to undermine any criticisms of their dominant policy view.

In contrast, where there are shifts in the balance of power over time (as has happened with the cigarette debates) or where the power of the corporate interests is low, then the debates are often more heated, with no one scientific world view dominating. Here, Collingridge and Reeve argue that the over-critical model of science will apply, and this is shown in Figure 16.2. If the power of corporate interests wanes, or where that power is not sufficiently strong to shape scientific debates, then the debates change into those where no single view of the underlying 'proof' is allowed to dominate. This is particularly problematic in those debates that draw upon multidisciplinary perspectives (as many risk debates invariably do) as there is a tendency for the evidential basis of the debates to become weaker as multiple perspectives are brought to bear on the arguments. Consequently, there is considerable debate between the various scientific 'camps' that leads to a heightened level of debate and criticism, and a loss of scientific autonomy owing to the competing interests involved.

The manner in which we move from one state to another in this framework is unclear, although there is some evidence to suggest that the underlying structures of capital may be influential in allowing corporate groups to 'influence'

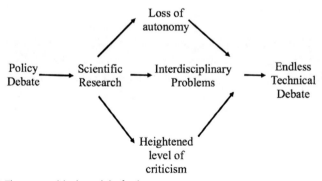

**Fig. 16.2** The over-critical model of science.
Reproduced from Collingridge & Reeve (1986), p. 32.

policy-makers and regulators (Smith, 1990). If this is the case, then there are potential problems when such power is exerted in an international context—especially where the power gradients that exist between wealthy multinational corporations and poorer countries and communities are steep. The debates in the 1990s around hazardous waste exports highlighted the willingness of some poorer countries to accept such material because of the relatively high sums of money that they were paid[4] (Smith, 1991; Smith & Blowers, 1992; Smith & Elliott, 1992). They also indicated the problems that host populations faced in mounting any meaningful resistance to these imports.

These issues raise some important questions for public health and risk communication. Firstly, if resistance towards such noxious activities is to be effectively mounted, then local populations must have access to information and the means of interpreting that information. There is a clear need to ensure that there is sufficient technical literacy available to such populations to interpret the extent of the risks that they face. As this is unlikely to be achieved from within the communities at risk (as they are, by definition, often amongst the poorest in those countries), then there is an opportunity for environmental groups (ranging from local to global non-governmental organizations) to take on a more proactive role by acting as agents for the powerless, perhaps at the risk of seeming to create new neocolonial relationships. An obvious problem here lies in the manner in which economic imbalances will serve as a driver for politicians to 'ease through' such activities. However, these issues can more easily be raised in the home countries of western multinationals where the share price of a company can be severely damaged by adverse media coverage, especially in the wake of accidents in developing countries.

Secondly, whilst it is clear that developing countries are unlikely to enact legislation that would restrict the import of wealth-generating (although noxious) industries, it is possible that pressure can be brought to bear on western governments to control these export activities more carefully. As the recent collapse of the western banking sector has sharply illustrated, there is no firm evidence to suggest that managers in western companies will behave in a responsible manner or will prioritize long-term sustainability over short-term gain. Unfortunately, as the debates around climate change suggest, certain

----

[4] It should be noted that there is also a trade in waste that is directed to Western countries, the UK being a prime example. This waste is usually sent for reprocessing and treatment rather than simply for disposal. By contrast, the export of hazardous waste and production activities from economically powerful to weaker countries is a process of exploitation rather than a trade that is driven by expertise and capability.

western governments also show a marked reluctance to enact legislation to address such issues until it is virtually too late.

Thirdly, if western companies are to export polluting activities abroad, then perhaps they should be made to invest in the health and educational infrastructures of those communities in which their plants are located. A socially responsible organization might well consider this to be a logical part of the process, certainly in terms of dealing with the wider issues of resilience in the local communities where their plants are located. Such a process would go some way to ensuring that the absorptive capacity of those populations at risk could be improved, although this does create some ethical issues.

Finally, a key requirement of any 'export' process should be the need to ensure that the hazards associated with the activity are effectively communicated to both local populations (and in a manner that is accessible to them) and to host governments. In an ideal world, we should seek to enact legislation that prevents the export of hazardous activities. Sadly, our world is far from ideal and there is no sign that the current processes of exploitation through risk transfers will cease as long as vested self-interest prevails. The lack of corporate social responsibility in a number of multinational corporations is likely to remain an important factor in this regard (Smith, 1993; Tombs & Smith, 1995).

## Conclusions

This chapter has highlighted a set of key policy issues around the export of hazardous activities and contextualized them within the wider process of globalization. The export of hazardous activities remains a problem despite attempts at international regulation via the Basel convention on the Control of Transboundary Movements of Wastes and their disposal (see http://www.basel.int). Whilst public policy can serve to reduce risks to some people in some places, it typically does so by enhancing the risk to other people in other places, albeit unintentionally. Such exports therefore remain a key policy issue and bring with them a series of concerns for public health, the manner in which governments and corporations communicate risk, and the capacity of local populations to comprehend the nature of the risks involved. Consequently, there continue to be considerable barriers to dealing with these problems of enhanced risk, not least of which is the manner in which economic power can be used as a principal driving force to export such hazardous activities and to provide a degree of legitimacy for that strategy. The consequence of this is that any effective solution to the problem will invariably need to be legislative in its scope and enacted on a global scale. Unfortunately, such global regulatory capacity is typically most noticeable by its absence, despite innovations such as the Basel convention. As a result, this issue is likely to remain on the policy agenda for years to come.

## References

Barnes, P. (2001). Regulating safety in an unsafe world (risk reduction for and with communities). *Journal of Hazardous Materials*, 86(1–3): 25–37.

Beck, U. (1992). *Risk society. Towards a new modernity* (M. Ritter, Trans.). London, Sage.

Browning, J. B. (1993). Union Carbide: Disaster at Bhopal. In: J. A. Gottschalk (ed.). *Crisis Response: Inside stories on managing under siege*. Accessed online at http://www.bhopal.com/pdfs/browning.pdf. Detroit, Visible Ink Press.

Coe, N. M., Hess, M., Wai-chung Yeung, H., Dicken, P. & Henderson, J. (2004). 'Globalizing' regional development: a global production networks perspective. *Transactions of the Institute of British Geographers*, 29(4): 468–84.

Cohen, M. J. (1997). Risk society and ecological modernisation alternative visions for post-industrial nations. *Futures*, 29(2): 105–19.

Collingridge, D. (1992). *The Management of Scale: Big organizations, big decisions, big mistakes*. London, Routledge.

Collingridge, D. & Reeve, C. (1986). *Science Speaks to Power: The role of experts in policy-making*. London, Francis Pinter.

Connors, W. (2008). 100 feared dead in Nigerian pipeline fire. *The New York Times*, 16 May 2008. http://www.nytimes.com/2008/05/16/world/africa/16nigeria.html. Accessed online 27 March 2009 at 1830 hours GMT.

Davis, D. (2002). *When Smoke Ran Like Water. Tales of environmental deception and the battle against pollution*. Oxford, Perseus Press.

Dicken, P. (2004). Geographers and 'globalization': (yet) another missed boat? *Transactions of the Institute of British Geographers*, 29(1): 5–26.

Douglas, M. & Wildavsky, A. (1983). *Risk and Culture*. Berkeley, University of California Press.

Edelstein, M. (1987). *Contaminated Communities: The social and psychological impacts of residential toxic exposure*. Boulder, Westview Press.

Epstein, S. (1996). *Impure Science. AIDS, activism, and the politics of knowledge*. Berkeley, CA, University of California Press.

Erikson, K. (1994). *A new species of trouble. Explorations in disaster, trauma, and community*. New York, W. W. Norton and Company.

Etkin, D. (1999). Risk transference and related trends: driving forces towards more mega-disasters. *Environmental Hazards*, 1: 69–75.

Featherstone, D. (2003). Spatialities of transnational resistance to globalization: the maps of grievance of the inter-continental caravan. *Transactions of the Institute of British Geographers*, 28(4): 404–21.

Fox, N. J. (1999). Postmodern reflections on 'risk', 'hazards' and life choices. In: D. Lupton (ed.). *Risk and Sociocultural Theory. New directions and perspectives*. Cambridge, Cambridge University Press, pp.12–33.

Giddens, A. (1990). *The Consequences of Modernity*. Cambridge, Polity Press.

Giddens, A. (1999). *Runaway World. How globalisation is reshaping our lives*. London, Profile Books.

Gigerenzer, G. (2002). *Reckoning with Risk. Learning to live with uncertainty.* London, Allen Lane, The Penguin Press.

Harvey, D. (1996) Justice, Nature and the Geography of Difference. Oxford: Blackwell.

Hazarika, S. (1987). *Bhopal. The lessons of a tragedy.* New Delhi, Penguin Books (India).

Holling, C.S. & Gunderson, L.H. (2002) Resilience and Adaptive Cycles. In: L.H. Gunderson and C.S. Holling (eds.) Panarchy. *Understanding Trasnformations in Human and Natural Systems.* Washington DC: Island Press, pp. 25–62.

Hudson, R. (2001). *Producing Places.* New York, The Guilford Press.

Hudson, R. (2002). Changing industrial production systems and regional development in the New Europe. *Transactions of the Institute of British Geographers,* 27(3): 262–81.

Hudson, R. (2009). The costs of globalization: producing new forms of risk to health and well-being. *Risk Management: An International Journal,* 11(1): 13–29.

Irwin, A. (1995). *Citizen Science: A study of people, expertise and sustainable development.* London, Routledge.

Irwin, A., Dale, A. & Smith, D. (1996). Science and Hell's Kitchen—the local understanding of hazard issues. In: A. Irwin & B. Wynne (eds). *Misunderstanding Science? The public reconstruction of science and technology.* Cambridge, Cambridge University Press, pp.47–64.

Jones, A. (2008). The rise of global work. *Transactions of the Institute of British Geographers,* 33(1): 12–26.

Lapierre, D. & Moro, J. (2002). *Five Past Midnight in Bhopal.* New York, Warner Books.

Lupton, D. (ed.) (1999). *Risk and Sociocultural Theory. New directions and perspectives.* Cambridge, Cambridge University Press.

Perrow, C. (1984). *Normal Accidents.* New York, Basic Books.

Phillips, J. (2000). The BSE Inquiry. *The report of the inquiry into BSE and variant CJD in the United Kingdom.* London, HMSO.

Rampton, S. & Stauber, J. (2001). *Trust us, we're experts! How industry manipulates science and gambles with your future.* New York, NY, Jeremy P. Tarcher/Putnam.

Routledge, P. (1997). The imagineering of resistance: pollok free state and the practice of postmodern politics. *Transactions of the Institute of British Geographers,* 22(3): 359–76.

Routledge, P. (2003). Convergence space: process geographies of grassroots globalization networks. *Transactions of the Institute of British Geographers,* 28(3): 333–49.

Shrivastava, P. (1987). *Bhopal. Anatomy of a crisis.* Cambridge, Mass., Ballinger Publishing Company.

Smith, D. (1990). Corporate power and the politics of uncertainty: Risk management at the Canvey Island complex. *Industrial Crisis Quarterly,* 4(1): 1–26.

Smith, D. (1991). The Kraken wakes—the political dynamics of the hazardous waste issue. *Industrial Crisis Quarterly,* 5(3): 189–207.

Smith, D. (1993). The Frankenstein factor—corporate responsibility and the environment. In: D. Smith (ed.). *Business and the Environment: Implications of the new environmentalism.* London, Paul Chapman Publishing, pp.172–89.

Smith, D. & Blowers, A. (1991). Passing the buck—hazardous waste disposal as an international problem. *Talking Politics,* 4(1): 44–9.

Smith, D. & Blowers, A. (1992). Here today there tomorrow: the politics of transboundary hazardous waste transfers. In: M. Clark, D. Smith & A. Blowers (eds). *Waste Location: Spatial aspects of waste management, hazards and disposal.* London, Routledge, pp. 208–26.

Smith, D. & Elliott, P. (1992). Hazardous waste and risk assessment. *European Environment*, 2(1): 1–4.

Smith, D. & Tombs, S. (1995). Self regulation as a control strategy for major hazards. *Journal of Management Studies*, 32(5): 619–36.

Tenner, E. (1996). *Why Things Bite Back. Technology and the revenge effect.* London, Fourth Estate.

Tombs, S. & Smith, D. (1995). Corporate responsibility and crisis management: some insights from political and social theory. *Journal of Contingencies and Crisis Management*, 3(3): 135–48.

Chapter 17

# Communication about persistent environmental risks: problems of knowledge exchange and potential of participative techniques

Sara Fuller (University of Durham),
Karen Bickerstaff (King's College London),
Fu-Meng Khaw (North Tyneside Primary
Care NHS Trust), & Sarah Curtis
(University of Durham)

This chapter reviews research on the potential for knowledge exchange and participative approaches in making risk communication more effective. We focus particularly on examples of communication concerning 'chronic', persistent risks associated with environments that are known to be contaminated, as well as 'potential' sources of environmental contamination such as industrial facilities in their normal operation and decommissioning. Communication relating to these rather 'routine' and unexceptional aspects of environmental risk may not be given as much attention and publicity as occasional, severe pollution events giving rise to crisis situations, but they may be important for the actors involved for several reasons.

One significant aspect of these chronic environmental risks is that they may be a direct and ongoing source of worry to lay sectors of society ('the public') in particular local settings, resulting in cumulative stress for members of the affected communities (Couch & Kroll-Smith, 1991; Edelstein, 2003; Boholm & Löfstedt, 2004). It is important from the point of view of the arguments presented here that these psychosocial impacts seem to be associated with a sense of powerlessness to intervene to address the causes of pollution. For example, Evans & Stecker (2004) review evidence that exposure to pollution due to noise, crowding or pollution can induce 'learned helplessness' which demotivates individuals and reduces their ability to work and learn effectively. In extreme cases, these effects are measurable; for example, researchers in an area of Australia (Higginbotham *et al.*, 2006) affected by open cast mining developed and tested the 'environmental distress scale', to record biosocial impacts of environmental disturbance, including *solastalgia*, which expresses the sense of loss, exacerbated by feelings of powerlessness associated with environmental changes affecting the area around one's home (Albrecht *et al.*, 2007).

Moreover, whilst much of the research focused on populations living adjacent to industrial facilities reveals an apparent lack of local disquiet or concern (Baxter & Lee, 2004; Burningham & Thrush, 2004), it has been argued that such 'silences' can mask anxieties that are not openly expressed for a variety of psychological, social, cultural, economic or political reasons (Wakefield & Elliott, 2000; Zonabend, 1993; Solecki, 1996; Simmons & Walker, 1999). It is a response that has been interpreted as borne of political–economic powerlessness, defending the subject's sense of security and protecting them from what would otherwise be unmanageable anxiety (Hollway & Jefferson, 1997; Wynne et al., 1993). For instance, Zonabend's (1993, p. 28) study of the everyday lives of the community adjacent to the nuclear reprocessing plant at La Hague reveals a desire—on the part of residents—to place the technological object at a certain, socially determined distance: 'You can't see the plant from my place . . . So we're all right'. The author argues that what is identifiable is a refusal to acknowledge risk, a form of 'active blindness' which amounts to a denial of danger. Zonabend also notes people's feelings of impotence in the face of risk, a situation in which the only realistic stance is one of silence.

Another issue is the sense of stigma that may be inflicted on communities in areas that are subject to ongoing risks of contamination (Edelstein, 2003; Zonabend, 1993; Flynn *et al.*, 2001)—particularly linked to industrial facilities or other undesirable technologies. Various authors (Bickerstaff, 2004; Bush *et al.*, 2001; McGee, 1999; Irwin *et al.*, 1999) have discussed the links between the social construction of the reputation of places and sense of individual or local collective identity defined by place (especially one's place of residence). Where society attributes a negative reputation to a place because of (a possible) environmental contamination, social discourses also tend, by association, to discredit the people living in these areas, and may also reduce residents' socioeconomic standing through processes such as housing markets (McCluskey & Rausser, 2003). Resisting these stigmatizing effects, people living in polluted areas, especially where the local economy depends heavily on the polluting activity, tend to construct the nuisance and health risks of environmental pollution differently to those outside the area; for example, by putting less emphasis on environmental conditions and stressing positive aspects of the social environment (Wakefield & McMullan, 2005; Bush et al., 2001; McGee, 1999). This may partly explain why, for example, Quandt et al. (2004) found that some participants in discussion of polluted environments tend to see their community as the norm, although it may in fact have worse than average conditions (see also the above discussion on psychosocial distancing). Thus the risks for human health and wellbeing may be social and psychological as much as physical.

Communication about relatively 'low level' and ongoing risks constitutes a significant element of professional practice for those for whom part of their routine workload is to communicate with wider society about the risks of environmental pollution. Through communication of these 'everyday', persistent risks, relationships are built up between affected publics and key professional and commercial organizations responsible for risk governance and communication, which may also be important on occasions when unusual risks arise or severe and urgent 'crisis' situations arise, as discussed in earlier chapters of this book. In the following discussion we consider research findings which suggest an important role for 'two-way', participative risk communication strategies and knowledge exchange in respect of risks of this type and we summarize findings from research on their potential and limitations, as well as the challenges they present.

## Our approach to review

The material used in this chapter is primarily drawn from a review and content analysis of publications concerning risk communication undertaken by some of the authors for the Health Protection Agency, North East. Full details of the review as a whole are available in the research report (Curtis *et al.*, 2008). In brief, the searches were carried out in the search engines Web of Science and Medline. The main search was conducted in March 2008 and some supplementary searches were completed by June 2008.The Medline search used archives running back to 1996, and although the Web of Science search was not time-limited, the selected publications were all published after 1990, reflecting the recent growth of research in this field. A summary of the search terms employed that are relevant to this chapter are given in Box 17.1. Of the 144 papers retained for this review, 72 were specifically concerned with communication relating to environmental pollution or general environmental health risks, and 25 of these explicitly argued in favour of some form of 'two-way' communication or participative strategy for engaging the public, together with public health professionals and other experts in processes of risk communication. This underlines the extent of agreement in research findings

## Box 17.1 Search terms to generate references to research relating to risk communication on environmental contamination

*Web of Science* search terms:

• Topic=(risk SAME communic*) OR (risk AND percept*)

• AND topic=(environment* SAME health*)

• Results refined by subject areas =(PUBLIC, ENVIRONMENTAL, and OCCUPATIONAL HEALTH OR ENVIRONMENTAL SCIENCES).

*Medline* search terms:

• Risk communic*.mp. [mp=title, original title, abstract, name of substance word, subject heading word] OR risk percept*.mp. [mp=title, original title, abstract, name of substance word, subject heading word]

• AND exp *environmental health.

concerning the importance of this aspect of risk communication. Several of the other papers discussed techniques of risk communication that might contribute usefully to effective two-way communication. We discuss these research findings in more detail below.

## The case for two-way participation in risk communication and knowledge exchange

As noted above, it is widely acknowledged in the published research that we reviewed that the process of communicating about risk should take the form of a 'two-way' exchange, rather than a one-way monologue on the part of 'experts' of what it is believed the community needs to hear.

Official advice on effective risk communication has been in circulation for some time, articulated at national and international levels. In England, the Inter-Departmental Liaison Group on Risk Assessment (ILGRA, 1998, p. 7) set out 'principles for good practice' which included the advice that:

> Regulatory bodies should identify and engage with all those interested in and affected by each risk issue . . . Their views and preferences should be incorporated into policy and practice.

Biocca (2005) discusses the Aarhus Convention, adopted in 1998 by the Pan-European Conference of Environment Ministers, which also called for participation in decision-making processes for citizens. Also, the World Health

Organization (2000) has issued guidelines for 'environmental risk assessment' that include recommendations which include better communication with stakeholders and increased transparency in risk assessment. Not only public bodies but also private organizations are encouraged to 'listen to stakeholders' affected by environmental risks. Gray (1995) considers that private companies who are potential polluters would do well to adopt a cooperative, rather than an adversarial, approach to the public, and Capriotti (2007) discusses using the internet to facilitate bidirectional communication between such companies and the communities likely to be affected.

In instrumental terms, it is argued that these more 'negotiated' methods of communication may be more effective in communicating risks and avoiding strident controversy or disproportionate pubic concern. Severtson et al. (2006) discuss the need to develop concrete information that meets the information needs of different public audiences. Williams (2004) points out that non-expert stakeholders need to be helped to understand scientific arguments to put risk information into a 'proper' (i.e. scientifically justifiable) perspective. Two-way communication may also be advantageous because such methods allow participants to 'clear the air' and negotiate their particular 'bargaining positions' (Leiss, 1995), and help to overcome problems of anxiety and apathy in response to environmental risks (McCallum et al., 1991). Weidemann and Schutz (1999) point out that risk communication over environmental hazards often involves an 'outrage' factor that requires consideration of conflictual positions of stakeholder groups. These are all reasons that help to explain why several authors (Kasperson et al., 1992; Klauenberg & Vermulen, 1994; Oleckno, 1995) suggest that methods that offer empowerment and negotiation for stakeholders may require a relatively long time to carry out, but are more successful in the long term.

The arguments for exchange through 'two-way communication' and participative strategies are not only justified in terms of these aims to make communication of information about risks to the public more 'effective' from the 'expert's' point of view. They rest partly on a political and moral argument relating to environmental justice and democratic representation of citizens and the importance for individual people of having the power to exercise influence over decisions relating to environmental conditions that affect them.

Expertise is constituted within institutions, and powerful institutions can perpetuate unjust ways of looking at the world unless they are continually put before and interrogated by lay persons (Jasanoff, 2003, p. 398). Research by Satterfield et al. (2004) suggests the importance of addressing the feelings of discrimination and injustice they found to be linked to high levels of concern about environmental risks in one's neighbourhood. Byrd *et al.* (2001) underline the importance of risk communication as a process to empower communities to make judgements based on information about risk that they can understand. Biocca (2005, pp. 263–5) also argues for 'communication among stakeholders' and a 'negotiated' approach to making choices about development and health, and for the idea of communication as a 'right', suggesting that citizens' rights in terms of risk communication should include 'the possibility to express one's own opinion in order to influence decision-making' (cf. Jasanoff, 2003). Other authors who emphasize the role of the audiences for risk communication as active participants and call for participatory methods include Griffin *et al.* (1998) and Hough *et al.* (2006). Frewer (2004) and Fox & Irwin (1998) also address the issue of power relationships involved in communication when they discuss the benefits of two-way exchange of information with stakeholders treated as equal partners in the process and institutions considering public views and societal values as part of their risk analyses.

Thus much of the risk communication literature emphasizes the importance of public involvement in developing sustained and interactive two-way communication strategies. We consider next the advice that is offered concerning 'what works' in terms of implementation.

## Ways to make information exchange and stakeholder participation more 'successful'

As implied from the discussion above, 'success' in information exchange and stakeholder participation could be defined in various ways, and this might be controversial. For example, should risks owing to environmental contamination be assessed in terms of reaching agreement that allows actually or potentially polluting activities to proceed or limits development that may be environmentally damaging? Are we concerned with the extent to which all stakeholders are able to 'understand' (or accept) scientifically based expert judgements about risk and the appropriate measures to take to prevent or mitigate risks, or is the crucial question one of empowerment of different stakeholders to have their views heard and balanced in an open debate which weighs scientific evidence and advance against other criteria? Whichever of these perspectives one chooses to adopt, paying attention to certain issues is likely to increase the potential for 'success'.

The risk communication literature highlights that a crucial factor influencing the success of risk communication strategies is sensitivity to the characteristics of the group receiving the message, one of which is socioeconomic status. Taylor-Clark *et al.* (2007) show that groups with low socioeconomic status perceive risk differently to other groups, and that addressing information gaps, defining the nature of environmental problems in health, and facilitating mobilization requires a shift away from a sole focus on individual level variables such as risk cognitions and perceptions, to larger structural conditions such as social class, communication inequalities, and social, health-related, and environmental policies. In relation to contaminated land, for example, this is clearly relevant because of the increasing evidence that people living in deprived communities are more likely to be subjected to environmental exposures arising from contaminated land. Byrd *et al.* (2001) also find significant differences in patterns of response between communities, with respondents in low income neighbourhoods having a poor understanding of risk and the possibility of a risk-free environment. Risk communication should therefore be sensitive to variations in attitudes and knowledge in different communities and social groups (discussed in the introduction) in order to make risk communication comprehensible to the audiences concerned. Other aspects of social position can also be important; for example, Satterfield *et al.* (2004) draw attention to differences in risk perception associated with race and gender, and these, as well as education, age group, and disabilities are characteristics that can also affect one's capacity to participate in discussion about risk. Dake (1992) points to social and cultural theories that highlight different sociocultural perspectives on risk likely to generate diversity in communication about risk, including hierarchical, egalitarian, individualist, fatalist, and autonomic points of view. Many other commentators (Vaughan, 1993; Griffin *et al.*, 1995; Wireman & Long, 2001; Cresswell & Foster, 2003; Foster *et al.*, 2003; 2004; Briggs & Stern, 2007; Payne-Sturges *et al.*, 2004; Tuler *et al.*, 2005) also recognize the diversity of stakeholders who should be informed about environmental health issues and the need for locally sensitive and adaptable structures as well as training and support for staff in agencies communicating risks. Different geographical settings may call for specific methods: for example, Larsson *et al.* (2006) discuss the need to adjust risk communication procedures for rural settings.

This diversity of audiences implies diversity of approaches and the crucial importance of matching the style of communication and exchange to the audience. It is recognized that communication should take varied forms that go well beyond merely 'sending out notices' (Prenney, 1993). Effective methods may include public meetings where audience concerns can be allayed (McComas, 2001), but Foster *et al.* (2004) comment that communicating to large numbers of people via public meetings can be problematic, so alternatives such as one-to-one, face-to-face feedback about risks with members of the communities that are affected may be required (Quandt *et al.*, 2004;

Payne-Sturges *et al.*, 2004; Renn, 2008). Gallagher & Jackson (2008, p. 617) noted that 'traditional' forms of risk communication may not be effective: 'when brownfields development is deployed in impoverished or underserved communities within larger cities, traditional tools such as public meetings and hearings may not be sufficient'. They note that, whilst involvement frameworks such as advisory committees and mediated negotiations can build trust, educate, and produce decisions that are more acceptable to citizens, public hearings may not engage community members living in poor neighbourhoods, and there is more success when community involvement processes go beyond formal meeting and hearing arrangements (Gallagher & Jackson, 2008).

Participative information exchange needs to be based on sharing of information, so one issue that requires careful consideration is the 'comprehensibility' of information that is presented by 'experts', since information produced for scientific audiences may not be readily understood by all participants. This was noted by Burger *et al.* (2008), who compared varying ways of presenting information in terms of the proportion of people studied who were able to give 'correct' answers about information conveyed in relation to environmental contamination. They noted that many of the participants in the study (who were college students in the US, and might be expected to have relatively good skills of assimilating and interpreting documents) had some difficulty in correctly interpreting complex information, especially when they were required to combine different sources of data. The authors recommend paying more attention to the ways that information is acquired, providing the same information in multiple formats and including a clear explanation of the intended message. Williams (2004) discusses the use of methods of risk analysis based on risk comparisons to help people interpret information on risk and put it into appropriate perspective.

Just as important, however, may be the development of ways for 'lay' participants to convey their views, and for decision-making processes to 'balance' the varying risk perceptions held by groups in the general public and scientific communities (Page, 1994; Garvin, 2001; Renn, 2004). Advances in research and in public health practice are providing examples of how this may be done.

Increasing attention has been given to analysing the factors that affect how stakeholders perceive and respond to risk as part of their involvement in decision-making processes. One such example is stakeholder processes related to the US Department of Energy's (DOE) clean-up of atom bomb production facilities and the US Department of Defense's base closure activities (Goldstein, 2005). The original attempts by the DOE to manage its environmental problems were heavily criticized. For many affected communities, information about their exposures had been shrouded in secrecy, difficult to understand, or simply unavailable or not relevant to their site-specific circumstances. The response to these communicational deficiencies has been to move towards a two-way communicative process involving citizen advisory groups (Goldstein, 2005). As a generic description, a citizen advisory board is selected by a sponsoring body from among citizens who are interested in or are in some way affected by a (potential) local or regional environmental impact. The subject matter is confined to an activity or decision and the members must be willing to approach the issues with an open mind. The process is deliberative, meaning that the essential activities are learning about the issues, scrutinizing various alternatives, and striving to reach a consensus resolution. However, even if consensus cannot be reached, a successful citizens' advisory board can narrow areas of disagreement, help affected parties recognize others' concerns, identify new options, and elucidate issues that remain to be resolved (Applegate, 1998). The process requires facilitation, not only in moderating discussion, but also in producing and communicating relevant information. These approaches demand much of participants, and the decision-maker (or sponsor) must accept the existence of such a group and its recommendations. The corollary is that the decision has not already been made. The decision-maker's investment in time, money, and openness to its critics will, in principle, lead to better informed public participation, improved relationships, and greater acceptance of difficult choices that have been made collaboratively.

Participative information exchange therefore requires suitable techniques for deciding which methods of communication are likely to be more effective, and implementing exchange and debate. Maibach *et al.* (2007) are among those calling for wider application of relatively innovative methods—among which they include social marketing, entertainment education, and media advocacy and interactive support systems. Effective participation also seems likely to be enhanced by what Brauer *et al.* (2004) discuss as the need to 'develop a relationship' with the public to communicate risks in ways that convey the information that people want to know. Wireman and Long (2001) suggest the need for risk communicators to undertake 'profiling' activities to 'get to know' the communities with which they are involved, and they imply the establishment of a continuing dialogue with communities of interest. Briggs & Stern (2007) similarly argue for active prior participation in the risk governance process of stakeholders who may have varying perceptions and expectations.

## What are the limitations and challenges of two-way risk communication?

Introducing greater levels of information exchange and participative discussion over issues such as environmental contamination brings particular challenges and, in spite of the plethora of research and advice spanning nearly 20 years, research continues to be published which highlights ongoing problems with current risk communication in relation to these kinds of risk.

Some of these studies date from the 1990s when the issues discussed here would have been less well understood. For example, Klauenberg & Vermulen (1994) review a risk communication programme in relation to the closure of waste sites and find that the public was typically only involved at the end of the process. Prenney (1993) reports a situation of community lead exposure where communication was influenced by the anger and resentment of the local community and the historical context. In such situations, an explicit recognition of social distrust may, through empowerment, risk clarification, and negotiation, be more successful in the long term (Kasperson et al., 1992).

Other studies are more recent, and are suggestive of continuing difficulties internationally in implementing principles and methods which are by now quite well publicized. Hough et al. (2006), in a study on brownfield sites, show that information from the local authority was alarmist and unhelpful, and, as the process was led by experts, the concerns of residents were not fully addressed. Furthermore, in a study which investigated how actors (private companies and local government agencies) concerned with the remediation of contaminated land view the task of interaction with local residents, Wiseen and Wester-Herber (2007, p. 181) commented that, although participants defined communication as a 'dialogue,' it 'usually took the form of one-way information campaigns with few ways for the public to interact or participate—reducing the communication to "risk information"'. This may suggest that actors may not have accurate perceptions of how well their efforts at communication incorporate effective participation for all those involved, and that their good intentions for 'two-way dialogue' are not always realized.

Although in the previous section we discussed various ways to make information from scientific evidence more 'accessible' to all stakeholders, there remain major difficulties in this respect. Understanding risks scientifically requires some degree of knowledge of science and scientific principles; this is very unevenly distributed in the population, so that achieving a 'level playing field' in terms of comprehension of the scientifically assessed risk is quite challenging. However, more seriously, the problem is made more difficult because the scientific evidence is often, even for scientists and experts, complex and difficult to interpret. The concept of 'exposure' to environmental pollutants, for example, is fraught with qualifications and caveats, so that the risks to human health of exposure depend at least as much on variable human behaviours and susceptibilities as on the actual level of contamination. It is often quite difficult to transfer scientific findings from one setting to another.

Comprehensive risk assessments require evaluation of a range of potential costs and benefits which are dependent on what are ultimately social rather than scientific judgements about risks (Garvin, 2001; Bickerstaff, 2004; Biocca, 2005). Many experts and academic writers admit that, at the end of the day, the precautionary principle may have to prevail in situations where knowledge is too incomplete to conclude whether or not risks are insignificant. We also note the concept of 'significant possibility of significant harm', which is used by local authorities to make the regulatory determination of 'contaminated land' under current legislation. This label for contaminated land has a specific definition in UK legislation. Whilst this 'label' may be helpful in qualifying local authorities to seek funding for remediation, it may, itself, cause alarm and distort risk perception.

Furthermore, Beck's (1999) assessment of the 'World Risk Society' suggests that, with respect to many aspects of environmental change and risk, we are faced with 'non-linear' knowledge which is not amenable to conventional scientific theorizing and empiricism. Beck argues for the development of a:

> ... public sphere in cooperation with a kind of 'public science' [that] would act as a secondary body charged with the 'discursive checking' of scientific laboratory results in the crossfire of opinions (Beck, 1999, p. 70).

This argument, if correct, is further endorsement of the need for a more participative information exchange in risk communication, but lays down a significant challenge to change our current views about 'evidence-based policy' in respect of risks to public health (Curtis, 2008).

We have noted above differences in the ways that communities perceive and respond to environmental risk. It is noted that people may be worried but they also may be curious or have other reactions that need to be considered; as Hough et al. (2006) note, residents may be concerned about housing prices and also about the ethics of selling their houses to other families when they are aware of land contamination. The remediation process is also relevant as Burger et al. (2008) note that both the extent of clean-up and future land use may be contentious in dealing with contaminated sites. Furthermore, participative methods often do not, at least in the short term, address issues of environmental injustice and power to prevent environmental changes that have already produced contamination. In a study of public response to a land decontamination project, Vandermoere (2008) illustrates that residents' distress was not related to the actual or perceived risk of the contamination to which they were exposed, but rather to their sense of lack of control over the source of decontamination and the remediation process. Indeed, whilst many see moves towards public and stakeholder participation and empowerment as evidence of progress and perceive real benefits in the changed relationships, the proliferation of activity brings with it new problems. One of the most obvious refers to whether there are demonstrable outcomes from some of these innovative processes, and the extent to which they mark a break with the traditional unidirectional approach that transferred very little real power to stakeholders and publics. These issues link to the emerging problem of 'consultation fatigue' for some stakeholder groups, with involvement in multiple deliberative processes placing an unsustainable demand on their resources, both organizational and personal (Simmons *et al.*, 2006, on activities relating to radioactive waste management in the UK). The danger is that current efforts may ultimately be rejected by some as, at best, little more than a legitimation exercise or, at worst, a cynical strategy of stakeholder co-option or exhaustion which does little to resolve the problems of institutional legitimacy associated with the management of chronic environmental risks.

Fundamental to many of these continuing difficulties, then, is the issue of trust in risk communication, which is significant and related to concern and care, openness and honesty, knowledge and expertise, commitment and level of information received (Peters *et al.*, 1997; on components of trust; see also Renn and Levine, 1991). In a study of citizen response to communication about cancer clusters, McComas and Trumbo (2001) observed that the higher the credibility assigned to the state health department or to industry, the lower is the perceived risk. Since trust is a major objective in risk communication and also a prerequisite for many other objectives, risk communicators' efforts need to more squarely embed an understanding of the meaning and implications of trust (Renn, 2008; Lofstedt, 2005). For instance, the long-term nature of chronic environmental risks such as contaminated land raises particular issues for communication around trust and power:

> Land contamination may affect local residents who have little or no control over the contamination and discover the problem after long periods of potential exposure. This may raise issues of trust between residents and local authorities to develop rapid policy solutions in order to deal with the contamination. These factors point to a need for political transparency and . . . risk communication (Hough *et al.*, 2006, p. 2).

## Conclusion

Almost all risk communication studies are quick to point out that risk communication is not a public relations problem (Renn, 2008). Advertisement and careful packaging of messages can help improve communication but they cannot overcome the psychosocial and structural contexts and constraints that we have alluded to in earlier sections of this chapter. Thus, in relation to environmental contamination, the challenges remain centred on the need to develop a strong understanding of community dynamics and the bases of community risk perceptions (McCallum *et al.*, 1991; Wireman & Long, 2001; Hough *et al.*, 2006), and to shift away from focusing on individual level variables to larger structural conditions such as social and political exclusion, communication inequalities, and social, health-related, and environmental policies (Taylor-Clark *et al.*, 2007). There is need to focus more on determining the importance of risk, its psychosocial as well as physical health expressions, and what information needs to be communicated. This demands a focus on developing and evaluating different models of engagement that facilitate dialogue between different stakeholder groups. In this regard, there is a need to better understand how risks and the significance of these risks are assessed by different stakeholders, including members of the public, and how agencies might organize and carry out risk communication in collaboration with other organizations representing relevant stakeholder groups. Although we have highlighted a number of critical research and praxis challenges with progressing this agenda, it is vital that risk communication incorporates a broad conception of risk—framed by processes of knowledge exchange and a 'realization that communication is a two-way process in which both sides have something to give and to learn' (Renn, 2008, p. 271).

## References

Albrecht, G., Sartore, G. M., Connor, L. *et al.* (2007). Solastalgia: The distress caused by environmental change. *Australasian Psychiatry*, 15: S95–8.

Applegate, J. S. (1991). Beyond the usual suspects: The use of citizen advisory boards in environmental decision-making. *Indiana Law Journal*, 73: 903–57.

Baxter, J. & Lee, D. (2004). Understanding expressed low concern and latent concern near a hazardous waste treatment facility. *Journal of Risk Research*, 7: 705–29.

Beck, U. (1999). *World Risk Society*. Cambridge, Polity Press (page references relate to the 2005 edition).

Bickerstaff, K. (2004). Risk perception research: socio-cultural perspectives on the public experience of air pollution. *Environment International*, 30(6): 827–40.

Biocca, M. (2005). Risk communication and the precautionary principle. *Human and Ecological Risk Assessment*, 11(1): 261–6.

Boholm, Å. & Löfstedt, R. (eds) (2004). *Facility Siting: Risk, Power and Identity in Land-use Planning*. London, Earthscan.

Brauer, M., Hakkinen, P. J., Gehan, B. M. & Shirname-More, L. (2004).Communicating exposure and health effects results to study subjects, the community and the public: Strategies and challenges. *Journal of Exposure Analysis and Environmental Epidemiology*, 14(7): 479–83.

Briggs, D. & Stern, R. (2007). Risk response to environmental hazards to health—towards an ecological approach. *Journal of Risk Research*, 10(5): 593–622.

Burger, J., Greenberg, M., Gochfeld, M. *et al.* (2008). Factors influencing acquisition of ecological and exposure information about hazards and risks from contaminated sites. *Environmental Monitoring and Assessment*, 137(1–3): 413–25.

Burningham, K. & Thrush, D. (2004). Pollution concerns in context: a comparison of local perception of risks associated with living close to a road and a chemical factory. *Journal of Risk Research,* 7: 213–32.

Bush, J., S. Moffatt and C.Dunn (2001) 'Even the birds round here cough': stigma, air pollution and health in Teesside, *Health & Place,* 7(1): 47-56.

Byrd, T. L., VanDerslice, J. & Peterson, S. K. (2001). Attitudes and beliefs about environmental hazards in three diverse communities in Texas on the border with Mexico. *Pan American Journal of Public Health,* 9(3): 154–60.

Capriotti, P. (2007). Chemical risk communication through the Internet in Spain. *Public Relations Review,* 33(3): 326–9.

Couch, S. R. & Kroll-Smith, J. S. (1991). *Communities at Risk: Collective Responses to Technological Hazards.* New York, Peter Lang.

Cresswell, T. & Foster, K. (2003). The deep end of effective risk communication: Experience of a local public: Health department in a complex and controversial environmental investigation. *Epidemiology,* 14(5): S131–2.

Curtis, S. (2008). How can we address health inequality through healthy public policy in Europe? *European Urban and Regional Studies,* 15: 293–305.

Curtis, S., Fuller, S., Khaw, F-M. & Foster, K. (2008). *Review of research evidence concerning factors influencing public interpretations and responses to risk communication.* Durham University/Health Protection Agency North East.

Dake, K. (1992). Myths of nature—culture and the social construction of risk. *Journal of Social Issues,* 48(4): 21–37.

Edelstein, M. (2003). *Contaminated Communities: Coping with Residential Toxic Exposure.* Boulder Co, Westview.

Evans, G. & Stecker, R. (2004). Motivational consequences of environmental stress. *Journal of Environmental Psychology,* 24(2): 143–65.

Flynn, J., Slovic, P. & Kunreuther, H. (eds) (2001). *Risk, Media and Stigma: Understanding Public Challenges to Modern Science and Technology.* London, Earthscan.

Foster, K., Pless-Mulloli, T. & Bush, J. (2003). Barriers to effective risk communication: Study of the role of a local public health department in a controversial environmental investigation. *Epidemiology,* 14(5): S132.

Foster, K., Pless-Mulloli, T. & Bush, J. (2004). *The role of the Health Authority Public Health Department in a controversial environmental health investigation.* School of Population and Health Sciences (Epidemiology & Public Health), University of Newcastle, February 2004.

Fox, C. R. & Irwin, J. R. (1998). The role of context in the communication of uncertain beliefs. *Basic and Applied Social Psychology,* 20(1): 57–70.

Frewer, L. (2004). The public and effective risk communication. *Toxicology Letters,* 149: 391–7.

Gallagher, D. R. & Jackson, S. E. (2008). Promoting community involvement at brownfields sites in socio-economically disadvantaged neighbourhoods. *Journal of Environmental Planning and Management,* 51(5): 615–30.

Garvin, T. (2001). Analytical paradigms: the epistemological distances between scientists, policy makers, and the public. *Risk Analysis,* 21(3): 443–55.

Goldstein, B. D. (2005). Advances in risk assessment and communication. *Annual Review of Public Health,* 26: 141–63.

Gray, P. C. R. (1995). Waste incineration—controversy and risk communication. *European Review of Applied Psychology-Revue Europeenne De Psychologie Appliquee*, 45(1): 29–34.

Griffin, R. J., Dunwoody, S. & Gehrmann, C. (1995). The effects of community pluralism on press coverage of health risks from local environmental contamination. *Risk Analysis*, 15(4): 449–58.

Griffin, R. J., Dunwoody, S. & Zabala, F. (1998). Public reliance on risk communication channels in the wake of a cryptosporidium outbreak. *Risk Analysis*, 18(4): 367–75.

Higginbotham, N., Connor, L., Albrecht, G., Freeman, S. & Agho, K. (2006). Validation of an environmental distress scale. *Ecohealth*, 3 (4): 245–54.

Hollway, W. & Jefferson, T. (1997). The risk society in an age of anxiety: situating the fear of crime. *British Journal of Sociology*, 48: 255–66.

Hough, R. L., Stephens, C., Busby, A., Cracknell, J. & Males, B. (2006). Assessing and communicating risk with communities living on contaminated land. *International Journal of Occupational & Environmental Health*, 12(1): 1–8.

Inter-Departmental Liaison Group on Risk Assessment (ILGRA). (1998). *Risk Communication: A guide to regulatory practice.*

Irwin, A., Simmons, P. & Walker, G. (1999). Faulty environments and risk reasoning: the local understanding of industrial hazards. *Environment and Planning A*, 31: 1311–26.

Jasanoff, S. (2003). Symposium: Breaking the waves in science studies. *Social Studies of Science*, 33: 389–400.

Kasperson, R. E., Golding, D. & Tuler, S. (1992). Social distrust as a factor in siting hazardous facilities and communicating risks. *Journal of Social Issues*, 48(4): 161–87.

Klauenberg, B. J. & Vermulen, E. K. (1994). Role for risk communication in closing military waste sites. *Risk Analysis*, 14(3): 351–6.

Larsson, L. S., Butterfield, P., Christopher, S. & Hill, W. (2006). Rural community leaders' perceptions of environmental health risks: improving community health. *AAOHN Journal*, 54(3): 105–12.

Leiss, W. (1995). Down and dirty: The use and abuse of public trust in risk communication. *Risk Analysis*, 15(6): 685–92.

Lofstedt, R. C. (2005). *Risk Management in Post-Trust Societies*. New York, Palgrave Macmillan.

Maibach, E. W., Abroms, L. C. & Marosits, M. (2007). Communication and marketing as tools to cultivate the public's health: a proposed 'people and places' framework. *Bmc Public Health 7*.

McCallum, D. B., Hammond, S. L. & Covello, V. T. (1991). Communicating about environmental risks—how the public uses and perceives information-sources. *Health Education Quarterly*, 18(3): 349–61.

McCluskey, J. J. & Rausser, G. C. (2003). Stigmatized asset value: Is it temporary or long-term? *Review of Economics and Statistics*, 85(2): 276–85.

McComas, K. A. (2001). Public meetings about local waste management problems: Comparing participants to non participants. *Environmental Management*, 27(1): 135–47.

McComas, K. A. & Trumbo, C. W. (2001). Source credibility in environmental health-risk controversies: application of Meyer's credibility index. *Risk Analysis*, 21(3): 467–80.

McGee, T. K. (1999). Private responses and individual action. Community responses to chronic environmental lead contamination. *Environment and Behavior*, 31(1): 66–83.

Oleckno, W. A. (1995). Guidelines for improving risk communication in environmental health. *Journal of Environmental Health,* 58(1): 20–3.

Page, S. D. (1994). Indoor radon—a case-study in risk communication. *American Journal of Preventive Medicine,* 10(3): 15–18.

Payne-Sturges, D. C., Schwab, M. & Buckley, T. J. (2004). Closing the research loop: A risk-based approach for communicating results of air pollution exposure studies. *Environmental Health Perspectives,* 112(1): 28–34.

Peters, R. G., Covello, V. T. & McCallum, D. B. (1997). The determinants of trust and credibility in environmental risk communication: an empirical study. *Risk Analysis,* 17(1): 43–54.

Prenney, B. (1993). Community lead-exposure. *American Journal of Industrial Medicine,* 23(1): 191–5.

Quandt, S. A., Doran, A. M., Rao, P. *et al.* (2004). Reporting pesticide assessment results to farmworker families: development, implementation and evaluation of a risk communication strategy. *Environmental Health Perspectives,* 112(5): 636–42.

Renn, O. (2004). Perception of risks. *Toxicology Letters,* 149(1–3): 405–13.

Renn, O. (2008). *Risk Governance: coping with uncertainty in a complex world.* London, Earthscan.

Renn, O. & Levine, D. (1991). Credibility and trust in risk communication. In: R. E. Kasperson & P. J. Stallen (eds). *Communicating Risk to the Public: International Perspectives.* Dordrecht, Kluwer, pp. 175–218.

Satterfield, T. A., Mertz, C. K. & Slovic, P. (2004). Discrimination, vulnerability, and justice in the face of risk. *Risk Analysis,* 24(1): 115–29.

Severtson, D. J., Baumann, L. C. & Brown, R. L. (2006). Applying a health behavior theory to explore the influence of information and experience on arsenic risk representations, policy beliefs, and protective behavior. *Risk Analysis,* 26(2): 353–68.

Simmons, P. & Walker, G. (1999). Tolerating risk: policy principles and public perceptions. *Risk, Decision and Policy,* 4: 179–90.

Simmons, P., Bickerstaff, K. & Walls, J. (2006). *CARL Country Report—United Kingdom.* Available at http://www.carl-research.org/docs/20070723141722BSCN.pdf.

Solecki, W. D. (1996). Paternalism, pollution and protest in a company town. *Political Geography,* 15: 5–20.

Taylor-Clark, K., Koh, H. & Viswanath K. (2007). Perceptions of environmental health risks and communication barriers among low-SEP and racial/ ethnic minority communities. *Journal of Health Care for the Poor and Underserved,* 18(4): 165–83.

Tuler, S., Webler, T. & Finson, R. (2005). Competing perspectives on public involvement: Planning for risk characterization and risk communication about radiological contamination from a national laboratory. *Health Risk & Society,* 7(3): 247–66.

Vandermoere, F. (2008). Psychosocial health of residents exposed to soil pollution in a Flemish neighbourhood. *Social Science & Medicine,* 66: 1646–57.

Vaughan, E. (1993). Individual and cultural-differences in adaptation to environmental risks. *American Psychologist,* 48(6): 673–80.

Wakefield, S. & Elliott, S. J. (2000). Environmental risk perception and well-being: effects of the landfill siting process in two southern Ontario communities. *Social Science and Medicine,* 50: 1130–54.

Wakefield, S. & McMullan, C. (2005). Healing in places of decline: (re)imagining everyday landscapes in Hamilton, Ontario. *Health & Place*, 11(4): 299–312.

Wiedemann, P. M. & Schutz, H. (1999). Risk communication for environmental health hazards. *Zentralblatt Fur Hygiene Und Umweltmedizin*, 202(2–4): 345–59.

Williams, P. R. D. (2004). Health risk communication using comparative risk analyses. *Journal of Exposure Analysis and Environmental Epidemiology*, 14(7): 498–515.

Wireman, J. R. & Long, G. C. (2001). Communicating risk in diverse communities. *Toxicology and Industrial Health*, 17(5–10): 298–301.

Wiseen, T. & Wester-Herber, M. (2007). Dirty soil and clean consciences: examining communication of contaminated land. *Water, Air and Soil Pollution*, 181: 173–82.

World Health Organization. (2000). Evaluation and use of epidemiological evidence for environmental health risk assessment: WHO guideline document. *Environmental Health Perspectives*, 108(10): 997–1002.

Wynne, B., Waterton, C. & Grove-White, R. (1993). *Public Perceptions and the Nuclear Industry in West Cumbria*. Lancaster, Lancaster University.

Zonabend, F. (1993). *The Nuclear Peninsula*. (J. A. Underwood, trans.) Cambridge, Cambridge University Press.

Chapter 18

# Geographical information systems as a means for communicating about public health

Christine E. Dunn (Department of Geography, Durham University)

## Introduction

Recent years have witnessed an upsurge in interest in techniques for analysing spatially referenced data; not least in this expansion has been the development of geographical information systems (GIS). The increasing availability of large volumes of digital, georeferenced data which can be positioned in space in computerized mapping systems, more affordable hardware and software, more user-friendly interfaces, and the onset of web-based tools for visualizing geographical information have played key roles in the widespread dispersal of this technology. Although the foundations for GIS were laid with software developments in the 1960s, the term 'GIS' really came into use only in the late 1980s, with the onset of initiatives such as the National Center for Geographic Information and Analysis in the USA and the development of commercial GIS packages such as Arc/INFO. GIS is now used in a wide variety of applications, extending far beyond those relating to public health, including urban planning, managing natural resources, services and facilities location, disaster management and emergency planning, environmental risk assessment, visualizing landscapes, geodemographics, and site suitability.

GIS has met with widely differing responses. It has been criticized, for example, as technologically deterministic and lacking the capabilities to meet public health needs (Jacquez, 2000). In the context of a specific public health application (malaria), it has also been described as making evidence-based response possible and moving mapping (of malaria) 'from a largely subjective science to one with quantitative foundations' (Hay *et al.*, 2000, p. 192). At its best, GIS has the potential to serve as an 'enabling technology'—an interdisciplinary framework through which different specialists (epidemiologists, statisticians, health geographers, and health service professionals) can work together to understand public health research questions from different but inter-related perspectives (Cockings *et al.*, 2004). GIS has a number of important constraints, however, and, to properly aid understanding of, and communication about, public health issues, it should not be used uncritically. With its focus on 'objective' information, the testing of hypotheses, and searches for statistical associations through quantitative analysis, the theoretical underpinnings of GIS are largely positivist. As a means of understanding and communicating about public health, and risks to health, therefore, GIS has important limits in terms of the type of health-related research to which it can be applied. It is best placed for the analysis of large, spatially referenced datasets on morbidity and mortality, and associated risk factors, often where those factors are related to the natural or built environment, and these applications provide the focus of this chapter. Other techniques and processes, considered elsewhere in this book, are more appropriate for disseminating ideas and information about social and cultural understandings of health, and more nuanced and individualized notions of risk. That said, developments over the past decade or so have embraced ideas around more 'socially aware' forms of GIS which have embraced notions of participation and environmental justice.

Some of the power of the technology of GIS lies in its ability to combine disparate types and sources of data, thereby allowing the user to explore and evaluate potential relationships between health outcomes and environmental risk factors. The literature contains a plethora of case studies which illustrate how GIS has been used to address specific questions about such relationships. The aim of this chapter is not to provide a comprehensive review of these studies (for a general overview of health applications of GIS, the reader is referred to Briggs *et al.* (2002), Cromley & McLafferty (2002), and Maheswaran & Craglia (2004)), but rather to use selective examples to illustrate the role which GIS can play in understanding and communicating about public health risks. The chapter considers some of the specific opportunities which a GIS-based approach offers but it also addresses some of the inherent assumptions and limitations of spatial representations of risks to health. The chapter begins by outlining the meaning of the term 'GIS', before going on to discuss issues of data quality and the challenges of representing population risk exposure. A range of case studies is drawn upon to illustrate some of the capabilities of GIS for identifying and illustrating spatial patterns of risks to health, in ways that can inform experts charged with communication of public health risks. The discussion then goes on to outline 'alternative' forms of GIS which enable wider user participation and which may be more directly applied to communication of risk to the public.

## What is GIS?

GIS provides a common framework for combining and analysing spatially referenced data about populations, their health, socioeconomic characteristics, and the environment in which they live (Cockings *et al.*, 2004). In this sense, GIS offers a promising framework for both understanding and communicating about notions of risks relating to public health. There are many different understandings of what GIS is, with many definitions of the term focusing on the specific functions and capability of the software. But hardware, data, and users are also critical components of running a GIS, as are the institutional, organizational, social, and political dimensions within which GIS is framed.

For the purposes of this chapter, a good working definition of GIS is 'a computing application capable of creating, storing, manipulating, visualizing, and analysing geographic information' (Goodchild, 2000, p. 6). GIS provides a means of evaluating geographical relationships through three main types of function: spatial analysis, data management, and visual display. Crucially, by enabling links between these functions, users are able to engage with information interactively. Thus, for example, a fundamental operation in GIS allows the user to 'point' to a position on a map display (the spatial data) and retrieve the descriptive (attribute) data which pertain to that location. By developing database queries, the user can instruct the GIS to display all locations which match the query; for example, residential addresses of children living within 1 km of a landfill site. This ability to query and analyse different types of information is facilitated by one of the concepts on which many GIS are based: that of data layers or planes. Unlike many conventional paper maps, which combine different types of features (vegetation, topography, hydrology, and settlements) in the same display, GIS separates out these different themes or features into commonly referenced layers. These can then be subsequently combined or overlaid in accordance with the aims of the inquiry.

Computer hardware forms an essential component of a GIS and, although in most cases this normally entails a desktop or laptop PC with peripherals such as a scanner and printer, more 'mobile' forms of GIS are becoming more widespread. These include personal digital assistants (PDAs) running off-the-shelf GIS software or larger tablet PCs which work with active pens. These handheld GIS can be an effective means of data collection and analysis in field situations. In addition, global positioning systems (GPS) can either operate as 'stand-alone' devices or can be embedded into other equipment such as mobile phones to allow real-time collection of locational data. Most are highly portable, some being designed to be wearable and no bigger than a wristwatch.

The types of information that GIS are able to handle and analyse have broadened beyond the confines of conventional map-based data around which early GIS were built. Aerial photographs, satellite images, voice and other sound clips, movies, scanned images, digital photographs, and mental maps, as well as 'traditional' data from mapping agencies, can all be incorporated into a single GIS package. In addition, representation of spatial data has become more complex, with fly-through animations, landscape visualizations, and interactive virtual environments. The recent onset of applications such as Google Earth, Google Maps, and WikiMapia has effected an explosion in the amount of geographical information to which 'non-expert' users have access. The Malaria Atlas Project (MAP) (Hay & Snow, 2006), for example, set up to map and predict global malaria risk, has developed a website which allows users to view malaria data for different countries using Google Earth (http://www.map.ox.ac.uk/). Other projects have a more interactive component and, with the potential involvement of large numbers of users, these web-based or internet GIS offer interesting possibilities for more democratic means of disseminating information, and a more inclusive approach to spatial decision-making (see, for example, Kingston et al., 2000). This type of GIS then has the potential to offer a useful interface for dialogue between 'experts' and 'non-experts', and opportunities for risk communication to operate in more than one direction.

## Data quality and representation: GIS as a tool to identify, analyse, and illustrate variation in risk

The data available to health researchers are inevitably selective, often for reasons of confidentiality, and are subject to certain limits of accuracy, precision, and completeness. These elements of 'data quality', which relate to both spatial and attribute data, can have significant impacts on the validity of the outputs from GIS and their interpretation. There may also be a temptation for inexperienced users to concentrate on using GIS to produce 'flashy' rather than meaningful outputs, essentially legitimizing 'bad' data and creating a false impression of accuracy and precision (Abbot et al., 1998).

Errors can arise not only in the data sources themselves (for example, errors in accuracy and completeness of routinely collected morbidity and mortality data), but also as a result of the fundamental ways in which GIS itself represents geographical information. GIS is limited by its attempts to represent the 'real world', in all its complexity, in digital form. Clearly data need to be abstracted, reduced, and simplified in some way. Most systems conceptualize spatial data either in terms of a raster or 'grid' of data cells (pixels), or as vectors comprising point, line, and area features. Inaccuracies in single layers of data can then be compounded when these layers are combined with others. The use of spatial boundaries to create areal zones in much public health-related research also creates well known difficulties since different findings can be generated by modifying the boundaries of these zones—the classic 'modifiable areal unit problem' (Openshaw, 1984).

Errors in GIS analyses can also arise as a result of assumptions about people's behaviour. In particular, it can be difficult to account for individual movements, both in terms of daily activities and longer term migration patterns. In this context, a fixed proxy for environmental exposure, often a residential home address, is usually used as the geographical location at which members of at-risk populations are assumed to be based. There are obvious limitations of using a fixed location at which, in reality, people spend only part of their time. In addition, the process of converting address-based data (e.g. postcodes) to a coordinate point (e.g. a grid reference) for mapping, known as 'geocoding', can generate locational errors which may have important ramifications for the ways in which findings are interpreted, and hence the validity of a study's conclusions. Such errors are particularly relevant for analyses which involve measuring distances between locations (Cromley & McLafferty, 2002) or 'point-in-polygon' operations (Schootman et al., 2007), and in this sense there is a need for studies to more openly declare measures of positional accuracy (Mazumdar et al., 2008).

The use of current residential address may also generate errors owing to the time lag between exposure to a hazard and disease notification. Drawing on data for the neuromuscular disease amyotrophic lateral sclerosis, Sabel et al. (2003) have shown how spatial cluster analysis for different times of the life cycle may yield different conclusions regarding the location of potential risk factors. In addition, in most environmental health studies which have access to environmental concentration data, the latter 'will often be used as a surrogate for both exposure concentration and dose' (Nuckols et al., 2004, p. 1012).

One setting in which problems of population migration have been partially circumvented is Denmark. Here, health data can be linked to individual level data on past and current residential addresses through a unique 10-digit central population register (CPR) number. Drawing on these data to explore relationships between airborne dioxin and cancer incidence in southern Jutland, Poulstrup & Hansen (2004) used an exposure simulation model to demarcate zones of exposure using data on pollutant emissions, meteorology, source stacks, and surrounding buildings and terrain. No account was taken of exposure in the workplace, however, and in this context developments in GPS technology, discussed above, are opening up opportunities for more accurate tracking of individuals over space and time, and therefore for more accurately assessing exposure at the individual level (Elgethun *et al.*, 2003).

Many traditional spatial explorations of public health data suffer from limitations because of the use of predetermined areal units such as those used to disseminate census data to define populations and their characteristics. These units, with well-defined boundaries, may be convenient for administrative and electoral purposes, but often have no direct relationship to factors which may help to explain public health or risks to health. GIS offers the flexibility of defining spatial zones which are tailored more specifically to suit the purposes of the study and the exposure risk of concern. The next section considers some of the ways in which GIS has been used to model risk exposure.

## Exploring spatial risk exposure and public health

To estimate population exposure to environmental hazards (for example, airborne emissions from industrial operations), it is a straightforward procedure in GIS to delimit a series of zones of increasing distance from the putative source(s). Spatial overlay using population data can then be used to determine residents potentially at risk. This type of proximity analysis provides only a crude approximation of population exposure, however, since it takes no real account of emission dispersion and the boundary demarcations are to some extent arbitrary. That said, it may have some value where, for example, meteorological data are unavailable or an exploratory visualization of the data is needed as a first step towards a more sophisticated analysis. In a study of the spatial epidemiology of Legionnaires' disease in Glasgow, Scotland, such an approach was used to explore infection risk for populations living at different distances and orientations from premises with cooling towers as potential sources of infection (Dunn *et al.*, 2007). Figure 18.1 demonstrates how spatial distance and simplified wind direction effects are represented in GIS by dividing the space into concentric circles, or 'buffers', and directional sectors. Cases of community-acquired, non-travel, non-outbreak Legionnaires' disease (CANTNOLD), along with population data, represented here as enumeration district (ED) centroid points, are then overlaid, maintaining their distance and position relative to cooling tower premises. This provides a single representation of disease cases and population in relation to one 'conceptual' cooling tower location. After aggregating the cases and population by sector, standardized rates and ratios can then be calculated for each sector. Even this straightforward use of GIS was found to add value to previous studies which had adopted more traditional epidemiological techniques to evaluating risk of infection.

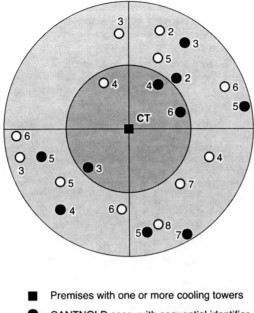

■    Premises with one or more cooling towers

●    CANTNOLD case, with sequential identifier

○    ED centroid, with sequential identifier

▨    Inner zone (0–500 m)

▨    Outer zone (500–1000 m)

**Fig. 18.1** 'Conceptual' cooling tower (CT) with an illustrative sample of Legionnaires' disease cases and enumeration district (ED) centroids overlaid. Source: Dunn et al. (2007).

By integrating predicted emission concentrations (for example, from air quality models), more realistic estimates of potential exposure can be determined by using GIS to generate a 'surface' of pollution contours (Figure 18.2). It is then possible to use this type of output in a number of ways. First, by overlaying data on household locations, the map provides a categorization of risk according to emission concentrations. Second, by entering $x$, $y$ grid coordinates for individual locations, a predicted air quality concentration value can be interpolated for specific addresses. Third, by linking the air quality contours to data on health outcomes for local populations (in this case, asthma), it is possible to explore potential associations between ill-health and pollutant concentrations and, where data are available, to adjust for potential confounding factors such as age, sex or cigarette smoking.

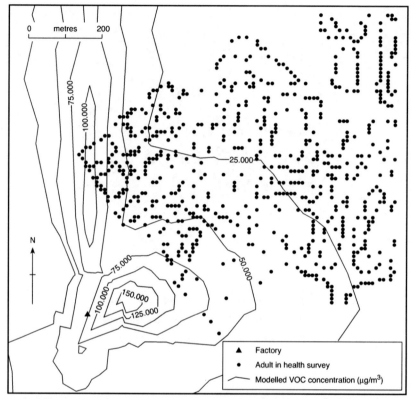

**Fig. 18.2** Location of asthma survey respondents' home addresses in relation to modelled levels of volatile organic compounds (VOCs) from a factory source in north-east England. Source: Dunn *et al.* (2001).

This representation of risk exposure is still essentially a static one which relies on imposed spatial boundaries, although modelled values of contamination can be calibrated by using monitored values (field measurements) where these are available (see, for example, Bellander *et al.*, 2001; Briggs *et al.*, 2000). Such estimates of population exposure can be valuable when used in combination with more conventional epidemiological approaches although, as Jarup (2004) reminds us, zones which are demarcated on a GIS map as being areas of exposure do not necessarily apply to the whole population, but only to those who have been exposed to the putative contaminant.

Techniques which avoid the need to use areal units altogether offer an alternative approach which can be used independently or in conjunction with GIS. These approaches rely on the availability of individual level data which are then expressed as point events through techniques such as spatial point pattern analysis (Diggle, 1983). Given the complexity of health–environment relationships, it may be argued that an integrating approach which draws on more than one spatial technique is most likely to reveal the most meaningful findings. A number of studies have therefore integrated GIS and point pattern analysis, often in the search for disease clusters (Bhopal *et al.*, 1992; Dunn *et al.*, 2001; 2007; Fotheringham & Zhan, 1996; Gatrell & Bailey, 1996; Gatrell *et al.*, 1996; Kingham *et al.*, 1995). One type of point pattern analysis, raised incidence modelling (Diggle & Rowlingson, 1994), can be used to assess the extent of clustering of point events (e.g. cases of a specific disease) around point source(s). In this approach, which treats risk as a quantity which varies continuously over the study area, the spatial distribution of disease cases is compared with that of a sample of suitable controls.

To explore the extent to which industrial toxic facilities are clustered in certain neighbourhoods and at different scales in San Francisco Bay, California, Fisher *et al.* (2006) adopt an approach which combines air quality dispersion modelling, GIS, and a spatial point pattern analysis based on Ripley's K function (Ripley, 1976). An intensity distribution of toxic release inventory (TRI) facilities shows several peaks, with two large clusters in the East Bay area being statistically significant (Figure 18.3).

GAM-K, a variant of Openshaw's geographical analysis machine (Openshaw & Turton, 1998) was used in an exploratory analysis of breast cancer clustering in Lancashire, England by Rigby & Gatrell (2000). Using data on residential postcodes for breast cancer patients, this technique has been used to reveal areas within the study region which can be used to suggest areas worthy of further investigation (Figure 18.4a). Presentation in three-dimensional form is used to assist with visual interpretation (Figure 18.4b).

A key benefit of GIS is its inherent ability to allow integration of data from disparate sources and relating to different spatial scales. Caution needs to be exercised here, particularly as differently scaled data normally imply different levels of accuracy. However, the ability to handle data for highly localized studies as well as continental or global applications provides a useful degree of flexibility in communicating about health and risk for different units of study. National and international systems for disease mapping have been established as a means of highlighting risk 'hotspots'. Thus, the UK Small Area Health Statistics Unit (SAHSU) developed a 'Rapid Inquiry Facility' (RIF) (Aylin *et al.*, 1999) to assess risks to health from environmental hazards. This has subsequently been expanded to a wider geographical scale through a European-wide programme of research, the European Health and Environment Information System (EUROHEIS) (Aylin *et al.*, 2002; Cockings & Jarup 2002), and through the Centers for Disease Control and Prevention (CDC) in the

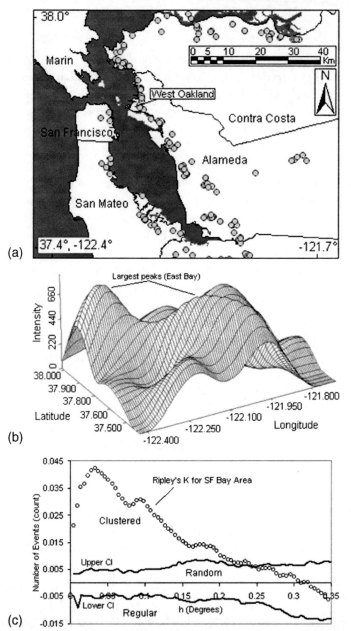

**Fig. 18.3 a** Toxic release inventory TRI (1999) facilities in the San Francisco Bay area.
**b** Intensity distribution for TRI (1999) sources in the San Francisco Bay area of points
per grid cell in longitude by latitude. **c** Ripley's K test for TRI (1999) facilities in the
San Francisco Bay area. The distribution above the upper confidence interval indicates clustering at the scales of degrees. The distribution between the confidence
intervals indicates a random spatial pattern. Below the lower confidence interval
would indicate a regular spatial pattern. The y axis represents the deviation of the
sample statistic from complete spatial randomness (CSR); the units are in
transformed count. Source: Fisher *et al.* (2006).

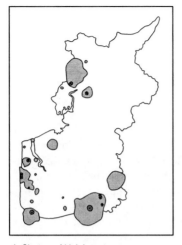 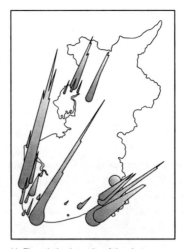

a) Clusters of high breast cancer
   incidence from a GAM-K search

b) The relative intensity of the clusters
   identified by the GAM-K search

**Fig. 18.4 a** Clusters of high breast cancer incidence from a GAM-K search. **b** The relative intensity of the clusters identified by the GAM-K search. Redrawn from Rigby & Gatrell (2000).

USA (Beale *et al.*, 2008). Using routinely collected health-related data in GIS, this system can be used to produce estimates of relative risk to a population, and to create disease cluster maps as well as 'smoothed' maps to account for sampling variability (Jarup, 2004). RIF is also now being developed to incorporate visualization of uncertainty in risk estimates (Beale *et al.*, 2008).

GIS can provide a useful platform for predicting the impact of global environmental change on risks to health and, in this sense, the onset of GIS has seen a renewed interest in the spatial mapping of malaria risk (Hay *et al.*, 2000), including predictive modelling. Thus, combining climate change models with GIS has allowed prediction of the impact of climate change on spatial ranges of mosquitoes and hence malaria transmission (Thomas *et al.*, 2004). Figure 18.5 demonstrates predicted future scenarios for 2025, 2055, and 2085 for malaria transmission in Africa.

Using GIS as an early warning system, fuzzy logic modelling was combined with a simulation model and expert system by Fleming *et al.* (2007) to predict risk of cholera outbreaks in southern Africa. This approach works on the basis of a set of environmental preconditions being met, notably growth of algal blooms, to stimulate growth of cholera bacteria. There are opportunities to extend this kind of approach to incorporate quantifiable population or socio-economic factors as Ali *et al.* (2002) did in a study which included educational status as a risk factor for cholera in Bangladesh.

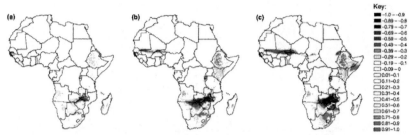

**Fig. 18.5** Projected changes in the climactic suitability for malaria transmission. These changes are projected for four consecutive months from observed climate (mean 1961–1990) to 30-year mean future climate centred on: **a** 2025; **b** 2055; and **c** 2085. Negative changes in fuzzy probability of climactic suitability for transmission indicate projected reduced transmission; positive changes indicate projected increased transmission; and zero indicates no change. Source: Thomas, C. J., Davies, G. & Dunn, C. E. (2004). Mixed picture for changes in stable malaria distribution with future climate in Africa. *Trends in Parasitology,* 20: 216–20, with permission from Elsevier.

GIS has also been used in attempts to determine the potential impact of 'linear' public health hazards such as overhead power lines (Blaasaas *et al.*, 2004; Kliukiene *et al.*, 2004), polluted rivers (Verkasalo *et al.*, 2004), road traffic accidents (Jones *et al.*, 2008), and traffic emissions and the implications for respiratory health (Brauer *et al.*, 2002; English *et al.*, 1999). Lovett *et al.* (1997) used GIS to predict transport routes for liquid hazardous waste in southern England using digital road networks, and then to calculate risks of pollution through waste spillages from tankers. By incorporating data from the UK Census of Population, GIS was used to estimate the number of residents living within 500 m of each road to determine potential population exposure to a vehicle accident. In using hydrogeological data to assess the vulnerability of groundwater to surface spillages of liquid waste, the authors identified and mapped a substantial vulnerability zone (categorized as 'extreme') close to Greater London. As acknowledged by the authors, more detailed and site-specific information is required to provide a more accurate assessment of the potential risks to health, but the analysis does provide a useful set of general hazard patterns worthy of further investigation. This qualified outcome is common to many studies of exposure mapping: the output should be regarded with a degree of caution and the user made aware of the limitations although, as an exploratory analysis, perhaps one to be followed up by using other techniques, such output has merit.

In an attempt to explore a range of risk measures for morbidity and mortality from road traffic accidents, Jones *et al.* (2008) use GIS to investigate the importance of a wide range of potential explanatory variables, including population characteristics (such as material deprivation), road features, topography, land use, and weather. Combining a GIS approach with multilevel statistical modelling, this work considers how public health policy interventions might be implemented to ameliorate the identified risk factors. These include physical interventions such as speed cameras and traffic calming measures, as well as stronger enforcement measures and policies to improve driving standards in neighbourhoods which are characterized by dangerous driving cultures.

By using GIS-based regression mapping to model spatial distributions of road traffic pollution, Briggs *et al.* (2000) consider the public health implications of urban traffic emissions in four UK cities. Data on traffic flows, land use, and altitude are integrated and used to predict nitrogen dioxide concentrations in the model which could then be used to inform air quality management strategies in local governments. Similarly, a land use regression model has been used to predict levels of small particulate matter (PM2.5) in Los Angeles (Moore *et al.*, 2007). This approach draws on both GIS and statistical software to generate an interpolated surface of pollution using inverse distance weighting. The model predicted particularly high levels of PM2.5 at freeway intersections which represent a potentially significant public health risk.

Similar approaches have been undertaken to explore the role of socioeconomic status in potential pollution exposure. Thus in Hamilton, Canada, one set of studies has shown that populations with lower socioeconomic characteristics were exposed to higher levels of particulate air pollution and, subsequently, that there were enhanced associations between mortality and air pollution in these groups, with concomitant implications for pollution control policies (Jerrett *et al.*, 2001; 2004). This use of GIS in the context of environmental justice has been a welcome recent addition to its range of applications and there have been calls for more focus on risk factors in these contexts (McEntee & Ogneva-Himmelberger, 2008). In a study of respiratory health risks for populations living near to major highways in Massachusetts, McEntee & Ogneva-Himmelberger (2008) used GIS in a 'hotspot' analysis to demonstrate the spatial commonalities between residents living in environmental justice neighbourhoods, and clusters of raised diesel particulates and asthma incidence. Similarly, proximity analysis using buffer zones has been used to show that those living closest to noxious land uses in the Bronx, New York City have a greater risk of being hospitalized for asthma than those living further away, and also have a higher likelihood of being poor and of minority status (Maantay, 2007).

These examples reflect broader developments over the past decade or so which have embraced ideas of more 'inclusive' forms of GIS through web-based platforms and/or citizen involvement. The implications of these developments for health-related applications are considered in the next section.

## Widening participation

GIS has traditionally been regarded as 'expert' technology with limits on user access. Although the uptake of GIS in health service environments has increased in recent years, it is still largely under-utilized in these settings (Cockings *et al.*, 2004; Higgs *et al.*, 2003; 2005; Houghton, 2004; Rushton, 2003; Smith *et al.*, 2003). The capacity of public health organizations to embrace a tool like GIS clearly depends on staff expertise, available financial resources, and software functionality, but there is also a need to 'raise awareness' amongst public health professionals and practitioners. Some authors have argued for enhancements of GIS software for improved health-related decision-making by those who lack expertise in GIS (e.g. Bedard *et al.*, 2003). Rushton (2003) has argued for more structured disease surveillance systems to provide improved decision support to public health workers. Others have proposed the need for more collaborative approaches which bring together researchers from different disciplines, technical professionals, and public health practitioners (Cockings *et al.*, 2004; Dunn *et al.*, 2007; Graham *et al.*, 2004). Some of this work has shown how public health workers welcome alliances with academic researchers, particularly in the case of more technically complex spatial techniques.

The growth of alternative manifestations of GIS through developments in web-based systems and participatory forms of GIS offers opportunities to widen access both to health practitioners and local communities. An approach which has potential for both public health professionals and citizens to highlight inequalities in local environmental health risks was adopted by Maclachlan *et al.* (2007) for the industrial city of Hamilton, Canada. Using open source software, a web–GIS was used to explore relationships between respiratory health, air pollution, and socioeconomic status. Health professionals were highly supportive, although concerns were expressed in relation to data confidentiality. Data sharing was a key objective in a study of beach quality in Portugal by Gouveia *et al.* (2004). Data which have been provided by citizens in multiple forms (images, sound, videos, and text) are subsequently sent to those with official responsibility for beach quality.

With a focus less on the technology and more on multiple framings of a specific, often local, issue, participatory forms of GIS (often labelled Participatory GIS or Public Participation GIS (Craig *et al.*, 2002; Dunn, 2007)) can be used to juxtapose official, 'expert' spatial data with local and/or indigenous geographical knowledge. By recognizing the salience of 'lay' as well as 'expert' information, Participatory GIS offers enhanced opportunities for understanding public perceptions of risks to health, and, indeed, for policy-makers to develop improved methods of risk communication. Thus, in a loose coupling of GIS and participatory methods, qualitative geographical information has been used to complement and enrich spatial risk data in a study of arsenic-contaminated groundwater in Bangladesh (Hassan et al., 2003; 2004). Participatory group mapping, semi-structured in-depth interviews, and focus groups were used to elicit information on local community practices, social stigma, and health outcomes while spatial interpolation (kriging) from point data on measured arsenic concentrations allowed production of a series of spatial risk maps. Concentrations were found to vary substantially over only a few tens of metres, presenting particular difficulties for the development of workable arsenic mitigation strategies. Community mapping exercises have also been used to produce spatial representations of citizens' views of local air quality in British cities (Cinderby & Forrester, 2005). This work has demonstrated how local knowledge can be highly spatially resolved where, for example, one side of a road junction was perceived to have worse pollution levels than the other.

A final example illustrates that, although local and indigenous spatial knowledge may not be 'accurate' in a Cartesian sense, it can be used to highlight relevant spatial understandings, thinking, and activities. Williams and Dunn (2003) combined participatory methods (group mapping and activity ranking exercises) with GIS in a study of risk to communities from landmine injuries in Cambodia. The study demonstrated how local people's understandings of risk from landmine injury can be mapped to help formulate more meaningful policies for injury reduction.

## Conclusion

GIS is potentially well placed for exploring and integrating some of the multiple facets of public health and risk where those risks have a well defined spatial dimension. Given the highly visual nature of GIS, it offers particular promise as a tool for risk communication. It provides opportunities to integrate and manipulate large and complex datasets, to map hazards at a range of scales, model the effects of environmental change, predict at-risk populations, and display research findings in intuitive ways. For GIS users to have confidence in the results of spatial analysis, however, an awareness of the limitations of the data and analytical processes is critical, particularly for those using it as a decision support tool.

Partnerships between academic researchers and public health professionals are essential if risks in relation to public health are to be more fully understood, and responded to appropriately. Recent developments in mobile spatial technologies, web-based resources, and community generated data have the potential to enrich these relationships and the ways in which risks to health are communicated.

## References

Abbot, J., Chambers, R., Dunn, C. *et al.* (1998). Participatory GIS: opportunity or oxymoron? *PLA Notes*, 33: 27–34.

Ali, M., Emch, M., Donnay, J. P., Yunus, M. & Sack, R. B. (2002). Identifying environmental risk factors for endemic cholera: a raster GIS approach. *Health & Place*, 8: 201–10.

Aylin, P., Maheswaran, R., Wakefield, J. *et al.* (1999). A national facility for small area disease mapping and rapid initial assessment of apparent disease clusters around a point source: the UK Small Area Health Statistics Unit. *Journal of Public Health Medicine*, 21: 289–98.

Aylin, P., Cockings, S., Ferrándiz, J. *et al.* (2002). EUROHEIS (European Health and Environment Information System)—applications and case studies. *European Journal of Public Health*, 12(4): (Suppl), 38.

Beale, L., Abellan, J. J., Hodgson, S. & Jarup, L. (2008). Methodologic issues and approaches to spatial epidemiology. *Environmental Health Perspectives*, 116: 1105–10.

Bedard, Y., Gosselin, P., Rivest, S. *et al.* (2003). Integrating GIS components with knowledge discovery technology for environmental health decision support. *International Journal of Medical Informatics*, 70: 79–94.

Bellander, T., Jonson, T., Gustavsson, P., Pershagen, G. & Järup, L. (2001). Using geographic information systems to assess individual historical exposure to air pollution from traffic and house heating in Stockholm. *Environmental Health Perspectives*, 109: 633–9.

Bhopal, R. S., Diggle, P. & Rowlingson, B. (1992). Pinpointing clusters of apparently sporadic cases of Legionnaires' disease. *British Medical Journal*, 304: 1022–7.

Blaasaas, K. G., Tynes, T. & Lie, R. T. (2004). Risk of selected birth defects by maternal residence close to power lines during pregnancy. *Occupational and Environmental Medicine*, 61: 174–6.

Brauer, M., Hoek, G., Van Vliet, P. *et al.* (2002). Air pollution from traffic and the development of respiratory infections and asthmatic and allergic symptoms in children. *American Journal of Respiratory and Critical Care Medicine*, 166: 1092–8.

Briggs, D. J., Cornelis de Hoogh, U., Gulliver, J. *et al.* (2000). A regression-based method for mapping traffic-related air pollution: application and testing in four contrasting urban environments. *The Science of The Total Environment*, 253: 151–67.

Briggs, D. J., Forer, P., Järup, L. & Stern, R. (eds) (2002). *GIS for Emergency Preparedness and Health Risk Reduction*. NATO Science Series. IV. Earth and Environmental Sciences, Vol. 11. Dordrecht, the Netherlands, Kluwer Academic Publishers.

Cinderby, S. & Forrester, J. (2005). Facilitating the local governance of air pollution using GIS for participation. *Applied Geography*, 25: 143–58.

Cockings, S. & Järup, L. (2002). A European health and environment information system for exposure and disease mapping and risk assessment (EUROHEIS). In: D. J. Briggs, P. Forer, L. Järup & R. Stern (eds). *GIS for Emergency Preparedness and Health Risk Reduction*. NATO Science Series. IV. Earth and Environmental Sciences, Vol. 11. Dordrecht, the Netherlands, Kluwer Academic Publishers.

Cockings, S., Dunn, C. E., Bhopal, R. S. & Walker, D. R. (2004). Users' perspectives on epidemiological, GIS and point pattern approaches to analysing environment and health data. *Health & Place*, 10: 169–82.

Craig, W., Harris, T. & Weiner, D. (2002). *Community Participation and Geographic Information Systems*. London, Taylor and Francis.

Cromley, E. & McLafferty, S. (2002). *GIS and Public Health*. New York, The Guilford Press.

Diggle, P. J. (1983). *Statistical Analysis of Spatial Point Processes*. London, Academic Press.

Diggle, P. & Rowlingson, B. (1994). A conditional approach to point process modelling of elevated risk. *Journal of the Royal Statistical Society, Series A*, 157: 433–40.

Dunn, C. E. (2007). Participatory GIS—a people's GIS? *Progress in Human Geography*, 31: 616–37.

Dunn, C. E., Kingham, S. P., Rowlingson, B. *et al.* (2001). Analysing spatially referenced public health data: a comparison of three methodological approaches. *Health & Place*, 7: 1–12.

Dunn, C. E., Bhopal, R. S., Cockings, S. *et al.* (2007). Advancing insights into methods for studying environment–health relationships: A multidisciplinary approach to understanding Legionnaires' disease. *Health & Place*, 13: 677–90.

Elgethun, K., Fenske, R. A., Yost, M. G. & Palcisko, G. J. (2003). Time–location analysis for exposure assessment studies of children using a novel global positioning system instrument. *Environmental Health Perspectives*, 111: 115–22.

English, P., Neutra, R., Scalf, R. *et al.* (1999). Examining associations between childhood asthma and traffic flow using a geographic information system. *Environmental Health Perspectives*, 107: 761–7.

Fisher, J. B., Kelly, M. & Romm, J. (2006). Scales of environmental justice: Combining GIS and spatial analysis for air toxics in West Oakland, California. *Health & Place*, 12: 701–14.

Fleming, G., van der Merwe, M. & McFerren, G. (2007). Fuzzy expert systems and GIS for cholera health risk prediction in southern Africa. *Environmental Modelling & Software*, 22, 442–8.

Fotheringham, A. S. & Zhan, F. (1996). A comparison of three exploratory methods for cluster detection in point patterns. *Geographical Analysis*, 28: 200–18.

Gatrell, A. C. & Bailey, T. C. (1996). Interactive spatial data analysis in medical geography. *Social Science and Medicine*, 42: 843–55.

Gatrell, A. C., Bailey, T. C., Diggle, P. J. & Rowlingson, B. S. (1996). Spatial point pattern analysis and its application in geographical epidemiology. *Transactions of the Institute of British Geographers*, 21: 256–74.

Goodchild, M. F. (2000). The current status of GIS and spatial analysis. *Journal of Geographical Systems*, 2: 5–10.

Gouveia, C., Fonseca, A., Camara, A. & Ferreira, F. (2004). Promoting the use of environmental data collected by concerned citizens through information and communication technologies. *Journal of Environmental Management*, 71: 135–54.

Graham, A. J., Atkinson, P. M. & Danson, F. M. (2004). Spatial analysis for epidemiology. *Acta Tropica*, 91: 219–25.

Hassan, M. M., Atkins, P. J. & Dunn, C. E. (2003). The spatial pattern of risk from arsenic poisoning: a Bangladesh case study. *Journal of Environmental Science and Health*, 38: 1–24.

Hassan, M. M., Dunn, C. E. & Atkins, P. J. (2004). Exploring risk from arsenic-contaminated drinking water in Bangladesh: GIS and participation. In: *Proceedings of the GIS Research*, UK *12th Annual Conference* (GISRUK), pp. 145–7. University of East Anglia, Norwich.

Hay, S. I. & Snow, R. W. (2006). The Malaria Atlas Project: developing global maps of malaria risk. *PLoS Medicine*, 3(12): e473.

Hay, S. I., Omumbo, J. A., Craig, M. H. & Snow, R. W. (2000). Earth observation, geographic information systems and *Plasmodium falciparum* malaria in sub-Saharan Africa. *Advances in Parasitology*, 47: 173–215.

Higgs, G., Smith, D. P. & Gould, M. I. (2003). Realising 'joined-up' geography in the National Health Service: the role of geographical information systems? *Environment and Planning C*, 21: 241–58.

Higgs, G., Smith, D. P. and Gould, M. I. (2005). Findings from a survey on GIS use in the UK National Health Service: organisational challenges and opportunities. *Health Policy*, 72: 105–17.

Houghton, F. (2004). Looking on from the sidelines: the use of Geographical Information Systems in Health Boards in Ireland 2003. *Area*, 36: 81–3.

Jacquez, G. M. (2000). Spatial analysis in epidemiology: nascent science or a failure of GIS? *Journal of Geographical Systems*, 2: 91–7.

Jarup, L. (2004). Health and environment information systems for exposure and disease mapping, and risk assessment. *Environmental Health Perspectives*, 112: 995–7.

Jerrett, M., Burnett, R., Kanaroglou, P. *et al.* (2001). A GIS-environmental justice analysis of particulate air pollution in Hamilton, Canada. *Environment and Planning A*, 33: 955–73.

Jerrett, M., Burnett, R. T., Brook, J. *et al.* (2004). Do socioeconomic characteristics modify the short term association between air pollution and mortality? Evidence from a zonal time series in Hamilton, Canada. *Journal of Epidemiology and Community Health*, 58: 31–40.

Jones, A. P., Haynes, R., Kennedy, V. *et al.* (2008). Geographical variations in mortality and morbidity from road traffic accidents in England and Wales. *Health & Place*, 14: 519–35.

Kingham, S. P., Gatrell, A. C. & Rowlingson, B. (1995). Testing for clustering of health events within a geographical information system framework. *Environment and Planning A*, 27: 809–21.

Kingston, R., Carver, S., Evans, A. & Turton, I. (2000). Web-based public participation geographical information systems: an aid to local environmental decision-making. *Environment and Urban Systems*, 24: 109–25.

Kliukiene, J., Tynes, T. & Andersen A. (2004). Residential and occupational exposures to 50-Hz magnetic fields and breast cancer in women: a population-based study. *American Journal of Epidemiology*, 159: 852–61.

Lovett, A. A., Parfitt, J. P. & Brainard, J. S. (1997). Using GIS in risk analysis: a case study of hazardous waste transport. *Risk Analysis*, 17: 625–33.

Maantay, J. (2007). Asthma and air pollution in the Bronx: Methodological and data considerations in using GIS for environmental justice and health research. *Health & Place*, 13: 32–56.

Maclachlan, J. C., Jerrett, M., Abernathy, T., Sears, M. & Bunch, M. J. (2007). Mapping health on the Internet: A new tool for environmental justice and public health research. *Health & Place*, 13: 72–86.

Maheswaran, R. & Craglia, M. (eds) (2004). *GIS in Public Health Practice*. Florida, CRCM Press.

Mazumdar, S., Rushton, G., Smith, B. J., Zimmerman, D. L. & Donham, K. J. (2008). Geocoding accuracy and the recovery of relationships between environmental exposures and health. *International Journal of Health Geographics*, 7: 13.

McEntee, J. C. & Ogneva-Himmelberger, Y. (2008). Diesel particulate matter, lung cancer, and asthma incidences along major traffic corridors in MA, USA: A GIS analysis. *Health & Place*, 14: 817–28.

Moore, D. K., Jerrett, M., Mack, W. J. & Künzli, N. (2007). A land use regression model for predicting ambient fine particulate matter across Los Angeles, CA. *Journal of Environmental Monitoring*, 9: 246–52.

Nuckols, J. R., Ward, M. H. & Jarup, L. (2004). Using geographic information systems for exposure assessment in environmental epidemiology studies. *Environmental Health Perspectives*, 112: 1007–15.

Openshaw, S. (1984). *The Modifiable Areal Unit Problem*, CATMOG 38. Norwich, Geo Books.

Openshaw, S. & Turton, I. (1998). *A smart spatial pattern explorer for the geographical analysis of GIS data*. Available online at http://www.ccg.leeds.ac.uk/projects/smart/. Accessed 10th August 2009.

Poulstrup, A. & Hansen, H. L. (2004). Use of GIS and exposure modeling as tools in a study of cancer incidence in a population exposed to airborne dioxin. *Environmental Health Perspectives*, 112: 1032–6.

Rigby, J.E. and Gatrell, A.C. (2000) Spatial patterns in breast cancer incidence in north-west Lancashire, *Area*, 32, 71–8

Ripley, B. D. (1976). The second-order analysis of stationary processes. *Journal of Applied Problems*, 13: 255–66.

Rushton, G. (2003). Public health, GIS, and spatial analytic tools. *Annual Review of Public Health*, 24: 43–56.

Sabel, C. E., Boyle, P. J., Löytönen, M. *et al.* (2003). Spatial clustering of amyotrophic lateral sclerosis in Finland at place of birth and place of death. *American Journal of Epidemiology*, 157: 898–905.

Schootman, M., Sterling, D. A., Struthers, J. *et al.* (2007). Positional accuracy and geographic bias of four methods of geocoding in epidemiologic research. *Annals of Epidemiology*, 17: 464–70.

Smith, D., Gould, M. I. & Higgs, G. (2003). (Re)surveying the uses of geographical information systems in health authorities 1991–2001. *Area*, 35: 74–83.

Thomas, C. J., Davies, G. & Dunn, C. E. (2004). Mixed picture for changes in stable malaria distribution with future climate in Africa. *Trends in Parasitology*, 20: 216–20.

Verkasalo, P. K., Kokki, E., Pukkala, E. *et al.* (2004). Cancer risk near a polluted river in Finland. *Environmental Health Perspectives*, 112: 1026–31.

Williams, C. & Dunn, C. E. (2003). GIS in participatory research: assessing the impact of landmines on communities in North-west Cambodia. *Transactions in GIS*, 7: 393–410.

## Chapter 19

# Exploring and communicating risk: scenario-based workshops

Simon French (Manchester University
Business School) & John Maule
(Leeds University Business School)

## Introduction

Finding effective ways of communicating risk is becoming increasingly important. We are living in an age where members of society are becoming increasingly sensitive to risk issues (Beck, 1992; Mythen, 2004). Failing to communicate effectively has led to adverse public reaction that, in turn, has led to lower public trust and confidence in authorities to manage and regulate effectively.

In the first edition of this book we reported on our work in the Department of Health on developing a series of research-led training seminars for senior health services personnel to improve their processes of risk communication (Bennett et al., 1999; French & Maule, 1999). The seminars were underpinned by some fundamental principles. First, the ideas presented were to be evidence-based and the nature of the evidence needed to be briefly addressed during the seminar. Second, a decision processes perspective was appropriate given that managing and communication of risk in organizations invariably involves making judgements and taking decisions. This allowed us to introduce the notion of 'value-focused thinking' (French et al., 2009; Keeney, 1992) and to stress the importance of setting objectives when developing a communications strategy. In addition, we were able to introduce a range of pencil and paper decision aids, including simple methods for identifying stakeholders and uncertainties, the use of decision trees to model different actions that were available, and the likely outcomes of taking those actions, and techniques underpinning the development of press releases. Third, participants needed to have opportunities to have first-hand experience of using the tools and techniques both to learn how to use them and to appreciate their usefulness. Fourth, all aspects of the seminar needed to be presented in the context of health settings so that participants appreciated the value of the content to their professional context. Fifth, following Fischhoff (1995), we emphasized the importance of taking account of how the public and other key stakeholders both perceive the risks involved and their expectations about how risk managers and regulators should act to manage and communicate the threats. Finally, the workshop participants had a broad and extensive range of backgrounds and professional responsibilities, were from central and regional offices, and included staff from the Press Office, and those responsible for formulating and communicating policy. Given that they already had a wealth of practical experience of risk communication, we needed a mechanism to capitalize upon this experience. To that end, we focused each workshop on a hypothetical but realistic scenario involving many aspects of risk communication. Since then we have developed and used similar formats in a series of training and research initiatives.

In this chapter, we reflect on what we learnt from these events, including how to design workshops and to develop scenarios. We also recognize that there have been some important changes in theory and research on risk perception and communication, and that our understanding of the underlying issues has developed from running related risk communication programmes in other contexts. Thus, the primary objectives of the chapter are to:

- Outline the underlying philosophy underpinning our understanding of risk communication and how that feeds into the design of training seminars
- Use our recent experience of running risk communication events to reflect on the changes necessary to the seminars in terms of content, focus, underlying philosophy, and techniques covered
- Identify some more recent developments in the literature on risk perception and communication, considering the implications of these in the context of the training seminar content.

## Language, risk communication, and perception

To understand our approach to public risk communication we need to discuss briefly our perspective on language. The philosophy of (public) language stemming from Wittgenstein's 'language games' and Searle's 'speech acts' emphasizes that an utterance or piece of writing is an act in a 'game of interactions' (Searle, 1969; Wittgenstein, 1953). From this standpoint, the primary purpose of the spoken or written word is to engender a change in the behaviour of the recipient, rather than the transfer of information. While we do not wish to become involved in philosophical debates about the foundations of language, we do commend this perspective as a very useful one in thinking about risk communication and the development of strategies for informing the public about risks. Of course, we recognize that any communication on a threat should be ethical, providing the public with an honest and unbiased assessment of the risks involved and any preventative or precautionary measure that might be necessary: we would not wish to follow a behavioural perspective on communications that leads us into the land of political 'spin'. However, we find it helpful to remember that any communication is an act in a language game with the public. To take the decision to commit to that act, the public body concerned should recognize that the act will have a variety of consequences for different stakeholder groups. There is some advantage, therefore, in structuring the development of public statements, their timing and content as a decision process that can benefit from the application of many management techniques used to support other kinds of decisions. Thus, our approach is much informed by our understanding of decision analysis (French et al., 2009). In the next section, we review briefly the content of the seminars and how these should change to take account of recent developments in risk perception and communication.

Our original set of seminars introduced delegates to some of the major research findings on perception and communication of risk, considering these from individual and social perspectives. The individual perspective included a brief discussion of research showing that the public and other stakeholders often conceptualize risk in ways that are different from those assumed by risk regulators and managers (Slovic, 1997); also noting that even these latter 'expert' groups often adopt different definitions of risk (Fischhoff et al., 1984; Moore, 1983). This provided an opportunity to review research from the 'psychometric' paradigm, showing that qualitative aspects of threats (e.g. the extent to which they were thought to be 'unknown to science' or 'dreaded') can influence public perception of risk. We drew on work by one of our collaborators at the Department of Health by presenting these aspects as a set of 'fright factors' (see Chapter 1) that risk managers and communicators were encouraged to review when predicting how people would respond to hazards. The more a hazard is associated with these factors—for example, the risk being involuntary, novel or inequitable—in the public's perception, the greater the public aversion. We also outlined the 'heuristics and biases' literature stemming from the seminal work of Kahneman and Tversky (Kahneman et al., 1982; Tversky & Kahneman, 1981). This included the effects of framing, e.g. that risk attitudes may depend on whether a message is framed positively or negatively, and that people often assess risk by means of simple judgemental heuristics, e.g. availability, representativeness or plausibility.

From the social perspective, we reviewed work identifying different cultural types within society (Douglas, 1992; Thompson et al., 1990) that determine how particular groups of people perceive and act in the face of risk, and the importance of trust and how it can be facilitated. Finally, we brought the work together in the context of the social amplification of risk framework (Barnett & Breakwell, 2003; Kasperson *et al.*, 2003; Kasperson, 1992). We used this framework to discuss those aspects of a risk situation likely to attract the attention of the media that, in turn, amplify or increase public interest and concern. Again, we drew on work by a colleague in the Department of Health who summarized the characteristics, dubbed 'media triggers', likely to induce media interest: (see Chapter 1). Common triggers include questions of blame, or the suggestion of an attempted 'cover-up'. This was a useful device for predicting those threats likely to be picked up and amplified by the media, thereby increasing public concern.

The delegates attending the seminars were generally unaware of this literature, and found it insightful and of practical help in understanding public perception of risk and how this can, on occasions, lead the public to act in ways that are at odds with prediction based on scientific risk assessments. Since running the seminars, this body of work has developed further (for reviews, see Edwards *et al.*, 2002; Berry, 2004; Maule, 2008; Fischhoff, 2008), though the primary findings and their implications for risk communication are broadly similar. However, there are some relatively new developments in the research literature that we advocate including in future training seminars.

## Distinction between system 1 and system 2 thinking

Since the early 1980s, psychologists have distinguished between two different forms of thinking (Chaiken *et al.*, 1989):

- System 2, characterized by conscious analytical thought that involves a detailed evaluation of a broad range of information, often based on a rule that is assumed to provide the 'correct' answer or solution

- System 1, often referred to as 'intuition' or 'gut reaction' that involves a superficial analysis/interpretation of the relevant information based on much simpler forms of thinking on the fringes or outside of consciousness.

While formal risk assessment techniques have the characteristics of system 2 thinking, the general public often use much simpler system 1 forms of thinking when assessing risks. For example, there is strong evidence to suggest that people determine how safe or risky a situation is according to whether they feel positively or negatively about the potential threat (Slovic *et al.*, 2004). These emotional reactions, which are either pre-programmed (e.g. fear of spiders) or learnt (e.g. fear of nuclear power), are automatic responses elicited outside conscious control, which makes them very difficult to change. There is also evidence to suggest that some threats, e.g. nuclear power, become stigmatized in that they consistently induce a negative emotional response, and this provides the continuing basis for how people assess risk in these situations (see, for example, Flynn *et al.*, 2001). Communications based on reasoned arguments about relevant statistics on safety, effective risk management practices, and so on are unlikely to influence people if their understanding is derived from this kind of system 1 thinking. It is important for risk communicators to recognize these different forms of thinking and to consider the implications of them for developing effective communications. If people are generally engaging with the situation using system 1 processes, then communicators may need to develop tactics that encourage a switch to system 2 thinking so that they process relevant statistical and scientific information about the threat. If this is not possible, then it may be necessary to develop ways of communicating pertinent to system 1 forms of thinking (see, for example, Visschers *et al.*, 2008).

## What information do people want?

Formal approaches to risk emphasize the importance of the impact of a possible threat and its likelihood of occurrence, so these have tended to be the factors that are addressed in risk communications. However, the general public and other stakeholders often require other kinds of information, and a failure to address these can considerably reduce the effectiveness of communications. For example, Lion *et al.* (2002) asked people to indicate what kinds of information they wanted, having been confronted by a relatively unknown risk. Interestingly, a small percentage of people said they did not want any information at all, because knowing about the threat might make one 'afraid to live'. Those that requested information indicated that they wanted, in order of priority, how one is exposed to the risk, its consequences (including the likelihood of negative consequences occurring), whether it is controllable, other people's experience with the risk, who is responsible for the negative consequences, and whether there are any advantages. While some of these issues would be covered by formal risk assessments, others such as controllability may not, and so are in danger of being overlooked. This list of priorities is likely to vary from threat to threat, so it is important to establish the information needs of the public directly for each type of threat.

## Mental models approach

The mental models approach (MMA) was emerging at the time we were developing the seminars, but was not sufficiently established to include in them.

The approach is founded on the suggestion that people represent the world internally in terms of small scale mental models of external reality and the actions they might take (Craik, 1943). The approach involves eliciting and comparing expert and lay mental models of a hazard to identify misunderstandings and errors in the lay models and then to construct risk communications that rectify these shortcomings (Morgan *et al.*, 2002). Cassidy & Maule (2009) argued that the MMA has a sound theoretical base, is user-centred, and there is evidence that it works (Cox *et al.*, 2003), though they do highlight some drawbacks. In particular, the MMA takes the 'expert' view as fact whereas, in reality, scientific knowledge is constantly evolving and is often contested even among experts themselves. This is likely to be particularly true for complex, new or poorly understood situations. Also, the approach places scientific knowledge as primal, with lay knowledge flawed and in need of correction, so tends to ignore relevant lay knowledge, understanding, and concerns. In addition, Cassidy's and Maule's research showed that there are situations where it is very difficult to elicit mental models (e.g. mental models of the food chain risks for chicken). To overcome this problem, they developed an icon-based methodology. This involved groups of individuals selecting pictures of key elements in the food chain (e.g. farms, lorries, production plants, and household fridges), sticking them in an appropriate order on a sheet of paper, drawing a line to indicate links between them, and then writing down, at appropriate points on the chain, what they consider the key risks to be and how these should be mitigated. A web-based implementation of this methodology was also developed (Zhang, 2008). The discussion generated while constructing the model and the final model itself provide a rich source of information for determining how people conceptualize a risk situation and the actions thought necessary to manage it (Cassidy & Maule, 2009). The strengths and weaknesses of MMA and techniques for eliciting lay and expert mental models should be a major element in training for risk communicators.

## Methods for communicating statistical risk information

Research shows that the public often misinterprets communications based on quantitative assessments. For example, Gigerenzer *et al.* (2005) showed that people often misinterpret risk when expressed as a percentage. Yamigishi (1997) observed that people are overly sensitive to the number of people at risk, viz. people judge that a threat of death expressed as killing 1286 people out of every 10 000 as more risky than a threat expressed as killing 24.14 people out of every 100 people, despite the contrary being the case. McDaniels (1988) showed such biases also occur in legislators, leading to imbalances in expenditure on preventing deaths from different hazards (see Berry 2004, Chapter 3 for a more extensive review). It is important to include recent suggestions on how to overcome these problems in training seminars.

One approach has involved using words or phrases rather than numbers. For example, EU legislation stipulates particular words to use when communicating the risk of side effects associated with medicines (EC Directive 92/27) (e.g. 'very rare' for the lowest band, 'very common' for the highest band). However, Berry *et al.* (2002) showed that people interpret the words differently from that assumed by risk regulators: e.g. whereas regulators defined 'very rare' as less than 0.01%, people gave a mean estimate of 4%. These and other studies suggest that words do not necessarily fare better than numbers as a means of conveying risk (see Maule, 2008 for a brief review). So communicators need to test out different modes in their own domain and context to determine which, if any, is better. A second approach has argued that communications using single event and conditional probabilities are inherently ambiguous and confusing to people (Gigerenzer & Edwards, 2003). These authors showed that people gave more accurate risk judgements when information was conveyed using a frequency format instead. A third approach has advocated the use of ladders, scales, and comparators that display by name and risk level (e.g. risk of dying over a specified period) the target hazard and a number of common hazards all presented in order of magnitude of the risk involved (Calman & Royston, 1997; Paling, 1997; Sandman *et al.*, 1994). While each of these approaches has limitations (Johnson, 2004; Lipkus & Hollands, 1999), with careful evaluation they can be useful ways of conveying risk information. Finally, some authors have advocated the use of graphical techniques to aid statistical understanding (Schirillo & Stone, 2005; Tufte, 2001), though evidence on their effectiveness in risk communication is rather mixed (Lipkus & Hollands, 1999). An evaluation of these techniques and some discussion of where and why they might be appropriate should be an integral part of training in risk communication.

## Soft modelling, risk management, and risk communication

We close this review by referring to one of our own papers, French *et al.* (2005). In this, we explored the use of soft modelling techniques—cognitive mapping, problem and issue structuring methods, soft systems, etc. (French *et al.*, 2009; Mingers & Rosenhead, 2004; Rosenhead & Mingers, 2001). We discussed how many techniques used to help explore and structure risk management issues are also very useful for developing risk communications. Indeed, we argued that the risk communication and risk management strategy should be developed and implemented together seamlessly (Carter & French, 2005; 2006).

## Design of workshops and scenarios

In our earlier chapter, we described a typical workshop, including the lay-out of an agenda. Over the intervening years, we have used several models for developing workshops and generating discussion. Generally, the workshops have three sessions, two in the morning, one in the afternoon, and a debriefing at the end.

Our aim in the first session of a workshop is to challenge the participants' intuitive responses to risk without losing touch with their values and emotions. It is important that risk managers and communicators understand the different ways in which others may react to a situation. If we are working with groups from varied backgrounds, we may begin with a session exploring the participants' own reactions to risk and uncertainty, using some of the standard heuristic and biases examples developed by Kahneman and Tversky (Bazerman, 2006; Kahneman *et al.*, 1982; Tversky & Kahneman, 1981). Such a session involves presenting participants with some behavioural and cognitive research findings, including system 1 and system 2 thinking, and reflecting on their own responses to the situation. At other times, we begin with the first phase of a hypothetical scenario, getting the participants to react to it in an unprompted manner and then reflecting back their reactions to them in the context of behavioural and cognitive theories. There are times when we work with pre-dominantly science-trained analysts. Such groups tend to respond to scenarios and cognitive examples with oversimplified system 2 thinking. Our aim then is to open up their thinking. So we might run the session as a facilitated decision conference (Eden & Radford, 1990; French *et al.*, 2009). We present the opening of the scenario to them, guiding them towards wider system 2 thinking using problem structuring methods and soft modelling interventions designed to encourage divergent thinking (Franco *et al.*, 2006; 2007; French *et al.*, 2009; Rosenhead & Mingers, 2001). We lay particular emphasis on identifying their values explicitly. We also seek to identify stakeholders and consider how these might behave, prompting the group to empathize with system 1 thinking, before presenting them with some cognitive and behavioural research findings.

By the end of the first session, we hope to have enhanced participants' understanding of responses to risk situations, helping them to recognize the different behaviours that may arise among the different stakeholders to a situation. In the second session, if the participants have been presented with the scenario, we continue with this, perhaps presenting a second phase. Otherwise, we introduce the scenario and explore their initial reactions to it. Either way, our aim in the second session is to introduce a range of problem structuring and soft modelling tools to help structure their thinking about the situation, how they will manage it, and what information they will seek. The range of such tools introduced will depend on the scenario, the approach that we followed in the first session, and the time available. In all cases, we emphasize value-focused thinking and stakeholder identification (French *et al.*, 2009; Keeney, 1992). For regulators developing societal risk management and communication strategies, these seem to us to be the two key matters that once were overlooked and even now may not be quite in the forefront of their thinking.

Thus in the first session, our aim is to facilitate the participants' understanding of system 1 thinking and how the various stakeholders may behave; in the second session we seek to mentor them to use simple system 2 thinking devices—problem structuring methods and soft modelling tools—in their management of situations. In the third session, we move them towards an explicit consideration of how they will communicate with the stakeholders. In other words, how from their perspective, now created by system 2 thinking, they will inform the public and stakeholders about the situation and how it is being handled, recognizing that the listeners are likely to use system 1 thinking. We may begin the third session by rolling the scenario on into another phase or continue with the current one. In this session, we seek to introduce two key sets of ideas and also to emphasize the decision-making perspective on communication.

The first set of ideas relates to understanding the media and the motivations of those working in it. Too often, the groups come to the workshops with an inherent distrust and, indeed, dislike of the media. They see them as seeking to 'get a story at all costs'. Thus we may take 'time out' from the scenario and discuss the media and what motivates reporters and editors—their need to be on or near the 'front page' is motivated as much by the pay and bonus structures in that industry as by reporters' desire for status. With this in mind, we seek to promote the idea of working with the media as partners. How can the risk communication be cast so that the message is fair and delivered as intended, but also achieves the reporters' objectives? We explore ideas of media triggers (see Chapter 1). Moreover, we may show the group how to cast the issue of the interaction with the media as a qualitative decision tree to help the group think further about how they will communicate with the public and stakeholders (French *et al.*, 2005).

The second set of ideas is around role-playing. Instead of thinking about what to communicate purely in the sense of conveying information, we ask the participants to think about how their communication will be heard, what behaviours it might encourage in different groups, and how this fits in with their broader communication objectives. We prime this discussion with presentations on fright factors (see Chapter 1) and different cultural theories of risk (Department of Health, 1998; Douglas, 1992; Thompson *et al.*, 1990).

In a sense, we encourage them to 'hold up what they are going to say against each stakeholder and ask: how will they hear this and will their actions be those that we intended?'

We often complete the session by getting the group to write a press release to give a concrete form to their learning.

In the final debriefing session, we reflect upon what has been learnt in the day. If two or more groups have been going through in parallel, we invite them to compare their experiences—this is particularly enlightening if the two groups are drawn from different stakeholders. We recommend further reading and sources of information. We ask that they do not lose their hypothetical scenarios 'on the bus home'. Despite headers and footers and possibly water-marks emphasizing that they are hypothetical scenarios, there is the potential to cause a 'scare' if they are read out of context!

We have said little about the scenarios per se. Examples of a scenario may be found in our earlier chapter (French & Maule, 1999) and in the exercises in our forthcoming book (French et al., 2009). In the appendix, we give a scenario used in a current executive education and change management programme for local government. Generally, we would repeat all the points that we made a decade ago; our experiences since then have confirmed our thinking. Most importantly, we find that discussion is better stimulated if we confound the risk issues with other factors that necessitated interaction with other stake-holders or which would capture disproportionate media interest. Thus, in the scenario in the Appendix, the issue is not just about the claim of poor hygiene in the kitchens but also relates to government policy and the celebrity status of Jamie Oliver, a celebrity UK chef who is in the forefront of a campaign for healthy eating, particularly in schools. We also find it wise to include refer-ences to named individuals and organizations, even though it takes consider-able effort to avoid libellous statements. For the participants in the workshop to react to a hypothetical scenario, it has to be realistic: it has to 'chime with their experience' so that they can build an emotional reaction to it. Including religious, moral or ethical issues can give the scenario a very effective edge in stimulating wide discussion.

## Experiences and research findings

We have used scenario-based workshops in a variety of educational contexts. Firstly, in our respective universities' degree programmes we have run them in MSc and MBA programmes. If they are part of a course running over a number of weeks, they may not be workshops per se, but rather a sequence of activities during a more conventional course. None the less, the thinking on the design of the sessions described above carries through. In some cases, we have been able to video sessions and use the replay to help the participants to recognize where they are using system 1 rather than system 2 thinking and also, an issue we have not discussed, where group dynamics are causing problems in the handling of the risk. We have run executive education courses for a multinational organization on the safety of its personal hygiene and food products using the same methodology. On an EU programme, one of us (SF) used similar workshops to train nuclear emergency managers. The other (JM) has used such workshops to investigate how the uncertainties associated with probabilistic atmospheric transport and dispersion models are communicated to gold commanders responsible for managing chemical, biological, radiological, and nuclear (CBRN) incidents.

Aside from training on risk management and communication, we have also used such workshops to help organizations in a process of change management. For instance, we used scenario-based workshops to help the nascent UK Food Standards Agency (FSA) plan its procedures and develop risk communication processes immediately prior to its taking on its full regulatory role in 2000. One of these involved helping the FSA build relationships with their key stakeholders. At Manchester Business School, there is a longstanding change management programme with a local authority, and scenario-based workshops have been a part of this. The scenario in the Appendix was developed for this programme.

As indicated in the introduction, scenario-based workshops can also be very effective tools in research on how to communicate risk. We were fortunate to be funded by the FSA for a research programme to explore the impact of different forms of risk communication (French et al., 2003). In this, we designed a methodology involving two different kinds of activities (Figure 19.1). Both activities involve presenting information over time about an evolving food risk

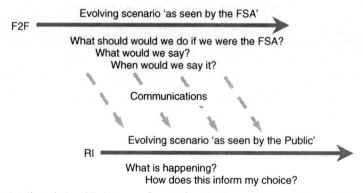

**Fig. 19.1** The relationship between face-to-face (F2F) workshops and remote interactions (RI) in the FSA project's methodology.

situation to research participants and recording their responses to it. However, the purpose and structure of each activity differed.

*Face-to-face workshops* (F2F) were designed to explore stakeholders' perceptions of the nature of evolving risk situations, their expectations of what the FSA should communicate, why they thought this form of communication was appropriate, how these views differed across different stakeholders, and the implications of this for effective communication of risk information. We ran these workshops pretty much to the format described in this chapter but without explicit presentation of any theory or research.

*Remote interactions* (RI) were designed to test predictions about the effectiveness of different communication strategies of the same information, at discrete stages of the evolving food risk situation. Different communication strategies were developed, based in part on the outcomes of the face-to-face workshops. The effectiveness of these strategies was tested by recruiting a sample from the general public and providing each with a booklet describing a hypothetical food risk situation in terms of one of the risk communication strategies, as it would have been conveyed to them via the media. This 'media coverage' was constructed by the researchers in conjunction with a media partner. Following the presentation of this information, participants were asked to complete a number of different activities designed to capture their: 'mental model' of the situation and their behavioural intentions.

In the F2F workshops, system 2 thinking predominated; in the RI, system 1 thinking was assumed to be more prevalent. This research led to a number of conclusions, among which we note the following.

- Different stakeholder groups do have different perceptions and are driven by different imperatives, but generally there were more similarities than differences in their views and expectations

- The majority of participants favoured early warning of a developing risk; however, a significant minority (around one-third in our studies) believe that a communication should be delayed until the situation has clarified. The former group felt that early communication built trust, while the latter were concerned about creating a 'scare' or jeopardizing commercial interests

- The act of communicating the currently understood facts is of primary importance

- Trust in the communicator is important and appears not only to affect how people evaluate a communication and how informed they feel but also to affect these aspects more than the actual content of the message itself

- The public are able to handle and react sensibly to descriptions of the uncertainty, both in qualitative and quantitative terms, and are not confused by the inclusion of relatively simple numerical representations of risk.

Recently, we have completed a research programme which investigated how to involve rural stakeholders in the management of food safety risks (Shepherd *et al.*, 2006). Our approach involved several scenario-based stakeholder workshops as components in exploring public participation in societal risk management. Thus, we moved the scenario-based workshop methodology into research on public participation. We are still evaluating much of the research, though it is true that the complexity of the issues was, to make an understatement, a challenge (Bayley & French, 2008b). One point that we noted early on is that in dealing with a major issue one may need a sequence of workshops, and the purposes of each of these will vary according to its position in the overall societal decision process: i.e. issue formulation → analysis → evaluation and decision (Bayley & French, 2008a). When the public and other stakeholders are participating in the process, the issue of communication is much more complex and may vary from stage to stage. Thus, the communication issues in public deliberations to identify issues and concerns in the formulation stage may be very different to those in the final stage, during which the authorities are seeking the public views on evaluating particular options and the decision to be taken.

## Conclusions and discussion

Since writing the chapter in the earlier edition of this book, our experience has made us recognize the importance of the interplay between system 1 and system 2 thinking in designing risk communications. The communicator should be writing from a system 2 perspective: surely we would expect our regulators to analyse and respond in some rational sense to a situation. But the listener is as, or more, likely to hear the message from a system 1 perspective as a system 2 one. So the communicator has to judge the effect of the message against that assumption. Thus we design scenario-based training workshops with this interplay in mind: we take the participants from system 1 perceptions of the world to a system 2 mode of thinking. Then we help them look back to a system 1 world when communicating with the public and stakeholders. In addition, thinking about communication as implementing a decision can add focus.

As we look to the future we are aware that there is much research needed in relation to public participation in societal risk management (Bayley & French, 2008b; French *et al.*, 2007). In particular, how do we handle risk communication issues in live debates, in which it is likely that all forms of system 1 and 2 thinking are active simultaneously? Moreover, the web now has a presence that it did not have 10 years ago. Current web technologies—'Web 2.0'—now support effective social networking and collaboration (Briggs *et al.*, 2003). How do we handle risk communication issues in such an environment? Whatever the answers, it is our conviction that scenario-based workshops, possibly conducted virtually, will provide a mechanism first to explore and then, when we have more understanding, to train and sensitize regulators and public bodies to risk communication issues.

## Acknowledgements

We are grateful to many colleagues for discussion and support in developing all the programme of training and research described above. Our work has been supported by a variety of contracts from the Department of Health, the UK Food Standards Agency, the Health Protection Agency, the EU FP5 and FP6 programmes, the European Science Foundation, the UK Research Councils Rural Economy and Land Use Programme, and by our own teaching commitments in Leeds University and Manchester Business Schools.

## Appendix: an example of a hypothetical scenario

Sloughborough Metropolitan Borough Council (SMBC) have just built and commissioned state-of-the-art kitchens with associated cafeterias and restaurants on a site in the north of the town near their own offices. The kitchens are close to:

- A senior and a junior school
- Some warden-controlled retirement homes and flats, owned and run by the Pericles Housing Association (PHA)
- SMBC's crèche facilities for its staff's children
- A day-patient treatment centre belonging to Sloughborough's Central Hospital Trust (SCHT).

SMBC have negotiated with PHA and SCHT an agreement that the kitchens will provide catering to the retirement homes and the day-patient centre in addition to the council, their crèche, and the schools. Moreover, they have contracted a local caterer, Higsons, to manage and run the kitchens. As part of the deal, Higsons will source a high proportion of their supplies from local farmers and market gardeners; and as little as possible of the catering will be based upon processed food.

Given the campaign by Jamie Oliver and the positive government response, SMBC are justly proud of this initiative. Last Thursday, the Prime Minister's Parliamentary Private Secretary, no less, on BBC's *Question Time*, referred to SMBC's successful embodiment of the government's objective of providing good food and nutrition to those in its care. On Friday, the local *Sloughborough Evening Post* rang up and asked to visit the kitchens with a view to publishing a report on the kitchens. They visited the kitchens yesterday morning and all seemed to go well.

However, last evening's *Evening Post* and today's national press carried articles under headings such as 'Poor Hygiene in Council Flagship Kitchens', 'Council Conned with Unhygienic Cheap Food', and 'Food Standards Agency should investigate Sloughborough Council Catering'. The articles pick up on two issues.

Firstly, the Food Standards Agency (FSA) have a long established campaign to persuade all caterers, housewives, and househusbands(!) to use separate knives and chopping boards for meat, fish, and fruit and vegetables to avoid cross-contamination between foodstuffs. They quote, for example, a case of salmonella food poisoning at a seaside hotel in which salad had been prepared on a board previously used to chop chicken prior to cooking. The reporter visiting SMBC's kitchens had seen three separate occurrences of such poor hygiene. In a couple of the newspaper articles, an FSA spokesperson refused to comment on the case without substantiated facts, but then said 'if true, it would be an example of poor kitchen hygiene'.

Secondly, after visiting the kitchens, the reporter returned surreptitiously and searched the dustbins, finding substantial evidence of the use of processed food from national and international suppliers. The proportion of freshly prepared food based on local produce may not be so high.

# References

Bayley, C. & French, S. (2008a). Designing a participatory process for stakeholder involvement in a societal decision. *Group Decision and Negotiation,* 17(3): 195–210.

Bayley, C. & French, S. (2008b). *Public Participation: Comparing Approaches.* (Submitted to Journal of Risk Research). Manchester M15 6PB, Manchester Business School.

Bazerman, M. (2006). *Managerial Decision Making.* New York, John Wiley and Sons.

Beck, U. (1992). *Risk Society: Towards a New Modernity.* London, Sage.

Bennett, P. G., Cole, R. A. & McDonald, A. (1999). Risk communication as a decision process. In: P. G. Bennett & K. C. Calman, (eds). *Risk Communication and Public Health: Policy, Science and Participation.* Oxford, Oxford University Press: pp. 207–21.

Berry, D. C. (2004). *Risk Communication and Health Psychology.* Maidenhead, Open University Press.

Berry, D. C., Raynor, D. K., Knapp, P. R. & Bersellini, E. (2002). Official warnings on thromboembolism risk with oral contraceptives fail to inform users adequately. *Contraception,* 66: 305–7.

Briggs, R. O., de Veerde, G.-J. & Nunamaker, J. F. (2003). Collaboration engineering with thinklets to pursue sustained success with GSS. *Journal of Management Information Systems,* 19(4): 31–64.

Calman, K. C. & Royston, G. H. (1997). Risk language and dialects. *British Medical Journal,* 315: 939–42.

Carter, E. & French, S. (2005). *Nuclear emergency management in Europe: a review of approaches to decision making.* ISCRAM 2005: Information Systems for Crisis Response and Management, Brussels.

Carter, E. & French, S. (2006). Are current processes for nuclear emergency management in Europe adequate? *Journal of Radiation Protection,* 26: 405–14.

Cassidy, A. & Maule, A. J. (2009). Risk communication and participatory research: using the visual domain to support group discussion of complex issues. In: P. Reavey (ed.) *Visual Psychologies: Using and Interpreting Images in Qualitative Research.* London, Routledge.

Chaiken, S., Liberman, A. & Eagly, A. H. (1989). Heuristic and systematic information processing within and beyond the persuasion context. In: J. S. Uleman & J. A. Bargh (eds). *Unintended Thought.* New York, Guilford: pp. 212–52.

Cox, P., Niewohner, J., Pidgeon, N., Gerrard, S., Fischhoff, B. & Riley, D. (2003). The use of mental models in chemical risk protection: developing a generic workplace methodology. *Risk Analysis,* 23(2): 311–24.

Craik, K. (1943). *The Nature of Explanation.* Cambridge, Cambridge University Press.

Department of Health. (1998). *Communicating About Risks to Public Health: Pointers to Good Practice.* London, HMSO.

Douglas, M. (1992). *Risk and Blame: Essays in Cultural Theory.* London, Routledge.

Eden, C. & Radford, J. (eds) (1990). *Tackling Strategic Problems: the Role of Group Decision Support.* London, Sage.

Edwards, A., Elwyn, G. & Mulley, A. (2002). Explaining risks: turning numerical data into meaningful pictures. *British Medical Journal,* 324: 827–30.

Fischhoff, B. (1995). Risk perception and communication unplugged: twenty years of process. *Risk Analysis,* 15: 137–45.

Fischhoff, B. (2008). Risk perception and communication. In: R. Detels, R. Beaglehole, M. A. Lansang & M. Gulliford (eds). *Oxford Textbook of Public Health,* 5th edn. Oxford, Oxford University Press: Chapter 8.9.

Fischhoff, B., Watson, S. & Hope, C. (1984). Defining risk. *Policy Sciences,* 17: 123–39.

Flynn, J., Slovic, P. & Kunreuther, H. (eds) (2001). *Risk, Media and Stigma: Understanding Public Challenges to Modern Science and Technology.* London, Earthscan.

Franco, A., Shaw, D. & Westcombe, M. (2006). Problem structuring methods I. *Journal of the Operational Research Society,* 57: 757–878.

Franco, A., Shaw, D. & Westcombe, M. (2007). Problem structuring methods II. *Journal of the Operational Research Society,* 58: 545–682.

French, S. & Maule, A. J. (1999). Improving risk communication: scenario based workshops. In: P. G. Bennett & K. C. Calman, (eds). *Risk Communication and Public Health: Policy Science and Participation.* Oxford, Oxford University Press: pp. 241–53.

French, S., Maule, A. J., Maule, S. *et al.* (2003). *Understanding Stakeholder Concerns in Relation to Communications on Food Safety: Summary Report.* Manchester, Manchester.

French, S., Maule, A. J. & Mythen, G (2005). Soft modelling in risk communication and management: examples in handling food risk. *Journal of the Operational Research Society,* 56: 879–88.

French, S., Rios Insua, D. & Ruggeri, F. (2007). e-participation and decision analysis. *Decision Analysis,* 4(4): 1–16.

French, S., Maule, A. J. & Papamichail, K. N. (2009). *Decision Making: Behaviour, Analysis and Support.* Cambridge, Cambridge University Press.

Gigerenzer, G. & Edwards, A. (2003). Simple tools for understanding risks: from innumeracy to insight. *British Medical Journal,* 327: 741–4.

Gigerenzer, G., Hertwig, R., van den Broek, E., Fasolo, B. & Katsikopoulos, K. V. (2005). A 30% chance of rain tomorrow: how does the public understand probabilistic weather forecasts? *Risk Analysis,* 25: 623–9.

Johnson, B. B. (2004). Varying risk comparison elements: effects on public reactions. *Risk Analysis,* 24: 103–14.

Kahneman, D., Slovic, P. & Tversky, A. (eds) (1982). *Judgement under Uncertainty.* Cambridge, Cambridge University Press.

Kasperson, R. E. (1992). The social amplification of risk: progress in developing an integrative framework. In: S. Krimsky & S. Golding, (eds). *Social Theories of Risk.* New York, Praeger.

Kasperson, J. X., Kasperson, R. E., Pidgeon, N. & Slovic, P. (2003). The social amplification of research: assessing fifteen years of research and theory. In: N. Pidgeon, R. E. Kasperson & P. Slovic, (eds). *The Social Amplification of Risk.* Cambridge, Cambridge University Press.

Keeney, R. L. (1992). *Value-Focused Thinking: a Path to Creative Decision Making.* Harvard, Harvard University Press.

Lion, R., Meertens, R. M. & Bot, I. (2002). Priorities in information desire about unknown risks. *Risk Analysis,* 22(4): 765–76.

Lipkus, I. M. & Hollands, J. G. (1999). The visual communication of risk. *Journal of National Cancer Institute Monograph,* 25: 149–62.

Maule, A. J. (2008). Risk communication and organisations. In: W. Starbuck & G. Hodgkinson (eds). *The Oxford Handbook of Organizational Decision Making.* Oxford, Oxford University Press.

McDaniels, T. (1988). Comparing expressed and revealed preferences for risk reduction: different hazards and question frames. *Risk Analysis,* 8: 593–604.

Mingers, J. & Rosenhead, J. (2004). Problem structuring methods in action. *European Journal of Operational Research,* 152: 530–54.

Moore, P. G. (1983). *The Business of Risk.* Cambridge, Cambridge University Press.

Morgan, G., Fischhoff, B., Bostrom, A. & Atman, C. (2002). *Risk Communication: A Mental Models Approach.* Cambridge, Cambridge University Press.

Mythen, G. (2004). *Ulrich Beck: a Critical Introduction to the Risk Society.* London, Pluto Press.

Paling, J. (1997). *Up to your armpits in alligators: how to sort out what risks are worth worrying about.* Gainesville, Florida, Risk Communication and Environmental Institute.

Rosenhead, J. & Mingers, J. (eds) (2001). *Rational Analysis for a Problematic World Revisited.* Chichester, John Wiley and Sons.

Sandman, P. M., Weinstein, N. D. & Miller, P. (1994). High-risk or low—how location on a risk ladder affects perceived risk. *Risk Analysis,* 14: 35–45.

Schirillo, J. A. & Stone, E. R. (2005). The greater ability of graphical versus numerical displays to increase risk avoidance involves a common mechanism. *Risk Analysis*, 25: 555–66.

Searle, J. R. (1969). *Speech Acts*. Cambridge, Cambridge University Press.

Shepherd, R., Barker, G., French, S. *et al.* (2006). Managing food chain risks: integrating technical and stakeholder perspectives on uncertainty. *Journal of Agricultural Economics*, 57(2): 313–27.

Slovic, P. (1997). Trust, emotion, sex, politics and science: surveying the risk-assessment battlefield. In: M. Bazerman, D. Messick, A. Tenbrunsel & K. Wade-Benzoni (eds). *Environment, Ethics and Behaviour*. San Francisco, New Lexington Press.

Slovic, P., Finucane, M. L., Peters, E. & MacGregor, D. G. (2004). Risk as analysis and risk as feelings: some thoughts about affect, reason, risk and rationality. *Risk Analysis*, 24(2): 311–22.

Thompson, M., Ellis, R. & Wildavsky, A. (1990). *Cultural Theory*. Boulder, Westview Print.

Tufte, E. R. (2001). *The Visual Display of Quantitative Information*, 2nd edn. Cheshire, CT, Graphics Press.

Tulloch, J. & Lupton, D. (2003). *Risk and Everyday Life*. London, Sage.

Tversky, A. & Kahneman, D. (1981). The framing of decisions and the psychology of choice. *Science*, 211: 453–63.

Visschers, V. H. M., Meertens, R. M., Passchier, W. F & de Vries, N. K. (2008). Audiovisual risk communication unravelled: effects on gut feelings and cognitive processes. *Journal of Risk Research*, 11: 207–21.

Wittgenstein, L. (1953). *Philosophical Investigations*. Oxford, Basil Blackwell.

Yamagishi, K. (1997). When a 12.86% mortality is more dangerous than 24.14%: implications for risk communication. *Applied Cognitive Psychology*, 11: 495–506.

Zhang, N. (2008). Doctoral Thesis: *Evaluation of e-Participation*. Manchester Business School. Manchester, University of Manchester.

Chapter 20

# Embedding better practice in risk communication and public health

Peter Bennett (Department of Health, London), Kenneth Calman (University of Glasgow), Sarah Curtis (University of Durham), & Denis Fischbacher-Smith (University of Glasgow)

This book has emphasized the lessons to be gained from analyses of communication about a diverse range of risks and in varying circumstances, each with a significant public health dynamic. Several issues emerge from the principles and cases set out in the preceding chapters.

These studies demonstrate the value of research as a means to *evaluate* processes of knowledge exchange and risk communication. Many professionals and lay members of the public are involved in such processes on a regular basis. Research should allow such groups to reflect on and evaluate their practice—an element often missing in policy discourse. Such reflection often only takes place when risk communication proves problematic—particularly when public criticism is directed at the communication process, by which time conflict will typically have become entrenched. Several of the examples discussed here have been of this type, and these may provide useful cautionary tales or lessons for 'fire fighting' situations when they arise. However, the chapters also contain key messages about how to help prevent crises from arising. Some of the difficulties that organizations face in crises may be due to a basic failure to manage the more routine communications about chronic risks (Reason, 1997; Turner, 1994): this undermines public trust and may provoke scepticism and cynicism concerning communication about the potential for major disasters (Smith & McCloskey, 1998). Ultimately, trust becomes a central issue in the process. This can be expressed in terms of the feelings that are held about the organization prior to any incident, the content of the message (and the manner in which the information is constructed), trust in the provider of the message, and the channel through which that message is transmitted.

Communication is part of a wider set of systems issues and so we need to consider how organizations can improve risk communication at a *systemic* level—as distinct from just managing crises better. Although generic official guidelines concerning good practice abound (e.g. FAO/WHO, 1998; Department of Health, 1997; US Department of Health and Human Services, 2002; Health Protection Network, 2008), the task of communicating effectively and sensitively about public health risks still seems challenging in many policy areas. Case studies such as those provided above can perhaps fill a gap, by helping those responsible for risk communication to see how general guidelines might be more effectively applied in real life.

The material in this book underlines the complexity of the issues around risk communication and the strategies that organizations adopt to deal with the task demands of the situations that they face. The strategic dynamics of the process are considerable and do not lend themselves to simple solutions. Organizations vary in structure and culture, have different responsibilities, and start with different problems. Each of these brings a different dynamic to bear on the issues around risk communication. Nevertheless, good practice can be fostered to some extent simply by bringing accepted knowledge on risk communication more fully to bear. Although this is far from an exact science, a significant amount is known, for example, about the nature of risk perceptions at an individual level, about how information tends to be processed, about the nature of trust, and about the factors that tend to amplify or attenuate concerns within societies. Earlier chapters have provided some illustration of these issues. Organizations genuinely seeking to communicate information or advice should not find themselves persistently surprised by responses that are actually quite well-researched and understood. At a more conceptual level, effective and honest communication calls for some appreciation of the various perspectives (and continuing controversies) on the nature of risk itself. Notably, it needs to acknowledge that risk is socially—not only scientifically— constructed, and that many risks are subject to fundamental (not just technical) uncertainties. Neither science nor society are in a position to have definitive knowledge—in some cases, even much robust and relevant knowledge—about some of the risks we may face (Beck, 1992; Giddens, 1990). This makes communication all the more challenging, especially if audiences are expecting clear, evidence-based, and unambiguous messages. Communication needs to be designed in ways that facilitate engagement in a discussion of the uncertainties, presented in ways that are comprehensible to non-experts.

There has been a tendency in the past to assume that orthodox scientific knowledge is always the most reliable and illuminating source of information on which to base risk communication. While it is vital to continue to communicate scientific findings effectively, several of the chapters in this book demonstrate how severe the limitations of knowledge can be. Even where expert consensus and clear scientific advice is available, *some* weight may need to be given to unorthodox views as this will allow the assumptions of the expert views to be challenged. Openness about the fallibility of knowledge is gradually growing, along with efforts to engage in public debate about uncertainty. This is especially important for risk communication (as well as risk response) strategies—although there is still a great deal that needs to be achieved in this regard. In practice, this recognition frequently leads to the use of the precautionary principle, pointing to where there is the 'possibility of significant harm', while acknowledging that the weight of scientific knowledge needs to be understood as inconclusive. The precautionary principle shifts the burden of proof around the hazards associated with activities to the risk generators. If adopted systematically, such an approach requires a shift in the ways that organizations deal both with uncertainty and with those who might be at risk (Calman and Smith, 2001). Even so, it is impossible to act in a completely 'precautionary' way toward all possible risks, and the precautionary principle has attracted criticism from some state actors (notably in the USA).

As already discussed, there is also a growing concern about risks that generate problems at an international level or where the hazards are more 'diffuse' (climate change being an obvious example). Until recently, public concern about these issues has been muted, partly because the threats may have seemed distant. However, this is rapidly changing, and risks are seen to transcend national boundaries and therefore require coordinated action to mitigate those risks. As this volume goes to press, the point has been amply demonstrated by the rapid international spread of human infection following the April 2009 outbreak of 'swine flu' in Mexico. While it is too early to tell how serious the eventual impact on health will be, the global nature of the threat is obvious, as is the need for a coordinated response. At least so far, that response seems to be forthcoming, though different countries are taking different steps to protect their respective populations. Who is going to take responsibility for 'coordinated' and 'coherent' risk communication as the various publics begin to take longer-term global issues like climate change more seriously?

## Improving risk communication as a decision-making process

The points just noted serve to emphasize that risk communication should not be seen in isolation but as an integral part of the decision-making process and its treatment of uncertainty. Risk communication itself involves making choices, whether in deciding what priority to give an issue, whom to consult, or what words to use. Usually all possible options to a decision problem carry risks that need to be factored into the final decision—for example, the approaches taken to warn people at risk, if not carefully expressed, may cause a panic that requires further intervention by decision-makers. They therefore, need to be aware of the (broadly defined) risks and opportunities of different options and to devise a coherent strategy on that basis. This requires attention to:

- The *internal* process of identifying issues, planning how to deal with them, taking action, and monitoring results. This will require organizations to acknowledge the uncertainty that exists within their assessments of risk (that is, ensure that their boundaries of consideration are wide enough to embrace the uncertainty in the evidence base)
- The management of *external* relationships with other stakeholders, e.g. through the setting up of consultation mechanisms, engaging with other interested parties, and building trust with the various communities of practice.

## Scanning, prioritization, and preparation

One approach to improving the 'internal' decision process is to use checklists of key factors to consider, and these can be helpful provided they are used to provoke thought rather than as a substitute for it. Checklists do, however, bring with them a set of problems as they can constrain the abilities of decision-makers to consider wider and more emergent issues. A key strategy that is adopted by some organizations relates to more in-depth, problem-structuring methods. For example, scenario-building, stakeholder analysis, classification of uncertainties, crisis simulations (Smart & Vertinsky, 1977; Smith, 2000) can be used in:

- Scanning exercises to identify and prioritize forthcoming issues
- Decision support workshops to help manage specific cases
- Development exercises using past cases or hypothetical scenarios (e.g. as described in the preceding chapter).

While the format of such exercises can be more or less elaborate, the aim should be to include those with expertise in different fields, e.g. on scientific topics or in dealing with the media. Indeed, the sharing of perspectives within the organization is often a significant byproduct. If further help is required, external advisers or analysts can bring fresh ideas to bear—although a strong working relationship with such groups is needed before the crisis emerges. Conversely, the sensitivity of some issues may make internal assistance more attractive. Staff will also start with greater knowledge of procedures and may be more immediately available.

Crisis conditions—combining time pressure, unexpectedness, and high levels of threat—almost always militate against effective decision-making and challenge the abilities of decision-making teams (Janis, 1989; Smart & Vertinsky, 1977; Smith, 2000). A key defence against crisis is the ability to spot possible difficulties in advance (Pauchant & Mitroff, 1992). Effective scanning will usually identify many potential issues, not all of which can—or should—be given equal attention. The 'Fright Factors' and 'Media Triggers' discussed in Chapter 1 can be used to set priorities. At a minimum, this process should provide greater opportunity for *internal* consultation between policy leads, managers, administrators, technical experts, medical staff, communications professionals, and others. The list will vary, but a variety of perspectives can be guaranteed and these differences should be seen as a central part of the process. Differences in viewpoint can be used constructively to foster a broader, more robust, view of the issues. Mismanaged, such disagreements can provide sources both of resentment and of confusing and contradictory public messages from different sources within the organization. The damage done to external credibility by poor internal coordination is difficult to overstate. Forward thinking will also be required in deciding when and how to engage with *external* stakeholders, and in ensuring that the necessary resources will be available. Deciding in favour of 'openness' will not make it simply happen—there has to be a clear commitment to action by senior members of the organization.

## Aims and stakeholders

A decision-based perspective should encourage constant attention to one key question: what are we trying to achieve? Answering it requires a clear view of who the relevant stakeholders are—those who are both affected by the issue and also those who may have some possible effect on it. The very exercise of listing stakeholders and their possible reactions can be highly informative in clarifying one's own aims. For example, these might include reassuring some sections of the public, persuading others to take certain actions, and securing support from other influential bodies. One way or another, communication should relate to the uncertainty inherent in decisions—whether already taken or still to be made—and recognize that there are likely to be different world views about the nature of that uncertainty. The term 'stakeholder' is used deliberately to direct attention beyond the intended *audience* for communication (that is, the receptors of the message) and to recognize that there are others who may have an interest in the issue. Politicians and the media are inevitably stakeholders in any major public health issue. So too are the public—though seldom as a homogeneous mass. Specific stakeholders might include different medical professions, charities and campaigning groups, various government departments and agencies, specific businesses, local authorities, and so on. Many issues also have strong international or European dimensions. It is therefore essential to consider, *as early as possible*, what other stakeholders could do and what might influence them, and to incorporate these factors into the organization's risk communication strategy.

At any given point—and certainly prior to major public announcements—a useful discipline is to formulate the *main* intended message and to check the construction of that message for sources of ambiguity. If this message is not understood and accepted, the communication must be counted as a failure and may escalate the issue still further. Some practitioners refer to this as a SOCHO—Single, Over-riding Communication Health Objective (cf. Murphy, 1997). Delivery may vary between audiences, there can also be subsidiary messages, fuller versions of arguments, and evidence made available and so on. But a clear priority has been chosen. Particularly where there is some complex science in the background, formulating a SOCHO will be difficult. The alternative, however, is much worse. If it is difficult to simplify, the answer cannot be to leave it to others and then accuse them of distortion! Emphasizing that the key message is itself a matter for decision should also signpost the need to keep it under review as the situation develops. The most inflexible choices are often those too 'obvious' to be questioned. Formulating the key message should also prompt one further check—that of whether the organization's behaviour is actually compatible with it. For example, if the intended message is of 'urgent investigation', is this demonstrably happening? Is the message 'don't panic' being delivered by an organization taking what look like desperate measures?

## Contingency planning and 'assumption busting'

Research on public perceptions of risk is neatly complemented by studies of its organizational mismanagement, in contexts as diverse as warfare, corporate policy, and engineering. A common pattern of failure is of otherwise able decision-makers (and their advisers) becoming constrained by a particular set of assumptions that ultimately allows lower-level events to escalate into a crisis (Mitroff *et al.*, 1989; Smith, 1990; Turner, 1976; Turner & Pidgeon, 1997). In such situations, uncertainties are often assumed away and alternative world views about the nature of risk ignored—often even in private. Lack of evidence for some effect may be translated into 'proof' of its non-existence, or issues defined in ways that simply omit significant public concerns. Caveats associated with scientific advice in relating laboratory to field conditions may be assumed away. Overconfidence and wishful thinking can be amplified when working in highly cohesive groups, in the process of 'groupthink' studied by

Janis and others (e.g. Janis, 1972; 1989; Esser & Lindoerfer, 1989; Moorhead *et al.*, 1991). By the time doubts finally surface, commitments have already been made, no contingency plans are in place, and there is a high risk that crisis will ensue. In the context of risk communication, the pattern can be seen in cases where a flawed message is repeated despite evidence that should have given pause for thought, eventually to be abandoned with maximum loss of credibility—and in some cases real damage to public health.

If an initial public position has to be modified, preparedness will limit the damage by allowing change to be both prompt and convincingly explained. There is therefore a need for early and determined challenge to key managerial assumptions. In the case of scientific assumptions, clues as to which assumptions to vary can be found by looking critically at the 'pedigree' of key evidence—how it was generated and by whom (Funtowicz & Ravetz, 1990). But sometimes even the highest pedigree assumptions turn out to be mistaken, and there is often a need to look at non-orthodox views. This is *not* to argue that all views should be accorded equal weight. Despite the attractions of a romantic view of science, most dissident views remain just that. Nevertheless, we should constantly ask *what if* the accepted view is mistaken. A useful concept here is that of *robustness* of decisions (Rosenhead, 2001). In the context of risk communication, a robust strategy is one that satisfies two criteria. Firstly, initial statements and actions should appear sensible in a wide variety of possible scenarios. Secondly, they should as far as possible leave future options open, to be taken as more becomes known about the issues.

Although there is sometimes a need to consider dramatic but unlikely scenarios without generating 'scare' headlines, there are strong arguments for at least acknowledging uncertainty in public, despite demands for certainty from public, media, and policy-makers alike. While not denying that there can be massive pressure for premature closure of debate, there is some evidence that the public is more tolerant of *uncertainty honestly admitted* than is often supposed. Indeed, a plethora of supposedly certain statements may only fuel the cynical belief that anything can be 'proven'. The risks of appearing closed-minded can also be great. On balance, acknowledging uncertainty often carries fewer dangers, even if it is not a route to instant popularity. The potential for swine flu to trigger a global human pandemic again provides a key illustration. In the UK, authorities have made strenuous efforts to communicate both the potential impact of a 'worst case' pandemic (previously recognized as the 'number one risk' to the nation on the government's risk register) and the uncertainties both as to when a pandemic might happen and how bad its consequences might be. This approach was maintained in the initial response to swine flu, and the indications (as of August 2009) are of public acceptance of the need to prepare for the "worst reasonable case". So far, there has been little hostile media coverage—although of course that could change rapidly.

How serious the health impact of this pandemic eventually is remains to be seen, as does the eventual public response. Whatever the outcome, it will be important to take the opportunity to learn—as regards communication just as much as risk management.

More generally, these arguments again support a *presumption* in favour of openness, so ensuring wider scrutiny of assumptions. Extending this to consider 'openness of process', as well as 'openness with information', offers further potential benefits. As well as being conducive to trust, two-way communication provides some chance of hearing something worthwhile. Those coming to the situation with a different perspective—particularly one involving experience on the ground—can prevent a too-easy consensus and may raise the 'obvious' question that turns out not to be so obvious. For example, this was reportedly one early effect of inviting 'lay' members to serve on governmental advisory committees. Open discussion also makes it easier to avoid acrimonious public debate as to with whom the 'fault' of uncertainty lies.

Success is likely to need a combination of measures designed to suit particular circumstances. However, the ideal endpoint would be for awareness of risk communication issues to become widely ingrained, and for attention to these issues to be an integral part of the organizational routine. Good practice would then be the rule rather than the exception.

## Conclusions

This book has sought to address a range of issues facing risk communication around a broad spectrum of public health concerns. At the same time, it has sought to show how these issues have evolved since the first edition of this collection was published. There is little doubt that the landscape in which policymakers and managers have to communicate risk has changed. The various public groups within our societies are also exposed to more diverse forms of information flows than were present even 10 years ago. Not all of it is accurate, and individuals now need to be able to filter, interpret, and make sense of the information that they are given in increasingly sophisticated ways.

Finally, and to return to the need for evaluation, each communication episode—'successful' or otherwise—represents an opportunity for organizational learning. Unfortunately, there are some significant barriers to such learning (Smith, 2001; Smith & Elliott, 2007). Consequently, issues are often recycled and any learning starts again from scratch, often at considerable long-term cost. Whilst this might be partly due to the manner in which the threats evolve and develop (Erikson, 1994; Smith, 2005), the challenge may partly reflect the nature of the human condition. The manner in which organizations fail to learn is likely to remain a significant policy issue for the next decade and beyond, and future discussion of risk communication will invariably return to this question. However, this book has been offered in the belief that while learning may be both imperfect and challenging, it need not be impossible.

## References

Beck, U. (1992). *Risk society. Towards a new modernity* (M. Ritter, Trans.). London, Sage.

Calman, K. & Smith, D. (2001). Works in theory but not in practice? Some notes on the precautionary principle. *Public Administration*, 79(1): 185–204.

Department of Health. (1997). *Communicating about risks to public health: pointers to good practice*. London, Department of Health.

Erikson, K. (1994). *A new species of trouble. Explorations in disaster, trauma, and community*. New York, W.W. Norton and Company.

Esser, J. K. & Lindoerfer, J. S. (1989). Groupthink and the Space Shuttle Challenger accident: Toward a quantitative case analysis. *Journal of Behavioral Decision Making*, 2: 167–177.

FAO/WHO. (1998). The application of risk communication to food standards and safety matters. Report of a Joint FAO/WHO Expert Consultation. Rome, 2–6 February 1998. *FAO Food & Nutrition Paper*, 70: i–iii.

Funtowicz, S.O. & Ravetz, J.R. (1990). *Uncertainty and Quality in Science for Policy*. Dordrecht, Kluwer.

Giddens, A. (1990). *The consequences of modernity*. Cambridge, Polity Press.

Health Protection Network. (2008). *Communicating with the public about health risks*. Health Protection Network Guidance 1, Health Protection Scotland, 2008.

Janis I. L. (1972). *Victims of Groupthink*. Boston, Houghton Mifflin.

Janis, I. L. (1989). *Crucial decisions: Leadership in policymaking and crisis management*. New York, NY, Free Press.

Mitroff, I. I., Pauchant, T. C., Finney, M. & Pearson, C. (1989). Do (some) organizations cause their own crises? Culture profiles of crisis prone versus crisis prepared organizations. *Industrial Crisis Quarterly*, 3: 269–83.

Moorhead, G., Ference, R. & Neck, C. P. (1991). Group decision fiascoes continue: Space Shuttle Challenger and a revised groupthink framework. *Human Relations*, 44(6): 539–50.

Murphy, C. (1997). Talking to the media. *Public Health Laboratory Service Microbiology Digest*, 14(4): 209–13

Pauchant, T. C. & Mitroff, I. I. (1992). *Transforming the crisis-prone organization. Preventing individual organizational and environmental tragedies*. San Fransisco, Jossey-Bass Publishers.

Reason, J. T. (1997). *Managing the risks of organizational accidents*. Aldershot, Ashgate.

Rosenhead, J. (2001). Robustness analysis: keeping your options open. In: J. Rosenhead & J. Mingers (eds) *Rational Analysis for a Problematic World Revisited*. Chichester, Sage.

Smart, C. & Vertinsky, I. (1977). Designs for crisis decision units. *Administrative Science Quarterly*, 22(4): 640–57.

Smith, D. (1990). Beyond contingency planning—towards a model of crisis management. *Industrial Crisis Quarterly*, 4(4): 263–75.

Smith, D. (2000). Crisis management teams: Issues in the management of operational crises. *Risk Management: An International Journal*, 2(3): 61–78.

Smith, D. (2001). Crisis as a catalyst for change: issues in the management of uncertainty and organizational vulnerability. In: British Bankers Association (eds). *E-risk: Business as Usual*: 81–8. London, British Bankers Association/Deloitte and Touch.

Smith, D. (2005). Dancing around the mysterious forces of chaos: exploring issues of complexity, knowledge and the management of uncertainty. *Clinician in Management*, 13(3–4): 115–23.

Smith, D. & Elliott, D. (2007). Moving beyond denial: Exploring the barriers to learning from crisis. *Management Learning*, 38(5): 519–38.

Smith, D. & McCloskey, J. (1998). Risk communication and the social amplification of public sector risk. *Public Money and Management*, 18(4): 41–50.

Turner, B. A. (1976). The organizational and interorganizational development of disasters. *Administrative Science Quarterly*, 21: 378–97.

Turner, B. A. (1994). The causes of disaster: Sloppy management. *British Journal of Management*, 5: 215–19.

Turner, B.A. & Pidgeon, N.F. (1997). *Man-made Disasters* (2nd edn). Butterworth–Heinemann.

US Department of Health and Human Services. (2002). *Communicators' guide for federal, state, regional and local communicators by the Federal Communicators Network*. Washington DC, FCN.

# Index